Community
Oral Health Practice
for the Dental Hygienist

Community Oral Health Practice
for the Dental Hygienist
Second Edition

Kathy Voigt Geurink, RDH, MA

Associate Professor
Department of Dental Hygiene
School of Allied Health Sciences
University of Texas Health Science Center at San Antonio
San Antonio, Texas

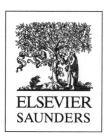

ELSEVIER
SAUNDERS

ELSEVIER
SAUNDERS

11830 Westline Industrial Drive
St. Louis, Missouri 63146

NOTICE

Dental hygiene is an ever-changing field. Standard safety precautions must be followed, but as new research and clinical experience broaden our knowledge, changes in treatment and drug therapy may become necessary or appropriate. Readers are advised to check the most current product information provided by the manufacturer of each drug to be administered to verify the recommended dose, the method and duration of administration, and contraindications. It is the responsibility of the licensed health care provider, relying on experience and knowledge of the patient, to determine dosages and the best treatment for each individual patient. Neither the publisher nor the author assumes any liability for any injury and/or damage to persons or property arising from this publication.

The Publisher

Previous edition copyrighted 2002

International Standard Book Number 1-4160-0096-8

Executive Editor: Penny Rudolph
Associate Developmental Editor: Julie Nebel
Publishing Services Manager: Patricia Tannian
Senior Project Manager: Anne Altepeter
Senior Designer: Amy Buxton

Printed in the United States of America
Last digit is the print number: 9 8 7 6 5 4 3 2 1

This text is dedicated to dental health professionals who have participated in community efforts to improve the oral health of all citizens. Oral health, as an integral component of the overall health and well-being of individuals, must be an entity available and attainable by all populations. Throughout my many years of working in the field of community oral health, I have observed the dedication and commitment of dental health professionals working toward this goal. They need to be commended and thanked and told to keep up their efforts. Many worthwhile programs and services have been provided, but there is still much to be done.

Contributors

Linda Altenhoff, DDS
Dental Director
Division of Oral Health, Texas
  Department of Health
Public Health Region 8
Headquarters: Austin, Texas
Oral Health Programs in the Community

Diane Brunson, RDH, MPH
Director, Oral, Rural, Primary Care
Colorado Department of Public Health
  and Environment
Clinical Assistant Professor
University of Colorado School of Dentistry
Denver, Colorado
Social Responsibility

Magda A. de la Torre, RDH, MPH
Assistant Professor
Department of Dental Hygiene
School of Allied Health Sciences
University of Texas Health Science Center
  at San Antonio
San Antonio, Texas
Cultural Competency

Kathy Voigt Geurink, RDH, MA
Associate Professor
Department of Dental Hygiene
School of Allied Health Sciences
University of Texas Health Science Center
  at San Antonio
San Antonio, Texas
*People's Health; Careers in Public Health for
  the Dental Hygienist; Oral Health
  Programs in the Community;
  Test-Taking Strategies and Community
  Cases*

Sheranita Hemphill, RDH, MPH, MS
Professor
Dental Hygiene Department
Sinclair Community College
Dayton, Ohio
Service-Learning

Beverly Isman, RDH, MPH, ELS
Dental Public Health Consultant
Davis, California
*Health Promotion and Health
  Communication*

Sherry R. Jenkins, RDH, BS
Clinical Professor
Department of Dental Hygiene
University of Texas Health Science Center
    at San Antonio
Program Dental Hygienist
School-Based Dental Program
Methodist Healthcare Ministries
San Antonio, Texas
Oral Health Programs in the Community

Sharon Logue, RDH, MPH
School Fluoride Mouthrinse Coordinator
Division of Dental Health
Virginia Department of Health
Richmond, Virginia
Careers in Public Health for the Dental
    Hygienist

Jane E.M. Steffensen, RDH, BS, MPH,
    CHES
Assistant Professor
Department of Community Dentistry,
    Dental School
University of Texas Health Science Center
    at San Antonio
San Antonio, Texas
Assessment in the Community; Measuring
    Progress in Oral Health; Oral Health
    Status and Trends

Stacy A. Weil, RDH, MS
Associate Director
Clinical Operations
Pharmaceutical Product Development
Austin, Texas
Research

Chapter 2 Mini-Profiles:

Diana Cudeii, BA, RDH, CDA
Dental Hygiene Education and
    Prevention Consultant
Inter Tribal Council of Arizona, Inc.
Phoenix, Arizona

Kathleen Mangskau, RDH, MPA
Director, Division of Tobacco Prevention
    and Control
Community Health Section
North Dakota Department of Health
Bismarck, North Dakota

Ginger Melton, RDH, BS
Dental Hygienist
Beazley Dental Center of the Portsmouth
    Community Health Center
Portsmouth, Virginia

Kathy Phipps, RDH, MPH, DrPH
Associate Professor
Integrative Biosciences
Oregon Health and Science University
Portland, Oregon
Oral Health Research Consultant
Morro Bay, California

Leonor Ramos, RDH
Hospital Dentistry Dental Hygienist
Department of Defense
United States Air Force
Wilford Hall Medical Center
Lackland Air Force Base
San Antonio, Texas

JoAnn Wells, RDH, BS
Human Services Program Coordinator
Statewide Education Coordinator
Virginia Department of Health
Division of Dental Health
Richmond, Virginia

Reviewers

Susan Callahan Barnard, RDH, MS
Assistant Professor
Bergen Community College
Paramus, New Jersey

Connie S. Grossman, MEd, RDH
Department of Dental Hygiene
Columbus State Community College
Columbus, Ohio

Charla J. Lautar, RDH, PhD
Associate Professor and Interim Chair
Department of Health Care Professions
Southern Illinois University at
    Carbondale
Carbondale, Illinois

Patricia A. Mannie, RDH, MS
St. Cloud Technical College
St. Cloud, Minnesota

Pamela Rettig, RDH, MS
Department of Periodontics and Allied
    Dental Programs
Indiana University School of Dentistry
Indianapolis, Indiana

**Kim S. Ritchhart, RDH, BS, MPA, PhD
    (ABD)**
Illinois Central College Faculty
Peoria, Illinois

Preface

"Why do I need to know anything about Community Oral Health?"

This is the question that many dental hygiene instructors hear from their students at the beginning of the Community Dental/Oral Health course. The purpose of this text is to provide students with information about community oral health that is relevant to dental hygiene. It is my intention that, through reading the chapters and participating in the suggested activities, dental hygiene students will find the answer to this question and will develop an understanding of the importance of this integral component of their education and future profession. Although this text is written specifically for dental hygiene students, it also is a valuable resource for all dental hygienists practicing their professional responsibility of improving the oral health of their community.

Community Dental/Oral Health is a required course for dental hygiene accreditation. The Commission on Dental Hygiene Accreditation states that the curriculum in dental hygiene schools must include content in the following general areas: general education, biomedical sciences, dental sciences, and dental hygiene science. These areas must be incorporated with sufficient depth, scope, sequence of instruction, quality, and emphasis to ensure achievement of the curriculum's competencies.

According to Accreditation Standard 2-14,

Dental hygiene science content must include oral health education and preventive counseling; health promotion; patient management; clinical dental hygiene; provision of services for and management of patients with special needs; **community dental/oral health;** *medical and dental emergencies, including basic life support; legal and ethical aspects of dental hygiene practice; infection and hazard control management; and the provision of oral health care services to patients with bloodborne infectious diseases.*

The American Dental Education Association (ADEA), Section on Dental Hygiene Education Competency Development Committee, developed dental hygiene competencies to assist dental hygiene schools in meeting accreditation standards. The competency statements are meant to serve as guidelines for individual programs in defining the abilities they want their graduates to possess. The competency statements are presented in the following five domains:

Core Competencies (C)
Health Promotion/Disease Prevention (HP)
Community (CM)
Patient/Client Care (PC)
Professional Growth and Development (PGD)

The ADEA Community Dental/Oral Health Competencies are as follows:

CM.1 Assess the oral health needs of the community and the quality of resources and services

CM.2 Provide screening, referral, and educational services that allow clients to access the resources of the health care system

CM.3 Provide community oral health services in a variety of settings

CM.4 Facilitate client access to oral health services by influencing individuals and organizations for the provision of oral health care

CM.5 Evaluate reimbursement mechanisms and their impact on the patient's or client's access to oral health care

CM.6 Evaluate the outcomes of community-based programs and plan for future activities

At the end of each chapter in this book, competencies from all domains that are relevant to the chapter content and knowledge application activities are listed. The complete document of competencies for entry into the profession of dental hygiene, approved and adopted by the ADEA House of Delegates in 2003, is located in Appendix B and on the Evolve website that accompanies this text. Therefore, the instructor and student will be able to relate the information within *Community Oral Health Practice for the Dental Hygienist* to the goal of developing competencies in the profession of dental hygiene.

Chapter 1 defines community oral health for students through examples of public health problems and solutions. The core public health functions and essential public health services are defined. Chapter 2, on careers in public health, enables students to envision the future use of the information they are learning about in the book and in the community course; it features dental hygienists who practice within the field of community oral health. Reviewing these featured career choices will allow the students to comprehend the relevance of the content in the forthcoming chapters.

Chapter 3, on assessment, and Chapters 4 and 5, on measuring oral health, emphasize the importance of these crucial steps in planning community oral health programs. Dental hygienists involved in public health need to be knowledgeable about and proficient in using the tools of assessment and measurement of oral health. *Healthy People 2010* oral health objectives are discussed as an important framework for assessment of community oral health programs. These chapters are appropriately placed within the book as a preparation for Chapter 6, on community oral health programs, which discusses planning, implementation, and evaluation phases of program development. Successful community oral health programs at local, state, and national levels are featured. Internet websites and updates on state oral health programs are included.

Chapter 7 covers statistics in a relevant, organized format, with application to community oral health. Criteria for reviewing dental literature are included. Chapter 8 explains theories of health promotion and identifies strategies for delivering health information to the public. The dental hygienist's social responsibility with respect to cultural competency and the dental hygienist's role in improving access to care for underserved populations are addressed in Chapter 9. A case study is provided to initiate discussion on the dental hygienist's roles, values, and beliefs. Chapter 10, on cultural competency, not only defines the term for students but also provides models of how to incorporate cultural competency into interactions with patients and in our community health promotion endeavors.

Chapter 11, Service-Learning, defines the importance of the collaboration between the needs of the community and the student's learning. The benefits of service-learning for the students, the community, the dental hygiene program, the academic institution, and the nation's oral health are discussed.

Chapter 12 provides the student with practice in answering community oral health test questions similar to those on the Dental Hygiene National Board Examination. These community cases test the student's understanding of content in the textbook. The practice test assists the student in successfully answering this type of question. Teachers who use this textbook should anticipate improved scores on the national board examination in the area of community oral health. Students are provided with the information they need to begin their profession with a positive attitude toward community dental health and a willingness to contribute to the oral health of all persons in their community.

A vocabulary of terms is unique to community oral health practice, and therefore a glossary is located at the end of the textbook for reference. The appendices contain websites for oral health resources, dental hygiene competencies, and valuable information for forming community partnerships and performing community health assessments.

New to this edition are sample community cases with test questions at the end of each chapter. These cases assist students in their mastery of the material in each chapter and provide additional practice in answering case-type questions similar to those on the Dental Hygiene National Board Examination. Instructors will find the answers/rationales on the newly developed Evolve website, which contains supplemental information and learning activities related to *Community Oral Health Practice for the Dental Hygienist.*

BIBLIOGRAPHY

Commission on Dental Accreditation: Accreditation Standards for Dental Hygiene Education Programs (approved July 1998; effective January 2000). Chicago, American Dental Association.

American Dental Education Association (ADEA): Competencies for Entry into the Profession of Dental Hygiene: ADEA Section on Dental Hygiene Education (approved March 2003 House of Delegates).

Kathy Voigt Geurink

ACKNOWLEDGMENTS

Over the course of preparing this text for publication, many people have provided their support, guidance, and assistance in researching information pertinent to oral health in the community. I want to acknowledge with sincere appreciation the following persons for their contributions and support:

Jane Steffensen
(colleague and contributor)

Jill Nield-Gehrig
(colleague and friend)

Ray Dunham
(network analyst, University of Texas Health Science Center at San Antonio)

Janna Lawrence
(Reference and Instructional Services Coordinator, Briscoe Library, University of Texas Health Science Center at San Antonio)

Faculty and staff
(Department of Dental Hygiene, School of Allied Health Sciences, University of Texas Health Science Center at San Antonio)

My family
(parents, Peg and Jim Voigt; husband, Terry; daughters, Kelly and Kimberly)

Contents

1

People's Health

Kathy Voigt Geurink, RDH, MA

Objectives

Upon completion of this chapter, the student will be able to:
- Define the terms *health, public health,* and *dental public health*
- Identify public health problems within a community
- Identify public health measures or solutions
- Define dental disease as a public health problem with public health solutions
- Explain the role of the government in public health solutions
- Discuss the 10 greatest public health achievements of the twentieth century
- Identify core functions of public health and the essential public health services
- Define six roles of the dental hygienist to determine how they relate to community oral health practice

Key Terms

Health
Public Health
Dental Public Health
Public
Community
Fluoridation

Department of Health and
   Human Services (DHHS)
Assessment
Policy Development
Assurance
Service Provider/Clinician

Health Educator/Wellness
   Promoter
Consultant/Resource Person
Consumer Advocate/
   Change Agent
Researcher
Administrator/Manager

OPENING STATEMENT

What Is Public Health?

- Influenza immunizations save lives and money.

- Vaccine research of human immunodeficiency virus (HIV) is a top priority to end the epidemic.

- Community water fluoridation is listed as one of the 10 greatest public health achievements of the twentieth century.

- Evidence links dental disease to life-threatening systemic diseases such as heart disease, respiratory ailments, and diabetes.

- The website of the world's largest tobacco company acknowledges that smoking tobacco causes serious health risks.

- Improved water sanitation controls infectious diseases.

- The White House and the American Dental Hygienists Association (ADHA) team together to provide dental insurance to children.

- Bioterrorism has put public health officials on alert for unusual diseases.

HEALTH, PUBLIC HEALTH, AND DENTAL PUBLIC HEALTH

Becoming familiar with the Opening Statement will set you on the right track to begin your journey in developing an understanding of the importance of people's health. The connection between people's health and community oral health will become apparent throughout the text. Thinking of specific examples, such as those in the Opening Statement, will enable you to envision what is meant by the topics of **health, public health,** and **dental public health.** It is also necessary to review the more formal definitions of these terms that occur in most texts on the topics. Various definitions exist for these terms; however, the following definitions should suffice for use within the scope of community oral health practice for the dental hygienist:

Health has been described by the World Health Organization (WHO) as follows: "Health comprises complete physical and social well-being and is not merely the absence of disease."[1]

Public health, as described by Winslow, is "the science and art of preventing disease, prolonging life, and promoting physical health and efficiency through organized community efforts."[2] It is concerned with lifestyle and behavior, the environment, human biology, and organizations of health programs and systems.[3] The **public** pertains to the community, state, or nation. Public health is people's health.[4]

Dental public health has been described by the American Board of Dental Health as *the science and art of preventing and controlling dental disease and promoting dental health through organized* **community** *efforts. It is that form of dental practice which serves the community as the patient rather than the individual. It is concerned with the dental education of the public, and applied dental research, and with the administration of group dental care programs as well as prevention and control of dental diseases on a community basis.*[2]

In this text, the terms *public health* and *community health* are used synonymously, and both refer to the "effort that is organized by society to protect, promote and restore the health and quality of life of the people."[3]

THE PUBLIC HEALTH PROBLEM AND THE PUBLIC HEALTH SOLUTION

Public Health Problem

Upon reading these definitions carefully, you are ready to view two concepts of importance to your comprehension of public or people's health: (1) the public health problem and (2) the public health solution. The public health problem, as perceived by the public, usually brings to mind an infectious disease such as acquired immunodeficiency syndrome (AIDS) or hepatitis. The spectrum of problems, however, is vast and more extensive than one might first realize. Examples of public health problems include:

1. Diseases caused by the pollution of the country's air and water systems
2. Chronic diseases of the expanding population of older adults
3. Inadequate funding for dental disease in indigent children
4. An increase in violence among youth of today

Studying examples of public health problems appears to be the easiest means of developing an understanding of what constitutes public health. Public health problems, as described by Burt and Ecklund, must meet the following criteria[5]:

1. A condition or situation that is a widespread actual or potential cause of morbidity or mortality
2. An existing perception that the condition is a public health problem on the part of the public, the government, or public health authorities

The history of public health demonstrates that once the problem is identified and knowledge and expertise have been developed to solve the problem, the community must unify to find social and political support to proceed with the public health solutions.

Public Health Solution

Examples of solutions to public health problems that most persons are familiar with include immunizations, tobacco cessation programs, **fluoridation** of drinking water, and seat belts and air bags in cars to prevent injuries and mortality. These public health solutions are concerned with health promotion and disease prevention. They address the problems of the community at large and are effective measures that follow seven characteristics (see "Guiding Principles").

GUIDING PRINCIPLES

Seven Characteristics of Public Health Solutions
- Not hazardous to life or function.
- Effective in reducing or preventing the targeted disease or condition.
- Easily and efficiently implemented.
- Potency maintained for a substantial time period.
- Attainable regardless of socioeconomic status.
- Effective immediately upon application.
- Inexpensive and within the means of the community.

Community water *fluoridation* has proved to be a safe, cost-effective solution for reducing dental decay in children. It is easily implemented by adding fluoride to the water supply, and it reaches all people regardless of socioeconomic status. It is effective immediately upon initiation and costs far less than the financial burden of restorative treatment. It meets all the seven characteristics to be considered an effective solution to the problem of dental decay.

DENTAL DISEASE AS A PUBLIC HEALTH PROBLEM

Dental Decay

Dental disease is a universal problem that does not undergo remission if left untreated. About 99% of adults have had tooth decay by the time they reach their early 40s. Sixty percent of adults over 75 years of age have had root caries.[6] The extent and severity of dental caries warrant the need for treatment and prevention programs throughout the United States. Dental decay, if left untreated, continues to escalate and results in expensive surgical procedures. Therefore it is important to focus on prevention of the disease.

Community water fluoridation is the perfect example of a dental public health solution to the problem of dental decay. Organized community efforts have brought fluoridated drinking water to more than 144 million people, and the results have shown a significant reduction in the amount of dental decay. Dental disease, however, still exists as a public health problem of the twenty-first century. More community dental health education needs to be performed with the implementation of additional dental health promotion and prevention programs.

Chapters 6 and 8 describe various programs and health promotion efforts that can be implemented and expanded upon within communities nationwide.

The 2000 Surgeon General's report on oral health emphasizes the need for these programs and addresses the importance of oral health to the general health of the public.[7] Dental disease is discussed as a dental public health problem of universal prevalence that can be alleviated, and even prevented, with future public health measures. Dental professionals, both those employed in the field of public health and those employed in private practice, must work together to educate the community and to provide the necessary programs to treat and prevent further disease.

Public Health/Private Practice

Programs to treat dental disease can be conducted on a *community* (public health) or *individual* (private practice) level. On the community level, the dental professional treats the community as a patient rather than as an individual. Table 1-1 demonstrates the similarities of community oral health practice to private practice. The community oral health steps parallel steps conducted in the private practice. Community oral health practice extends the role of the dental hygienist in private practice to include the people of the community as a whole. The public health facility (e.g., hospital, community clinic, school, or agency), rather than the private dental office, becomes the environment in which the service of oral health care is provided. The patient's dental examination parallels the community survey as a means of assessment of the situation or problem.

The treatment plan and the plan for the community are similar; both include the many facets of preparation, such as determining various methods, strategies, and costs of choosing a plan that will work best for the patient or community. The treatment and the program operation occur during the actual implementation of the plan. Payment for dental services is equated with program funding. Various methods of payment are often explored in both cases.

Evaluation of the treatment is similar to the program appraisal and should occur during the implementation and at the end of the treatment or operation.[5] This comparison should help the private practice hygienist become comfortable with the concepts of community program planning, implementation, and evaluation (see Chapter 6).

Table **1-1**   **Comparison of components in private practice and public health**

Private Practice	Public Health
Patient	Community
Exam	Survey
Diagnosis	Analysis
Treatment planning	Program planning
Treatment	Program implementation
Fee/payment	Budget/financing
Patient evaluation	Program evaluation

GOVERNMENT'S ROLE IN PUBLIC HEALTH

Government Agencies

As a dental hygienist, you may contribute to the health of people in the community through participating in community health promotion activities. You may choose to present an educational presentation at a school or conduct a cancer screening at a facility for older residents (see Chapter 8). The more formal public health programs, however, generally fall under the aegis of the government. Both prevention and the delivery of services are concerns within the programs developed by government agencies.

The federal government's role in participating in dental health-related activities falls under the jurisdiction of the **Department of Health and Human Services (DHHS).** *Healthy People 2010,* a publication of the DHHS, lists health objectives for the United States, including oral health, that need to be achieved by the year 2010 (see Chapter 4).

The Public Health Service (PHS) is one of four major agencies within the DHHS. The PHS promotes health standards, ensures that the highest level of health care is available for all citizens, and cooperates with other nations on health projects. There are eight operating agencies under the PHS (Figure 1-1). Agencies that are important because they are involved in oral health programs include the following:

- Centers for Disease Control and Prevention (CDC)
- Health Resources and Services Administration (HRSA)
- National Institutes of Health (NIH), National Institute of Dental and Craniofacial Research (NIDCR)
- Agency for Healthcare Research and Quality (AHRQ)[8]

At the state level, public health agencies have been charged with the task of developing oral health programs within their state. These programs usually include educational programs for children under 18 years of age. Restorative and emergency services are often included through community clinics. Screening and data collection for needs assessments are also conducted at this level.

At the local level, dental programs vary throughout the nation. As a result of a decline in funding at all levels, there has been less involvement at this level in recent years, and fewer data have been collected to determine needs.[9]

National Initiatives

Whether an oral health program has national, state, or local impact, its objectives should be tied in with the National Initiatives. National Oral Health Initiatives have the common goals of:

- Promoting oral health
- Improving the quality of life
- Eliminating oral health disparities

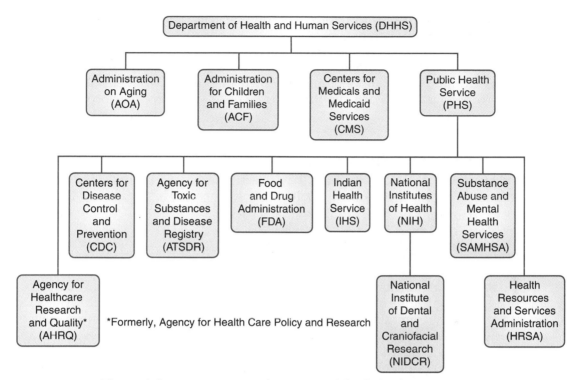

Figure 1-1 Departments and agencies of the federal government.

The 2000 Surgeon General's Report, *Oral Health in America,* is a 300-page document with a focus exclusively on oral health issues. The major message of the Report is that oral health is essential to the general health and well-being of all Americans and can be achieved by all Americans; however, there are profound and consequential disparities within the U.S. population.[7] Several federal, state, and local initiatives developed in response to the Surgeon General's Report, including *Healthy People 2010* and the 2003 National Call to Action to Promote Oral Health. *Healthy People 2010* is a comprehensive set of disease prevention and health promotion objectives that contains an oral health focus area and 17 oral health objectives.[10] The National Call to Action to Promote Oral Health was a combined effort of a broad coalition of public and private organizations and individuals who generated five principal actions and implementation strategies to be undertaken to ensure that all Americans achieve optimum oral health. As health care providers we are called to participate in the following five actions:

- Change perceptions of oral health
- Overcome barriers by replicating effective programs
- Build the science and accelerate science transfer

- Increase oral health workforce diversity, capacity, and flexibility
- Increase collaborations [11]

The successful execution of the five actions requires partnerships and collaborations focused on the common goals. The public, health care providers, policy makers, communities, and anyone interested in the improvement of oral health must work together to achieve the vision, goals, and objectives of the National Initiatives.

Core Functions of Public Health

Federal, state, and local programs have been charged to improve the health of the people through assessment, policy development, and assurance. These core

BOX 1-1   CORE FUNCTIONS OF PUBLIC HEALTH AGENCIES AT ALL LEVELS OF GOVERNMENT

Assessment
- Every public health agency regularly and systematically collects, assembles, analyzes, and makes available information on the health of the community, including statistics on health status, community health needs, and epidemiologic and other studies of health problems. Not every agency is large enough to conduct these activities directly; intergovernmental and interagency cooperation is essential. Nevertheless, each agency bears the responsibility for seeing that the assessment function is fulfilled. This basic function of public health cannot be delegated.

Policy Development
- Every public health agency exercises its responsibility to serve the public interest in the development of comprehensive public health policies by promoting use of the scientific knowledge base in decision making about public health and by leading in developing public health policy. Agencies must take a strategic approach, developed based on a positive appreciation for the democratic political process.

Assurance
- Public health agencies assure their constituents that services necessary to achieve agreed upon goals are provided, either by encouraging actions by other entities (private or public sector), by requiring such action through regulation, or by providing services directly.
- Each public health agency involves key policy makers and the general public in determining a set of high-priority personal and community-wide health services that governments will guarantee to every member of the community. This guarantee should include subsidization or direct provision of high-priority personal health services for people unable to afford them.

Reprinted with permisson from The Future of the Public's Health in the 21st Century, National Academy of Science, Washington, DC, National Academy Press, 2002.

public health functions of **assessment, policy development,** and **assurance** were identified in an Institute of Medicine (IOM) report in 1988. This report states that the core public health functions were developed to protect and promote health, wellness, and the quality of life and to prevent disease, injury, disability, and death.[12] Box 1-1 presents these core functions.

The public health functions have been further delineated since the publication of the IOM report. Through a consensus development process, a number of organizations and agencies produced a document entitled *Public Health in America.* This document lists essential public health services necessary to accomplish the core public health functions (Box 1-2). Successful provision of these services requires collaboration among private and public partners within the community and across various levels of government. These services are essential to achievement of healthy people in healthy communities.[13]

Building on the framework of the core public health functions and the essential public heath services, the Association of State and Territorial Dental Directors (ASTDD) developed guidelines for state oral health programs within state health departments (see Chapter 6). The core public health functions, the essential public health services, and the essential public health services for oral health provide

---

Box 1-2   Essential Public Health Services in the United States

Public Health

- Prevents epidemics
- Protects against environmental hazards
- Prevents injuries
- Promotes and encourages healthy behaviors
- Responds to disasters and assists communities in recovery
- Ensures the quality and accessibility of health services

Essential Public Health Services

- Monitor health status to identify community health problems
- Diagnose and investigate health problems and health hazards in the community
- Inform, educate, and empower the public about health issues
- Mobilize community partnerships to identify and solve health problems
- Develop policies and plans to support individual and community health efforts
- Enforce laws and regulations that protect the public's health and ensure safety
- Link policies to needed personal health services
- Ensure a competent public health and personal health care workforce
- Evaluate effectiveness, accessibility, and quality of personal and population-based health services
- Conduct research for new insight and innovative solutions to health problems

From Public Health in America. Washington, DC, Public Health Functions Steering Committee, 1994.

guidance for dental public health professionals working at national, state, and local levels.

FUTURE OF DENTAL PUBLIC HEALTH

What Needs to Be Done

Over the years, the number of dental public health programs at federal, state, and local levels has declined as a result of tight budgets and diminishing resources. Dental disease persists as a public health problem that can be alleviated and, possibly, eliminated. The knowledge exists, but because of restraints and a lack of resources, this knowledge is not being applied toward the goal of communities free from dental disease. The ongoing need to emphasize the importance of oral health has never been stronger. It is the responsibility of the dental health professionals to emphasize the connection of oral health to people's general health to the policymakers of our nation. Corbin and Marten's report[14] on the future of dental health states that although oral health needs are documented, oral health is given a low priority by health planners. The report emphasizes goals to meet for improved dental public health (see Guiding Principles).

GUIDING PRINCIPLES

> **Goals to Be Met to Improve Dental Public Health[14]**
> - Earn support from the public
> - Earn support from the policymakers
> - Earn support from program administrators
> - Earn support from the dental community
> - Ensure recruitment and professional development of dental public health personnel
> - Ensure collaboration with colleagues

Going in the Right Direction

Although the dental profession must continue to seek legislation and funding for health programs and to educate the public on the relationship of oral health to general health, the profession appears to be moving in the direction of success. A 1999 report by the CDC[15] lists the 10 most important public health accomplishments of the twentieth century. This list is encouraging and supportive to the efforts of all public health professionals (see Guiding Principles).

The 10 Greatest Public Health Accomplishments of the Twentieth Century[15]

- A significant decline in deaths from coronary heart disease and stroke as a result of behavior modification, a decrease in smoking, and early intervention programs
- The 1964 Surgeon General's acknowledgment of tobacco as a health hazard and resultant antismoking campaigns that have changed the public health perceptions about the habit
- Vaccination, which has helped to eradicate smallpox and to manage diseases such as measles, rubella, and tetanus
- Improved motor vehicle safety, with greater emphasis placed on personal responsibility for reducing motor vehicle–related fatalities caused by drinking and reckless driving
- Control of infectious diseases, which has been aided by improved water sanitation and better understanding of the science of microbiology
- Safer workplaces that have contributed to a higher standard of living and a 40% reduction in job-related injuries and fatalities
- Safer and healthier foods as a result of less microbial contamination as well as fortification of foods with supplements and vitamins
- Healthier mothers and babies, thanks to improved prenatal care and greater access to care
- Better access to family planning information and greater use of contraceptives, which has improved the socioeconomic status of United States citizens
- Fluoride in drinking water, which reaches 144 million people safely and is an inexpensive method of preventing tooth decay independent of a person's socioeconomic status

---

Dental hygienists play an important role in assessing and prioritizing dental health needs in the community. They have a responsibility to participate in the activities that will list community oral health practice as an important achievement in the twenty-first century. Social responsibility and the dental hygienist's commitment to the community are discussed in Chapter 9.

The dental hygienists who have chosen careers as state dental directors or public health educators contribute to the advancement of dental public health, but much more needs to be accomplished by all members of the dental hygiene profession. Through various roles, dental hygienists can affect the oral health of all people (Box 1-3).

BOX 1-3   SIX ROLES OF THE DENTAL HYGIENIST

1. Service provider/clinician
2. Health educator/wellness promoter
3. Consultant/resource person
4. Consumer advocate/change agent
5. Researcher
6. Administrator/manager

From Public Health in America. Washington, DC, Public Health Functions Steering Committee, 1994.

SIX ROLES OF THE DENTAL HYGIENIST

Definition of Roles

The following roles of the dental hygienist demonstrate the various opportunities for the profession to be involved in improving people's health. Future chapters cover the knowledge and skills necessary to develop these roles. Chapter 2 describes the skills necessary to become actively involved at various levels and further describes career opportunities involving the six roles that the hygienist may play within the field of public health. Herein, as an introduction, are their definitions.

Service provider/clinician. The dental hygienist assesses oral health conditions and develops a plan to manage oral diseases. Treatment is then provided.

Health educator/wellness promoter. Preventing disease and promoting oral health through the presentation of scientific information on topics such as fluoridation make this role crucial to the improvement and enhancement of oral health.

Consultant/resource person. The dental hygienist is the liaison between the community and the dental profession. In this role, the dental hygienist determines the appropriate program or activity that will serve the needs of the community.

Consumer advocate/change agent. In this role, the dental hygienist must have the knowledge and skills to work legislatively to promote change and advance the health of the public through legislation, public policy, research, and science. As a consumer advocate, the dental hygienist represents individuals or large groups of consumers and informs them of quality services and products.

Researcher. As a researcher, the dental hygienist determines which methods of prevention work best for the people served by the profession. This includes evaluating products and techniques and sharing the findings.

Administrator/manager. In both the private office and in the public health arena, the dental hygienist administers and manages programs. Within the administrator role, many functions of the other roles are required.

Common Goal in All Roles

The goal of dental public health is optimal oral health for all citizens and universal access to comprehensive dental care. To accomplish this goal, dental hygienists perform duties within the six roles listed. Both dentists and dental hygienists have entered the field of public health by accepting employment within programs that include health promotion, community disease prevention, and provision of dental care to selected groups of people.

Dentists become recognized specialists in the field of dental public health through specialty certification with the American Board of Dental Health. In most states, dental hygienists have no required formal or specialty education to work within this field in the community, although some have pursued advanced degrees in public health or community health. Further education prepares the dental hygienist to work with underserved populations who continually face barriers to health care. These barriers, such as inadequate geographic and financial access, pose challenges to the dental and dental hygiene profession.

In an attempt to reach underserved populations (see Chapter 2), some states are permitting less restrictive dental hygiene supervision for dental hygienists working in the community. In 1998, the California legislature recognized a new title, the Registered Dental Hygienist in Alternative Practice Settings (RDHAP). The purpose of the title is to qualify dental hygienists to practice community oral health with less supervision in underserved areas. The dental hygienist who has a concern for the improvement and protection of the oral health of the whole population can participate in community oral health practice at a level of personal choice.

In June 2004, the ADHA House of Delegates, addressing the problem of access to health care, approved the creation of the Advanced Dental Hygiene Practitioner (ADHP) credential. This credential is designed to allow dental hygienists to provide diagnostic, restorative, and therapeutic services directly to the public. Those dental hygienists who receive the ADHP credential will have graduated from an accredited dental hygiene program and also completed the ADHA-approved advanced educational curriculum. This credential is being developed to improve and enhance the oral health care delivery system. Because dental supervision is not required of the ADHP, it will open doors for dental hygienists to work in places such as school systems, hospitals, and nursing homes and with underserved populations throughout the country.[16]

SUMMARY

An understanding of people's health includes learning the basic terminology to define health, public health, and dental public health. People's health is the health of the public living within a community, state, or nation. Identifying public health problems and solutions provides dental hygienists with the knowledge to explore this field of health further and a means by which they might become involved. The government's role in people's health is mentioned briefly as an introduction to the programs to be discussed in more detail in future chapters. Comparison of private practice to community oral health practice demonstrates the similarities and prepares dental hygienists for the planning, implementation, and evaluation phases that constitute public health programs. As health care providers, with many roles and responsibilities, dental hygienists have a calling and a duty to serve the community in which they live.

Applying **Your Knowledge**

1. Bring articles to class from the daily news or current magazines that present a public health issue, and discuss what the problem is and how it is being addressed. (Use the seven characteristics described in this chapter to evaluate the issue.)
2. Choose a government public health program and further investigate its purpose and success in accomplishing this purpose. (See websites for state oral health programs, Chapter 6.)
3. Choose one of the six roles of the dental hygienist and explain how dental hygienists improve the oral health of their community through this role.
4. Research and report on the creation of the ADHP (Advanced Dental Hygiene Practitioner). What is required for this advanced education and how does an ADHP affect access to oral health care?

DENTAL HYGIENE COMPETENCIES

Reading the material within this chapter and participating in the activities of Applying Your Knowledge will contribute to the student's ability to demonstrate the following competencies:

Health promotion and disease prevention

HP.1 Promote the values of oral health and general health and wellness to the public and organizations within and outside the profession.
HP.4 Identify individual and population risk factors and develop strategies that promote health-related quality of life.

Community Case

In your new position as a Dental Health Consultant at the State Health Department, you are asked to conduct a statewide screening project to determine the oral health status of school-age children. After you collect and analyze the data from the statewide survey, you are to determine what oral health programs you would like to plan that will address the needs of children in your state.

1. Which core public health function is addressed through the screening project?
   a. Assurance
   b. Assessment
   c. Policy development
   d. Essential public health services
   e. Planning
2. If dental caries in school-age children is the problem you want to address, what public health solution would be best for this problem?
   a. School fluoride mouth rinse
   b. Grade-specific oral health education program
   c. School sealant program
   d. Community water fluoridation
   e. Fluoride varnish applications
3. Which one of the major agencies within the Department of Health and Human Services would have the most possibilities for funding the project you select to conduct?
   a. PHS (Public Health Service)
   b. ACF (Administration for Children and Families)
   c. CMS (Centers for Medicare and Medicaid)
   d. AOA (Administration on Aging)
   e. HP 2010 (*Healthy People 2010*)
4. The survey you conduct relates to which private practice function?
   a. Diagnosis
   b. Treatment
   c. Exam
   d. Evaluation
   e. Treatment planning
5. Your participation in the screening survey and data collection/analysis falls mainly under which one of the roles of the dental hygienist?
   a. Administrator
   b. Change agent
   c. Researcher
   d. Service provider
   e. Consultant

REFERENCES

1. Constitution of the World Health Organization. Geneva, World Health Organization, 1946, p 3.
2. Winslow CE: The untitled fields of public health. Mod Med 2:183, 1920.
3. Block LE: Dental public health: An overview. In Gluck GM, Morganstein WM (eds): Jong's Community Dental Health, 5th ed. St. Louis, Mosby, 2003.
4. Knutson JW: What is public health? In Pelton WJ, Wisan JM (eds): Dentistry in Public Health, 2nd ed. Philadelphia, WB Saunders, 1955.
5. Burt BA, Ecklund SA: Dentistry, Dental Practice, and the Community, 5th ed. Philadelphia, WB Saunders, 1999.

6. Allukian M, Horowitz A: Effective community prevention programs for oral diseases. In Gluck GM, Morganstein WM (eds): Jong's Community Dental Health, 5th ed. St. Louis, Mosby, 2003.

7. Oral Health in America: A report of the Surgeon General. Rockville, Md, U.S. Department of Health and Human Services, National Institute of Dental and Craniofacial Research, National Institutes of Health, 2000.

8. Gluck GM, Morganstein WM: Jong's Community Dental Health, 5th ed (Appendix). St. Louis, Mosby, 2003.

9. Kuthy R, Odum JG: Local dental programs: A descriptive assessment of funding and activities. J Public Health Dent 48:36, 1988.

10. Healthy People 2010: Understanding and Improving Health (Conference ed, 2 vols). Washington, DC, U.S. Department of Health and Human Services, 2000.

11. A National Call To Action To Promote Oral Health. Rockville Md, U.S. Department of Health and Human Services, Public Health Service, Centers for Disease Control and Prevention and the National Institutes of Health, National Institute of Dental and Craniofacial Research. NIH Publication No. 03-5303, May 2003.

12. Institute of Medicine Committee for the Study of the Future of Public Health, Division of Health Care Services: A Vision of Public Health in America: An Attainable Ideal in the Future of Public Health. Washington, DC, National Academy Press, 1998.

13. Public Health in America. Washington, DC, Public Health Functions Steering Committee, 1994.

14. Corbin SB, Marten FR: Future of dental public health report—preparing dental public health to meet the challenges: Opportunities of the 21st century. J Public Health Dent 54:80, 1994.

15. American Dental Hygienists Association: Lifestyle, Public Health Top Ten. Access 13:7, 1999.

16. The Advanced Dental Hygiene Practitioner. Access 8:18, Sept.-Oct. 2004.

2

Careers in Public Health for the Dental Hygienist

Sharon Logue, RDH, MPH
Kathy Voigt Geurink, RDH, MA

Objectives

Upon completion of this chapter, the student will be able to:

- Explain public health career options for dental hygienists
- Differentiate between career options available independently and through community agencies
- Discuss public health careers as a means of addressing the problem of access to oral health care
- Define skills and educational requirements for various roles in public health
- Explain the relationship of private practice activities to public health activities
- Identify specific careers, categorized by the six roles of the dental hygienist

Key Terms

Alternative Practice
Primary Prevention
General Supervision
Shortage Areas

Follow-up/Referral
Health Education
Networking
Social Marketing

Technical Assistance
Legislative/Policy Changes

OPENING STATEMENT

Career Possibilities
- Public health hygienist at a local health department
- Statewide coordinator for a school-based fluoride mouth rinse program
- Dental hygienist at a Veterans Administration hospital
- Dental hygienist working with a state migrant farm worker program
- Dental hygienist at a state correctional facility
- State dental director in a state health department
- Dental hygienist with a university hospital department
- Dental health educator with a school system
- Dental hygienist on a dental sealant team
- Dental hygienist in the U.S. Public Health Service
- Dental hygienist contracting for service in a nursing home
- Consultant to a Head Start program

COMMUNITY ORAL HEALTH PRACTICE AS A CAREER

Public health careers for dental hygienists run the gamut from high-level administrative posts to providing oral hygiene care for elderly residents in a nursing home or providing dental education for school-age children. In the public health field, some dental hygienists have an associate's degree or certificate, a bachelor's, a master's, or a doctorate degree. Many dental hygienists with advanced degrees working in public health began their public health careers with the minimum level of education. They chose to continue their education as their interests developed, their challenges expanded, and their desire grew to do more for the oral health of their community. A career in community oral health practice offers a variety of rewarding experiences that tend to feed the desire to make a difference in the oral health of all people.

We have provided a career chapter in the beginning of this text to allow you to make a connection with the role you might play in performing the functions discussed in the successive chapters. In private practice the individual patient is your focus; in public health the community is your patient. Your responsibilities will advance beyond individual clinical care, although in many positions individual care still remains a very important duty. Public health takes you into the realm of program development, implementation, and evaluation and offers an opportunity to work with various populations, other professionals, agencies, financing mechanisms, and rules and regulations.

FUTURE TRENDS FOR DENTAL HYGIENISTS IN PUBLIC HEALTH

The Problem of Access to Oral Health Care

In a national report entitled *Oral Health in America*, the Surgeon General reviewed the profound disparities among specific population groups in oral health status and access to dental care.[1] Dental disease has been a chronic problem among low-income populations.[2] Federal agencies and state governments are addressing these gaps in access to oral health care through legislation and policy development. Examples of some actions created through these processes are shown in "Guiding Principles."

GUIDING PRINCIPLES

Creating Access to Oral Health Care through Legislation and Policy Development[2,3]
- Allocating additional funds for dental services
- Expanding treatment for special populations
- Creating volunteers and donated dental services
- Providing service programs
- Additional dental benefits through existing public insurance programs
- Extending educational loans and loan forgiveness for dental professionals
- Creating tax credits for providers
- Forming career ladders for dental providers
- Increasing flexible licensure requirements
- Increasing the scope of the dental hygienist's duties
- Expanding coverage for provider services

Some of these developments may increase the demand for dental hygienists in community oral health practice.

Alternative Practice Settings

Public health settings are categorized as **alternative practice** settings (i.e., providing oral hygiene services outside the private office in a "nontraditional" setting). Examples of the setting might be a community clinic, a mobile van, a school, a hospital, or a nursing home (Figures 2-1 and 2-2). The delivery of dental services offered in private practice does not reflect the need for services for those without

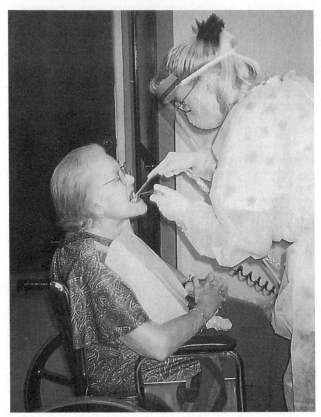

Figure 2-1 A dental hygienist is providing oral hygiene care to a resident of a nursing home.

means or without the capability of accessing care. In an alternative setting, dental care can be brought to people in need. Dental hygienists can provide preventive services in these settings, reaching large numbers of people who might not otherwise receive care.

Preventive services, or **primary prevention,** are more effective, less costly, and involve less technology than secondary or tertiary prevention (Box 2-1). Methods such as fluoride mouth rinse programs, nutritional counseling, dental health education to community groups, and oral hygiene services and instruction are at the primary level. Often primary prevention strategies do not require a dentist.[4] Therefore, with less restrictive supervision, the dental hygienist can perform functions at this level and reach underserved populations.

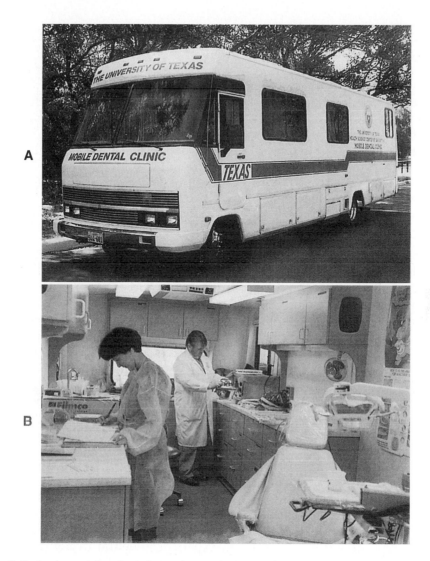

Figure 2-2 **A,** A mobile dental van is used as an alternative practice setting. **B,** Inside treatment area, mobile dental van.

Public Health Supervision

Regulatory Changes

Because of the need for services in places such as schools, nursing homes, and migrant health centers, dental hygienists are initiating oral health programs in

BOX 2-1   LEVELS OF PREVENTION

- **Primary prevention** prevents the disease before it occurs. This level includes health education, disease prevention, and health protection. (Dental prophylaxis, sealants, and water fluoridation are examples.)
- **Secondary prevention** eliminates or reduces diseases in the early stages. (Restorations such as amalgams or composites are examples. This level requires more technology and is more costly than primary prevention.)
- **Tertiary prevention** limits disability from disease in later stages and requires rehabilitation and surgical procedures. (Dentures, implants, and bridge work are examples. This level is most costly and requires highly trained professionals to treat the disease.)

these alternative settings. They are also filling positions beyond those connected with public health agencies. To create such positions, dental hygiene regulatory changes are being discussed and are now under way throughout the United States. Most states allow the dental hygienist to practice under **general supervision** (i.e., the dentist need not be on site, but the patient must have been one of record or must have been seen by the dentist previously). Between 1991 and 1999 seven states passed laws to permit less restrictive dental hygiene supervision, allowing for dental hygienists to reach underserved populations. Table 2-1 illustrates these states, including Colorado, which since 1987 has allowed unsupervised practice in all settings, and Washington, which since 1984 has allowed unsupervised practice in alternative settings, provided that the dental hygienist refers the patient to a dentist for further treatment. In a more recent example Virginia legislation went into effect July 2002 to allow dental hygienists to practice under general supervision. Conditions for duties to be delegated to a dental hygienist include a written prescription for the treatment that specifies the time period for filling the prescription, with a time period that cannot exceed 7 months. The Arizona Dental Hygienists Association in April 2004 supported two bills that would create a collaborative practice. This proposal would allow an experienced dental hygienist with a bachelor's degree to enter into a collaborative agreement with a dentist to provide unsupervised services in a variety of public health settings. In a 2001 American Dental Hygienists' Association (ADHA) Access to Care Position Paper, the ADHA confirmed its position that dental hygienists who are graduates from an accredited dental hygiene program can be fully used in all public and private practice settings to deliver preventive and therapeutic oral health care safely and effectively. "Licensed dental hygienists, by virtue of their comprehensive education and clinical preparation, are well prepared to deliver preventive oral health care services to the public, safely and effectively, independent of dental supervision."[5] In June 2004, the ADHA House of Delegates, addressing the problem of access to health care, approved the

Table 2-1   States that permit less restrictive dental hygiene supervision

Year	State	Condition
1999	New Mexico	Dental hygienists practicing in a cooperative working relationship with a consulting dentist without general supervision may be certified "collaborative dental hygienist."
1998	California	Registered dental hygienists in alternative practice (RDHAP) provide service in facilities and professional shortage areas with a prescription from a dentist or a physician.
1997	Oregon	Limited-access dental hygiene permit to treat patients in alternative settings; RDH must refer the patient annually to a licensed dentist available to treat the patient.
1997	Connecticut	Pilot program to allow an RDH to practice in specific settings without supervision.
1995	Maine	Public health supervision with permit to practice in specified alternative settings with a dentist who consults at the end of the project or annually but without general supervision.
1993	New Hampshire	Public health supervision with authorization of a dentist in an alternative setting; dentist reviews records annually.
1991	Michigan	RDH permitted to treat the underserved, provided that the dentist is available for review and consultation.
1987	Colorado	Unsupervised practice allowed in all settings.
1984	Washington	Unsupervised practice allowed in alternative settings, provided that the dental hygienist refers patient to a dentist for dental treatment and planning.

Data from Schroder K: States permitting unsupervised practice/less restrictive supervision. American Dental Hygienists Association, Division of Governmental Affairs (personal communication, 1998). Reprinted in J Dent Hygiene 74:118, 2000.

creation of the Advanced Dental Hygiene Practitioner (ADHP) credential. As stated in Chapter 1, this credential will allow dental hygienists to provide diagnostic, preventive, restorative, and therapeutic services directly to the public. Those dental hygienists who receive the ADHP credential will have graduated from an accredited dental hygiene program and will also have completed an ADHA-approved advanced educational curriculum. This credential is being designed to improve and enhance the oral health care delivery system. Because dental hygienists with the ADHP credential do not have to be supervised by a dentist, the door will open for them to work in school systems and nursing homes, and with underserved populations throughout the country. The ADHA website www.adha.org/governmental_affairs posts the most current state legislative news on oral health.

In determining the necessity of regulatory changes, one must consider many factors, such as

1. The ratio of dentists to people.
2. The number of dentists and dental hygienists in the state.
3. The number of low-income adults and children who need dental care.

These factors contribute to defining dental health professional **shortage areas.** Statistics compiled from the 2000 Synopsis of State and Territorial Dental Health Programs provide information necessary in determining the available workforce of dental professionals and of community health departments and clinics.[6] The workforce numbers, compared with population size, are useful in determining professional shortage areas and the need for community oral health programs. Inadequate access to health care caused by professional shortages and geographic and financial barriers prevents people from attaining improved health status and improved quality of life. The dental profession, in realizing the need for reaching these underserved populations, is initiating preventive programs conducted by dental hygienists in various states.

Public Health Supervision in Maine

In the state of Maine, data were collected and analyzed between May 1995, when the law allowed dental hygienists to practice without general supervision in alternative settings, and November 1998. Of 761 Registered Dental Hygienists in Maine, 38 dental hygienists were granted public health licensure to conduct community oral health programs. Twenty-three (60%) of the dental hygienists were with a public health agency; 15 (40%) were applicants seeking board approval for programs in their own communities to address specific oral health needs (Box 2-2).[7] All nonagency dental hygienists were volunteers or unpaid. Although being a volunteer is an important concept in public health, the trend for dental hygienists to enter this arena will increase notably with the development of expanded payment mechanisms.

It is interesting that some dental hygienists, initially volunteers, have found creative ways to be reimbursed for working in alternative settings. Writing grants, seeking school board funds, collecting Medicaid payments through an accepted provider, or contracting with a facility, in states that allow it, are a few of the innovative reimbursement plans currently being used. With the less restrictive dental

BOX 2-2   APPLICANTS FOR PUBLIC HEALTH LICENSURE IN MAINE

Dental hygienists licensed in Maine	761
Dental hygienists granted public health licensure	38
Dental hygienists with an agency or a school	23
Dental hygienists initiating their own projects	15

Box 2-3   Six Roles of the Dental Hygienist

1. Service provider/clinician
2. Health educator/wellness promoter
3. Consultant/resource person
4. Consumer advocate/change agent
5. Researcher
6. Administrator/manager

From Public Health in America. Washington, DC, Public Health Functions Steering Committee, 1994.

hygiene supervision and the increased number of dental hygienists seeking public health work, funding changes in the way of direct payment may be further explored in the future.

Dental hygienists in public health positions use a variety of skills in implementing community oral health programs that have positive effects on their communities. In this chapter we further define the six roles of the dental hygienist (Box 2-3) as they apply to specific career options for the dental hygienist. Most public health jobs require a combination of skills defined in multiple roles. Positions held by dental hygienists working in public health are included to inspire and illustrate the variety of career possibilities.

CAREERS IN DENTAL HYGIENE PUBLIC HEALTH

Service Provider/Clinician

In this familiar role, the public health dental hygienist provides clinical services to a targeted population, including assessment of oral health conditions and delivery of periodontal and preventive care. Often the population served in a public health dental clinic has had limited access to dental care, has been excluded from dental benefits under employer insurance, and is often described as having lower socioeconomic status. Socioeconomic status includes factors such as income, education, and occupation. Populations of low socioeconomic status generally are at increased risk for dental disease.[8] These factors and different social and cultural values can influence use of dental services offered in public health clinics. Additional skills needed by the clinician include the ability to assess the perceived dental needs of the patient and to recognize the social and economic barriers to successful oral health outcomes. Examples of barriers to accessing dental services may include transportation problems, geographic distances, missed work hours, or lack of day care services for children.[9]

The clinician must know effective preventive strategies for populations who are at high risk for dental caries. Topical and systemic fluorides, dental sealants, and fluoride varnishes are preventive therapies to be considered for clinical care in public health settings. Health education classes and oral hygiene instructions need to be adapted for the community audience. The dental hygienist may require additional preparation, including health education courses that reinforce teaching methods. Public health dental programs address health problems that affect a large number of people and design solutions to work within the social and cultural contexts of communities. These programs influence individual and group behaviors and practices.

Alternative settings for dental clinics may be in fixed facilities or operatories at local health departments, in stationary school trailers, or in mobile dental vans that can be moved to various schools within a geographic area. Some states have school-based dental programs with dental teams who use portable dental equipment for placing dental sealants. Other regions have dental programs partnering with Boys and Girls Clubs who have received funds to offer dental services to uninsured children with the use of portable equipment. Clinical dental hygiene positions are available in other community settings, including hospitals, nursing homes, and prison facilities. These locations offer the clinician additional challenges of complex medical histories and patients with physical or mental disabilities. Federal and state agencies have established clinical dental hygiene positions (e.g., the Indian Health Service, Community and Migrant Health Programs, military bases). In addition, clinical care programs in communities may be supported by nonprofit volunteer or religious organizations. In nonprofit and in publicly funded programs, these clinicians must be accountable with the most cost-effective way to provide quality dental services to the most people.

Public health dental hygienists may be asked to participate in the ongoing assessment of the prevalence of dental disease. This task is essential for public health program planning and evaluation. Clinical dental hygiene skills are used in conducting dental surveys and screenings for targeted populations. For example, a dental hygienist may be the coordinator who organizes a community-wide screening of school-age children. The dental hygienist selects and uses appropriate supplies, portable equipment, and infection control procedures and communicates with school personnel and parents to create the screening schedules for schools. Knowledge of dental indexes, data collection, and reporting of dental findings are essential.

In addition, with any screening program there must be a **follow-up/referral** component. Alerting the community to the problems discovered is part of the assessment; however, without the plan for action, the collection and presentation of data are ineffective. The plan for action includes a system to provide prevention and treatment for the documented needs.

Educational requirements for a public health clinical position may vary from an associate's degree to a bachelor's degree. If the public health job requires more administrative or consulting skills (see later), an employer may require more work experience or a master's degree.

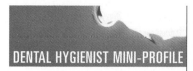

DENTAL HYGIENIST MINI-PROFILE *Service Provider/Clinician*

Name: Ginger Melton, RDH, BS

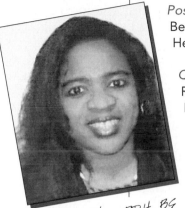

Ginger Melton, RDH, BS
Dental Hygienist, Service
Provider, and Clinician

Position and place of employment: Dental Hygienist; Beazley Dental Center of the Portsmouth Community Health Center; Portsmouth, Virginia

Qualifications and experience required for this position: Registered Dental Hygienist, Virginia Dental Hygiene License, at least 2 years of work experience; community education experience preferred.

Main dental hygiene role(s) fulfilled in this position: Service provider/clinician

Duties performed in this position

Provide dental health education, preventive dental services, and administrative services for the department. Provide oral hygiene services and dental education to children at school sites using the "Beazley Smile Mobile," which is a 40-foot, two-operatory, Mobile Dental Unit. Screen and refer children and adults to the appropriate program for dental care. Coordinate care for indigent adults at the Beazley Dental Center. Educate families about oral hygiene care.

Personal comment

As a public health dental hygienist, I face many challenges that are rewarding and motivating for me. In my clinical role, I provide much needed dental education, preventive services, and some administrative services. I am very proud of being able to provide dental care on the Beazley Smile Mobile. It is an outreach to this community like no other. Also, with the new laws governing supervision in my state, I am allowed to provide preventive care to the children without the dentist being on site. This is a milestone for our program. I am also able to use the Smile Mobile to screen and to provide dental awareness at health fairs and community events. This is very significant when you have a population that sees dental care as secondary. My challenge is to get the community to understand the importance of oral health and the prevention of disease.

Health Educator/Wellness Promoter

As in private practice, an important role of the public health dental hygienist is that of health educator. **Health education** is the process in which the client is encouraged to become responsible for personal oral health and is informed of scientifically based methods for preventing dental diseases. Beyond dental health education, though, is the promotion of total wellness. The community dental health educator must reinforce the relationship of oral health to total health.

Early childhood caries may be the result of infant feeding practices that are related to nutritional issues. Improved dietary habits by adults may mean less risk of dental decay and less risk of other chronic diseases. The dental hygienist working at the community level always needs to consider the larger picture of wellness in creating education programs. For example, current research indicates a possible relationship among periodontal health, cardiovascular health, incidence of premature births, and diabetes. Programs planned to intervene in these chronic diseases must be expanded to include oral health education.[10]

The team approach is always essential in public health. Dental health educators can participate in **networking** with other health professionals (i.e., they can share information about a common population). Working with public health nutritionists or Early Head Start Program staff could open channels to implement a fluoride varnish program targeting infants to toddlers. School nurses may have a unique perspective on the dental needs of schoolchildren, and sharing this information is helpful in program planning. Networking means that health statistics, resources for educational materials, and general community information are exchanged among dentists, physicians, dental hygienists, nurses, and nutritionists. As noted at a symposium (Children, Our Future) in 1998,[11] "the lack of integration of oral health into overall health adds a significant barrier to improving children's health outcomes." All health professionals must understand the impact of oral disease on systemic health. Effective networking among dental hygienists and other health professionals increases the awareness and importance of the relationship of oral health to general health. Community education, therefore, can be designed to include several health messages for a target group. This team approach is comprehensive and cost-effective.

Public health education programs have built upon the success of commercial marketing techniques by means of **social marketing** to promote the adoption of a behavior to improve health. Social marketing refers to using the effective advertising tools from commercial marketing to influence a valued health behavior change. Dental hygienists can use social marketing concepts to develop a public awareness campaign, to create educational materials, or to improve dental services.

An effective health educator researches the target population to identify the community's needs and concerns about dental health. A town forum or smaller focus groups may be organized to learn about the community's ideas on dental issues. Dental hygienists must study and understand the community to develop the appropriate message; they then monitor health education programs and, finally, readjust programs to meet changing trends. Mass media, the means of communication that reaches large numbers of people, can be a marketing tool. Skills in writing newspaper or newsletter articles and developing television and radio public service announcements can be valuable assets in a public health education position. Even the development of an oral health website can be a job responsibility.

Dental health educators may work statewide on preventive programs or may work with smaller, targeted populations at the county or community level. Examples of oral health education programs include:

- A spit tobacco intervention program related to prevention of oral cancer
- Promotion of dental sealants for schoolchildren
- Education about prevention of early childhood caries (baby bottle tooth decay) in cooperation with public health nutritionists
- A dental poster contest for third-graders
- Adoption of fluoridation in a community
- Promotion of mouth guards for athletes in a school district

The months of February (National Children's Dental Health Month) and October (Dental Hygiene Month) provide excellent opportunities for oral health educational activities. Health fairs are events that can reach the general public and provide information on numerous dental topics. Wellness fairs in local shopping malls or community centers provide an opportunity for public health and private dental professionals to offer exhibits together. The American Dental Association in partnership with Crest dental products company has promoted their "Give Kids A Smile!" program during February, where on a specific day dental professionals can provide free dental care to the community. Oral health educators can also collaborate with local dental hygiene components on National Children's Dental Health Month plans.

The successful dental health education program is planned to target a specific dental concern or a need identified in a population. Dental health educators in the community need organizational skills, current scientific knowledge, excellent communication skills, creativity, and flexibility to meet the challenges of community health improvement (see Chapter 8). Educational requirements for health educator positions may vary from a 2-year degree to a graduate degree, depending on specific job requirements.

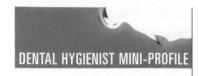

DENTAL HYGIENIST MINI-PROFILE

Educator/Wellness Promoter

Name: Leonor Ramos, RDH

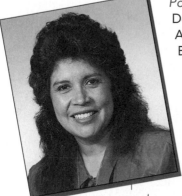

Leonor Ramos, RDH
Dental Hygienist, Educator,
and Wellness Promoter

Position and place of employment: Hospital Dentistry Dental Hygienist; Department of Defense; United States Air Force; Wilford Hall Medical Center; Lackland Air Force Base, Texas

Qualifications and experience required for this position: Registered Dental Hygienist, graduated from an accredited school of dental hygiene. Broad-based knowledge of complex medical and pathologic conditions and their impact on overall health. Experienced in providing appropriate clinical techniques and instructions for oral care and able to perform complex functions that differ with the needs of each medically compromised patient. Exceptional judgment, organizational skills, and leadership qualities preferred.

Main dental hygiene role(s) fulfilled in this position: Educator, clinician

Duties performed in this position

Educator

Educate hospitalized patients on oral hygiene care, provide numerous in-service presentations to various medical professionals on the oral management of medically compromised patients.

Clinician

Provide preoperative and postoperative preventive oral care for patients hospitalized for urgent surgery who require dental clearance before their surgery per our hospital's protocol. Included are patients receiving organ transplants, bone marrow transplants, and major orthopedic joint replacements; chronically ill patients; patients with hematologic disorders; patients with poorly controlled diabetes; patients in intensive critical care units; and terminally ill patients who need palliative oral care. Dental examination with x-rays and cleaning is required to reduce the incidence of secondary infections or graft rejections and thus reduce the incidence of extended hospitalization and patient mortality/morbidity.

Personal comment

I am currently serving in my thirtieth year of full-time work in the dental hygiene field. Over the years I have partnered with both the medical and dental community in various health care initiatives. It was through this involvement that I realized total patient care is best achieved when a network of health care providers work toward a common goal. This interdisciplinary cooperation inspired me to initiate both a clinical and a hospital dentistry rotation for second-year dental hygiene students. I also initiated the development of guidelines for health care providers of patients with cancer, with focus on their oral management. The monograph, entitled "Oral Health in Cancer Therapy," is made possible through the Oral Health Education Foundation.

In promoting these guidelines, it is my hope that more collaborative efforts be developed between dental and medical facilities. As others in the community embrace this concept, it will be beneficial to network with local cancer associations, legislators who focus on Medicare and Medicaid oral care reimbursements, and medical and dental school advisory boards.

Consultant/Resource Person

A public health dental hygienist may be asked to be a resource person for dental information and provide **technical assistance** at the local, state, or federal level. Technical assistance refers to the use of professional skills and a knowledge base to provide guidance to nondental community members interested in developing preventive programs. In this role the dental hygienist acts as a consultant to community agencies, schools, or other health professions on dental issues. Oral health education for persons who will deliver the dental message to other adults and children is an example of a "train the trainer" activity. Oral health education can be targeted to Head Start Programs, nursing homes, and day care staffs; parent organizations; schoolteachers; coaches; school nurses; and nutritionists.

Another example of the resource/consultant role might involve representing the dental profession on local committees, such as the American Cancer Society, the American Heart Association, Head Start Health Advisory committees, local health partnership coalitions, and dental professional organizations. Committee options are unlimited. On a regional level, dental hygienists can be employed part time to be consultants and to review Head Start programs for compliance with program standards. State public health programs that monitor community water fluoridation may have dental hygienists who provide technical assistance to water engineers or to community leaders initiating a council vote on fluoridation. A school system considering starting a school-based fluoride mouth rinse program may ask for supportive testimony at a school board meeting from a dental hygienist.

As resource persons, dental hygienists can help guide the public on the appropriateness of available dental health educational materials. Given the existence of many information clearinghouses, the dental hygienist needs organizational skills to maintain current directories of dental resources. The Maternal and Child Health National Oral Health Clearinghouse is an example of a directory with dental educational materials appropriate for many community preventive programs. Public health dental programs must always be cost-effective, and national clearinghouses may often be good sources of quality materials at reasonable prices.

With communication technology constantly changing, knowledge of current dental websites for references is essential in this role. Websites are a resource not only for professionals but also for consumers at all income levels who are gaining access to this form of communication. A dental hygienist can provide technical assistance by

1. Creating a web page containing information on oral health.
2. Maintaining a lending library of dental brochures, videotapes, and educational displays available to the public.
3. Developing culturally appropriate educational materials to meet the needs of community groups.

Dental schools and dental hygiene education programs may request guest lectures on community oral health from a resource person. Student interactions with public health staff can only add to an increased understanding of public health policies and their positive impact on society. A dental hygienist may coordinate an extramural public health rotation for dental hygiene students and get them involved in health promotion activities. Educational requirements for a consultant/resource person may range from a bachelor's degree to a master's degree.

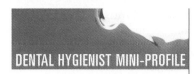

DENTAL HYGIENIST MINI-PROFILE *Consultant/Resource Person*

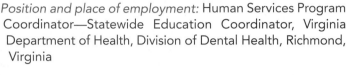

Name: JoAnn W. Wells, RDH, BS

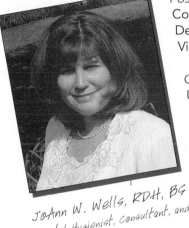

JoAnn W. Wells, RDH, BS
Dental Hygienist, Consultant, and
Resource Person

Position and place of employment: Human Services Program Coordinator—Statewide Education Coordinator, Virginia Department of Health, Division of Dental Health, Richmond, Virginia

Qualifications and experience required for this position: Undergraduate degree in dental hygiene. Preferred: Master's degree in an educationally related area or with a strong emphasis in health education and at least 1 year of work experience.

Main dental hygiene role(s) fulfilled in this position: Consultant/resource person

Duties performed in this position

Act as a consultant for Head Start Programs, Statewide Head Start Health Advisory Committee, Early Child Care Educators, Governor's Child Health Task Force, Virginia's Alliance of Adolescent and School Health, the Virginia Dental Association's Mission of Mercy, and Virginia's Partnership for Achieving Successful Schools.

Plan and present workshops on oral health education including early intervention with fluoride varnish, nutritional information, and basic dental health facts. As a resource person, assist workshops through the Department of Education for teachers, school nurses, health care providers, WIC/nutritionists, and dental public health and nursing staff at local health departments. Present programs to dental/dental hygiene students on Public Health Dentistry in Virginia. Review and evaluate appropriate oral health educational materials for distribution to other community agencies and to individuals. Complete translation services of all educational brochures.

In collaboration with the Virginia Dental Association's national campaign "Give Kids a Smile Day," conduct consultation with local dental components. Assist with National Children's Dental Health Month Activities sponsored by the Virginia Dental

Association, the Department of Pediatric Dentistry and Division of Dental Hygiene at the Virginia Commonwealth University School of Dentistry.

Personal comment

My concern is for the dental health of children and the educational achievement of young people. The recognition that education and health are intertwined has resulted in considerable interest in school health programs that engage the entire community. My experience as a consultant/resource person with school administrators, school nurses, schoolteachers, parents, and caregivers is to focus on the child's oral health to achieve a common vision.

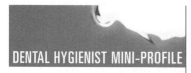

DENTAL HYGIENIST MINI-PROFILE *Consultant/Resource Person*

Name: Diana Cudeii, BA, RDH, CDA

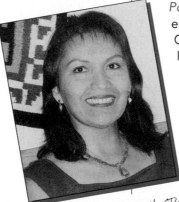

Diana Cudeii, BA, RDH, CDA
Dental Hygienist, Consultant,
and Resource Person

Position and place of employment: Subcontractor (self-employed) as a Dental Hygiene Education and Prevention Consultant with the Inter Tribal Council of Arizona (ITCA) Inc., an organization based in Phoenix, Arizona.

Qualifications and experience required for this position: Bachelor's degree in dental hygiene and an Arizona dental hygiene license are required. A Master's of Public Health (or equivalent degree) and/or experience in dental public health is desirable. Experience with Tribal programs and/or working in the Public Health Service or Indian Health Service are desirable. Travel will be required as determined by program needs and responsibilities.

Duties performed in this position

The purpose of this position is to assist the Director of the Dental Support Center in developing, implementing, and evaluating dental health programs for the tribes located in Arizona as well as Indian Health Service programs in the Phoenix and Tucson Service Areas.

- Develop, implement, and evaluate training programs for staff on periodontal disease prevention and intervention at clinical and community levels. Emphasis will be on public health-based interventions (sealants, fluoride varnish, etc.) and their effectiveness.
- Conduct assessments on periodontal health status and community and staff needs.
- Develop and implement culturally appropriate training programs for staff and community on dental prevention and education topics.
- Assist with recruiting Native American students into the dental professions, including Career Days.
- Deliver dental health presentations at conferences, community wellness fairs, and school events.
- Promote opportunities of working as a dental health care provider with the Native populations at colleges, universities, and dental schools.
- Other special projects as designated by the Dental Director.

The work consists of complex operatives of a professional nature that require independence, creativity, self-direction, and the ability to work with team members.

Contacts with individuals or groups from within and outside the ITCA dental support center are in a moderately unstructured setting. The purpose of contacts is to negotiate, clarify, or resolve matters involving significant issues. Through effective communication, technical consultation is provided to dental health professionals, laypersons, private vendors, and others.

Personal comment

I was born and raised in the community of Shiprock, New Mexico, on the Dine' (Navajo) Reservation. I received my dental assisting certification from the University of New Mexico in Albuquerque in 1984 and my dental hygiene education at the University of Texas Health Sciences Center at San Antonio in 1992. I have worked in private dental practices in Texas, Arizona, and Colorado, and various state, county, tribal, Indian Health Service, and urban community clinics in Arizona, New Mexico, Colorado, and North Dakota.

The Native philosophy teaches that life is envisioned as a journey to a long and healthy life. On this journey, one experiences meaning, purpose, and responsibility. As a population that is used as a measurement for statistics from dental decay to diabetes, the Native population has begun to take responsibility for their own health. They are establishing fitness/health programs to combat the infectious diseases of the body. Our knowledge about the risks and causes of the diseases that have inflicted our tribal people and how to prevent or delay the illnesses has increased. The Native world combines tradition, culture, spirituality, and humor to boost people's sense of well-being and to reconnect and revive the balance and harmony with the elements of the universe. A connection has to exist among the healer (health care provider), patient, and creator for holistic healing to occur. Working with tribal communities, you have to participate in their community activities from tribal pow-wows to community celebrations. These events provide the opportunities to educate leaders, elders, youth, parents, and educators of the community about effective tribal based dental intervention strategies. These programs empower the community to address their dental needs, to implement dental preventive programs, and to become more active in their own health care delivery system. The intergenerational home setting of Native families provides open communication for passing on healthy habits to decrease the rate of early childhood decay, periodontal diseases, diabetes, cancer, and heart diseases. Through my journey I have been blessed in my professional career to meet and share experiences and knowledge with health care providers truly committed in not only improving the health status but also in preserving the social, cultural, and spiritual well-being of our Native people.

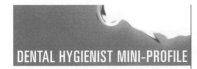

DENTAL HYGIENIST MINI-PROFILE *Consultant/Resource Person*

Name: Sharon Logue, RDH, MPH

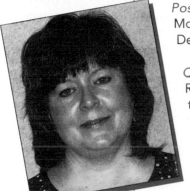

Sharon Logue, RDH, MPH
Dental Hygienist, Consultant, and
Resource Person

Position and place of employment: School Fluoride Mouthrinse Coordinator; Division of Dental Health; Virginia Department of Health; Richmond, Virginia

Qualifications and experience required for this position: Registered Dental Hygienist (RDH) with a current license to practice dental hygiene in the Commonwealth of Virginia and knowledge of dentistry with emphasis on prevention and oral disease. As a result of the prescriptive nature of fluoride and the involvement in oral health surveys, the RDH is required. Communication and presentation skills and the ability to work independently are necessary. Experience in teaching and group presentations and the ability to work effectively with school personnel and community agencies when implementing preventive programs are preferred.

Main dental hygiene role(s) fulfilled in this position: Consultant/resource person

Duties performed in this position

Provide on-site training and monitoring for the school-based fluoride mouth rinse program in the 50 counties currently participating. Program guidance to schools includes working with school nurses, teachers, administrators, parent volunteers, and students. Training and consultation are also provided for program expansion. Coordinate mouth rinse supply ordering statewide with the contracted vendor and track the budget. Annually update information to be included in the fluoride mouth rinse training packet. Provide oral health information on other preventive topics to communities. Coordinate school oral health surveys to evaluate effectiveness of the fluoride mouth rinse program.

Personal comment

My experiences in public health with oral health education and promotion have been rewarding and challenging. Working with the school-age population is always fun! Communication and organizational skills are very important in developing and implementing successful community-based programs. I have found that assessing the "big picture" of oral health needs in a population is always needed, followed by creative thinking in developing strategies to meet those needs. The variety of tasks in public health and the networking that occurs with different agencies and health professionals are enjoyable.

Consumer Advocate/Change Agent

With the community considered to be a "patient," the public health dental hygienist assesses the dental needs and concerns of the population. After exploring the available dental resources, the dental hygienist identifies any "gaps" in oral health services for specific populations. A gap refers to the inability of a group of individuals to receive, or have access to, oral health services. For example, an indigent group of older adults may lack finances to obtain dental care. The dental hygienist might represent these individuals in seeking community resources and in developing special programs. Once consumer issues are brought to the attention of local media or powerful citizens, changes can occur and problems can be solved. The consumer advocate sees problems related to achieving optimal oral health and attempts to develop a solution.

As a dental professional, the hygienist can be a leader for the consumer and can be asked to be a vocal advocate for oral health. Dental hygienists who serve on state dental boards are evaluating skills of recent graduates, thus protecting the public and acting as a consumer advocate. The role of consumer advocate/change agent may not be a full-time position but may be part of another role in the dental hygiene profession. A request for expert testimony on dental issues might come from state legislative bodies or boards of health. In this role the dental hygienist is working to advance the health of the public through **legislative** and public **policy changes**.

Legislative activity to change dental hygiene supervision laws is a task of the dental hygienist in the role of change agent. The ADHA cites restrictive supervision laws for dental hygienists as a barrier to access for oral health care. Dental hygienists working under *direct supervision* (i.e., a dentist must be physically present during procedures performed by a hygienist) is limited in performing preventive services for segments of the population who do not have access to regular oral health care, such as the poor, elderly, and disabled. Through the role of change agent/consumer advocate, dental hygienists have changed supervision from *direct* to *general* in many states. As a result of legislative involvement by dental hygienists in California, certification of the Registered Dental Hygienist in Alternative Practice (RDHAP) was initiated in 1998. The RDHAP is a licensed dental hygienist who provides unsupervised dental hygiene services in settings such as schools or institutions as prescribed by a dentist or physician.[12]

Dental hygienists who become consumer advocates/change agents may have several years of experience in their profession and have the ability to visualize the "big picture." A specific educational degree beyond being a Registered Dental Hygienist may not be needed in this role. An effective consumer advocate/change agent is knowledgeable, confident, and eager for all citizens to have optimal oral health.

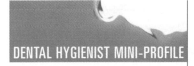

DENTAL HYGIENIST MINI-PROFILE *Consumer Advocate/Change Agent*

Name: Kathleen Mangskau, RDH, MPA

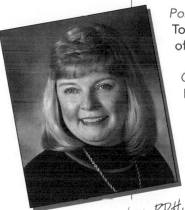

Kathleen Mangskau, RDH, MPA
Dental Hygienist, Consumer Advocate, and Change Agent

Position and place of employment: Director, Division of Tobacco Prevention and Control; North Dakota Department of Health; Bismarck, North Dakota

Qualifications and experience required for this position: Master's degree in public health, public administration, business, or related behavioral science field and 4 years' experience in program administration, policy development, and community intervention.

Main dental hygiene roles fulfilled in this position: Administrator and change agent (primary); educator and consultant (secondary)

Duties performed in this position

Planning, organizing, directing, controlling, and evaluating a statewide comprehensive tobacco prevention and control program. Essential functions include planning and evaluation, policy making, management, education, consultation, fiscal control, and human resource management. Primary duties include grants and contracts management, policy, development, advocacy, and implementation.

Personal comment

My background and experience as a clinical dental hygienist and state dental director prepared me for my role as the Director of the Division of Tobacco Prevention and Control.

As a clinical dental hygienist, I knew changing personal behavior is often difficult. Dealing with nicotine addiction and promoting environmental change are very challenging and at the same time rewarding. In addition to public education, community inter-vention, strategic use of media, and policy and environmental change and evaluation are key strategies needed to effectively change risk behaviors. Just as public health dental hygienists must counter the attacks of anti-fluoridationists, tobacco control advocates must counter the attacks and influence of the tobacco industry. Understanding how public education, science, and politics influence community actions becomes a key role for a change agent.

Researcher

As a researcher, a dental hygienist uses scientific methods and knowledge to identify and pursue a specific area of interest (see Chapter 7 for a discussion of the scientific method used in research). Dental hygienists employed in the research arena work in settings that vary from state health departments to universities to private industry.

In a state health department dental program, the epidemiology of dental diseases is a likely area of interest. Knowledge of dental indexes to survey the prevalence of dental diseases is required, and biostatistical skills for analyzing data are important. Funding for state dental programs is becoming difficult to maintain, given the trend toward government downsizing in some states. Being accountable for public funds is an essential part of program evaluation. Dental data must be continually gathered to evaluate and demonstrate the effectiveness of public health programs in improving oral health and reducing barriers to oral health care.

In a research position, the dental hygienist coordinates a statewide needs assessment. For a dental survey of this size, the dental hygienist must select a sample of appropriate size across the state and obtain permission to examine a specific population. If an oral health needs assessment involves the caries rates for children, the researcher may work through the school system to arrange for the children to be examined. Dental examiners are trained to use the dental indexes through a calibration exercise to ensure that valid data have been obtained by the survey. Ultimately, the dental data analysis is important for future public health program planning. Epidemiologic research is crucial in maintaining existing oral health programs or in initiating new ones.

Research positions are available at many university or dental school settings. For example, a dental hygienist might be hired to participate in a periodontal research project to study the effectiveness of a new antimicrobial product, a microbiology department might seek dental hygienists as research associates, or a dental hygienist at a Veterans' Affairs hospital might study therapeutic procedures for patients with head and neck cancer.

Certainly, dental product companies have ongoing research to scientifically determine the effectiveness of new methods and products to prevent and treat oral diseases. A dental hygienist working as a researcher has an appropriate background in basic science and dental science to join a research team. Dental hygienists choosing research positions may work part time as a researcher, with the remainder of the job description being one of the previously discussed roles. Educational requirements for research positions may require a bachelor's degree. The specific background needed for research positions varies with the employer.

DENTAL HYGIENIST MINI-PROFILE | *Researcher*

Name: Kathy Phipps, RDH, MPH, DrPH

Position and place of employment: Associate Professor; Oregon Health & Science University; Portland, Oregon

Qualifications and experience required for this position: Doctoral degree with experience in research; postdoctoral research fellowship recommended. With research experience, candidate may be in the process of doctoral degree completion.

Main dental hygiene role(s) fulfilled in this position: Researcher

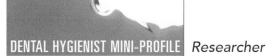
Kathy Phipps, RDH, MPH, DrPH
Dental Hygienist and Researcher

Duties performed in this position

Research is concerned with epidemiology, or the study of disease trends in populations. With an RDH background, oral epidemiology is the area of research that is emphasized. For example, the present researcher is studying the impact of fluoride on skeletal health (osteoporosis).

Assisting local, state, and federal agencies in tracking the oral health status of people in their jurisdictions is also a function of the position.

Research interests may be expanded from dentistry to medicine. This researcher is a co-investigator for a major 7-year research project looking at risk factors for osteoporosis, cardiovascular disease, and prostate cancer in older men.

Primary duties of the epidemiology aspect include writing grant proposals, developing research protocols, analyzing research data, and writing manuscripts. Research assistants actually work with the study participants and collect the data.

Personal comment

I am a graduate of the dental hygiene program at Oregon Health & Science University with a Bachelor of Science degree in Dental Hygiene. At the same time, I also attended classes at Portland State University and received a Bachelor of Science degree in general science with an emphasis in public health studies.

After receiving my bachelor degrees, I practiced dental hygiene for about 1 year. I then applied to graduate school and received a scholarship to attend the Program in Dental Public Health, School of Public Health at the University of Michigan. My emphasis during the master's program was in health care administration. I returned to the state of Oregon and worked as a health administrator and social service manager for an agency serving senior citizens.

I was away from dentistry for about 6 years and decided that it was time to return to the field. I applied for and received funding to complete my doctoral degree at the University of Michigan. I became interested in fluoride and started doing my research on fluoride and osteoporosis while still in graduate school.

Since that time, I have had three research projects funded by the National Institute of Dental and Craniofacial Research. The results of these projects have been published in the *Journal of Dental Research* and the *British Medical Journal*.

Although research my not sound glamorous or exciting, it has given me an opportunity to experience many different aspects of life. For example, I have done research in Russia and remote villages in Alaska, I have made presentations to dentists and hygienists in both the United States and the United Kingdom, and I am on several advisory panels for the National Institutes of Health and the Centers for Disease Control and Prevention.

Administrator/Manager

The expanded coordination needed for community-wide oral health programs creates the need for a dental hygienist to be an administrator/manager. In this role the hygienist is an initiator who develops, organizes, and manages oral health programs to meet the needs of targeted groups of people. Planning skills may be required for local, state, or federal oral health programs. If the oral health program is implemented for a large population or within a large geographic area, supervision of other professional and technical staff may be required.

The type of oral health program managed depends on the needs of the population. For example, a hygienist may manage a statewide school-based fluoride mouth rinse program funded from state revenues or from a federal grant. In this position the dental hygienist needs the following:

1. Knowledge of how systemic and topical fluorides work to prevent dental caries.
2. Good communication skills to establish a working relationship with school superintendents, principals, and teachers.
3. Organizational skills to plan a budget, to order supplies, and to keep records.
4. Knowledge of evaluation procedures to account for the cost versus the program effectiveness.

To assess the dental caries rate among participating schoolchildren, one ideally conducts a dental survey before and after initiating this preventive program. Writing skills are important for summarizing survey results and program successes and for soliciting for additional grant funds.

An administrator or manager may often have additional roles, as previously discussed. The administrator may be required to provide some consulting, to become an advocate for changing public policy, or to be involved with social marketing for a new oral health initiative. Educational requirements of this administrative role are usually several years of experience and a bachelor's or master's degree in a related field such as public health or health administration (Figure 2-3).

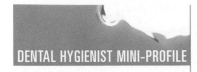

DENTAL HYGIENIST MINI-PROFILE

Administrator/Manager

Name: Diane Brunson, RDH, MPH

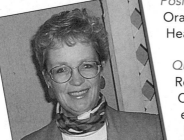

*Diane Brunson, RDH, MPH
Dental Hygienist, Administrator,
and Manager*

Position and place of employment: Section Director for Oral, Rural, Primary Care; Colorado Department of Public Health and Environment

Qualifications and experience required for this position: Registered Dental Hygienist licensed in the state of Colorado. Three years' experience in dental hygiene, education, and/or planning. Master's degree in Public Health preferred. Three years' experience in dental public health. Experience in program administration, community education, and planning.

Main dental hygiene role(s) fulfilled in this position: Administrator/manager (primary); Change agent, consultant, and educator (secondary). Position also offers opportunities for research and clinical responsibilities.

Duties performed in this position

Assessing oral health status of state residents; identifying contributing risk factors and barriers to accessing care; working with key stakeholders to identify policy changes to improve oral health; planning, directing, and evaluating a statewide oral health program in oral disease prevention and health promotion (i.e., fluoridation and school-based/school-linked sealant programs); supervising staff; and fiscal accountability in managing program budgets.

Personal comment

I really enjoy the variety, flexibility, and creativity that public health has to offer. In an administrative role, I have access to the policy makers who make decisions every day that affect their constituents, so I derive satisfaction when those decisions include improving oral health.

JOB DESCRIPTION
ORAL HEALTH PROGRAM DIRECTOR

SUMMARY: The Dental Health Program Director is responsible for planning, developing, directing, and evaluating a statewide dental health program in oral disease prevention/health promotion according to the long-term goals of the department and the delegated duties in the Division of Maternal and Child Health.

ESSENTIAL DUTIES AND RESPONSIBILITIES include the following. Other duties may be assigned.

Planning and evaluation
- Develops Dental Health Program goals, objectives, and work plans.
- Conducts community and statewide assessment of dental health and dental health–related problems and resources to determine current needs:
  a. Plans and conducts surveys. Analyzes and disseminates results.
  b. Uses secondary data.
  c. Directs special projects in dental health and prepares and analyzes reports of findings.
- Monitors and evaluates oral health prevention projects.

Management
- Uses data to document, monitor, and evaluate dental health services, costs, and outcomes
- Supervises application of and implementation of and contract performance under state and federal grant programs.
- Analyzes and summarizes program data.
- Prepares progress, quarterly, annual, and other administrative reports.
- Develops administrative and operational relationships with other state and local health, human services, and education units.
- Recommends staffing needs to division director.

Education
- Interprets and disseminates current scientific information on oral health prevention and treatment to professionals in health and human service agencies, educational institutions, and the general public.
- Develops, updates, and evaluates dental health education materials for use in health agency programs.
- Arranges, plans, and conducts in-service and training programs for program staff, health professionals, educators, volunteers, and the public.
- Prepares monthly program communication to dental health staff.
- Participates in professional development activities (reading journals, attending professional meetings, etc.)

Consultation
- Provides oral health consultation and technical assistance to administrators, policymakers, other dental personnel and professionals in the health agencies, other human service professionals in related agencies, and educators in academic institutions.

Figure 2-3 Sample of typical job description for oral health program director.

Continued

Policymaking
- Establishes and revises policies and procedures for the Dental Health Program in compliance with Health department policies and federal rules, regulations, and guidelines.
- Advises senior policymakers and administrators on dental health related issues.
- Reviews and comments on proposed federal or state laws, regulations, standards, and guidelines being promulgated by legislators or regulatory agencies.
- Provides leadership and advocacy for oral health issues.

Fiscal control
- Prepares and controls the operating budget for the Dental Health Program.
- Oversees approval of dental health special initiative grants to local entities.
- Prepares grant proposals and contracts to obtain external funding and technical assistance to evaluate and expand dental health services.

Supervision
- Supervises and evaluates program administrative support staff.
- Supervises and evaluates regional dental health consultants.
- Recruits, orients, trains, supervises, and evaluates work performance of contract staff and volunteers for special projects.

Figure 2-3 Sample of typical job description for oral health program director.

SUMMARY

Various career options exist for dental hygienists in the public health arena. The public health career options offer many challenges and opportunities for the dental hygienist to become actively involved in providing optimal oral health for the community. The trend of less restrictive dental hygiene regulation to facilitate the dental hygienist's desire to provide preventive treatment to underserved populations is explored. Data collected on population numbers related to dental manpower and community programs are mentioned and can be located at the website for the Association of State and Territorial Dental Directors (http://www.astdd.org).

Public health career options and public health positions for dental hygienists are available in a variety of settings. Within the primary setting of your dental hygiene career, you may choose to develop skills to work as a clinician, educator, researcher, consultant, consumer advocate, or administrator. The skills and education necessary to fulfill these roles have been delineated in the chapter.

Applying **Your Knowledge**

1. Check with your state health department to determine whether public health or community dental hygiene positions are available in your community. Obtain a job description and evaluate the skills needed for this position using the six roles described in the chapter.

2. Research all available dental resources in your community for older adults who are unable to afford or travel to private dental offices. Whom would you contact to find out the location of these dental services? Write a job description for yourself to treat elderly residents unable to have access to care in private offices.
3. Review dental supervision laws in your state, and determine whether there is a need for change. Which populations might benefit from a change? How might you be involved in initiating a change?
4. Participate in a community rotation/service project that is considered an alternative practice setting.

DENTAL HYGIENE COMPETENCIES

Reading the material in this chapter and participating in the activities of Applying Your Knowledge will contribute to the student's ability to demonstrate the following competencies:

Core competencies

C.8 Communicate effectively with individuals and groups from diverse populations verbally and in writing.

Community involvement

CM.3 Provide community oral health services in a variety of settings.

Professional growth and development

PGD.1 Identify alternative career options within health care, industry, education, and research, and evaluate the feasibility of pursuing dental hygiene opportunities.
PGD.2 Develop management and marketing strategies to be used in nontraditional health care settings.
PGD.3 Access professional and social networks and resources to assist entrepreneurial initiative.

Community Case

In your position as the oral health education coordinator for the Division of Dental Health, State Health Department, you are assigned the task of developing an educational campaign promoting oral health as part of overall health. You need to collaborate with other health professionals within the health department system to accomplish your goal.

1. One of the first steps in planning your educational campaign would be:
    a. Use your public health directory to contact each health division
    b. Define the target population for your educational campaign

      c. Develop the educational materials yourself and distribute to focus groups

      d. Develop strategies other than mass media because of the expense

2. You decide to set up a committee to help develop the "healthy mouth, healthy body" campaign, and invite a public health nurse, nutritionist, and chronic disease health educator to join. This step is an example of:

      a. Networking to pool resources and skills

      b. Taking steps toward policy changes

      c. A dental hygienist working under general supervision

      d. Secondary prevention strategies

3. A parent who is president of a local school PTA has contacted your public health office and needs information about how her school can participate in the school fluoride mouth rinse program offered at other schools. In responding to this request, your role would most likely be categorized as:

      a. Administrator/manager

      b. Consumer advocate/change agent

      c. Consultant/resource person

      d. Service provider/clinician

REFERENCES

1. Oral Health in America: A Report of the Surgeon General. Rockville, Md, U.S. Department of Health and Human Services, National Institute of Dental and Craniofacial Research, National Institutes of Health, 2000.
2. Oral Health: Dental Disease Is a Chronic Problem Among Low-Income Populations. Washington, DC, U.S. General Accounting Office, 2000.
3. State of the States: Overview of 1999 State Legislation on Access to Oral Health. Washington, DC, Center for Policy Alternatives, 1999.
4. Warren RC: Oral Health for All: Policy for Available, Accessible and Acceptable Care. Washington, DC, Center for Policy Alternatives, 1999.
5. Access to Care Position Paper 2001: American Dental Hygienists' Association, 2001. http://www.ncdha.org/access_to_care.htm.
6. Synopsis of State and Territorial Dental Public Health Programs: Association of State and Territorial Dental Directors (ASTDD) Home Page, 2000. http://www.astdd.org.
7. Beaulieu E: Dental Hygiene public health supervision changes in Maine law. J Dent Hyg 74:117, 2000.
8. Brick P: Working in public health. Access 7:12, 1993.
9. Capilouto E: Improving the oral health of at-risk children. J Health Care Poor Underserved 2:132, 1991.
10. Berthold M: Profiles in public health: Dental hygienists reach out. Access 12:13, 1998.
11. Mouradian WE: Introduction and Overview of Children's Oral Health: A forgotten area. Symposium: Children, Our Future. Seattle, 1998.
12. American Dental Hygienists Association, Division of Governmental Affairs, Stateline. Access 12:32, 2000.

3

Assessment in the Community

Jane E.M. Steffensen, RDH, BS, MPH, CHES

Objectives

Upon completion of this chapter, the student will be able to:

- Explain the importance of assessment as a core public health function
- Describe the roles of public health professionals in assessment
- Discuss the basic terms and concepts of epidemiology
- Describe the conceptual models that illustrate the determinants of health
- Identify the determinants of health that affect the health of individuals and communities
- Identify the specific stages of a planning cycle
- Discuss a community oral health improvement process
- Describe the main steps followed and key activities undertaken in a community oral health assessment
- Compare and contrast the different methods of data collection that can be used in community health assessments

Key Terms

Assessment	Determinants of Health	Assess
Epidemiology	Mandala of Health	Plan
Host Factors	Systematic Approach to	Implement
Agent Factors	Health Improvement	Evaluate
Environmental Factors	Planning Cycle	

Community Oral Health
  Improvement Process
Community Oral Health
  Assessment

Community Profile
Data Collection

Quantitative Data
Qualitative Data

OPENING STATEMENT

National Leading Health Indicators

Indicators	**Related Statistic***
• Access to health insurance	• 16% of children and adults (under 65 years) do not have health insurance
• Access to personal health care	• 12% of children and adults do not have a source of ongoing primary health care
• Prenatal care	• 17% of pregnant women have not received prenatal care during the first trimester
• Immunizations	• 75% of young children (aged 19 to 35 months) are fully immunized
• Physical activity	• 67% of adults are not physically active on a regular basis
• Overweight and obesity	• 31% of adults are obese
• Tobacco use	• 22% of adults smoke cigarettes
• Substance abuse	• 20% of adolescents have used alcohol or illicit drugs during the past month
• Mental health	• 23% of adults with recognized depression have received treatment
• Injury and violence	• 101,537 deaths per year caused by unintentional injuries
• Environmental quality	• 41% of Americans are exposed to harmful air pollutants
• Responsible sexual behavior	• 14,477 deaths per year from HIV/AIDS[†]

Statistics 2000-2002 from http://www.cdc.gov (accessed June 2004).
[†]*HIV, Human immunodeficiency virus; AIDS, acquired immunodeficiency syndrome.*

PUBLIC HEALTH PRACTICE

Professional work in community health is dynamic because the environment changes continuously. Community health is affected by social, demographic, political, economic, and technologic changes. In this milieu public health practitioners perform a broad array of duties focused on entire populations, with the overarching goal that people are healthy and live in healthy communities.[1,2] The mission of public health is to "fulfill society's interest in assuring the conditions in which people can be healthy."[3,4] Public health carries out this mission through organized, interdisciplinary efforts that address health problems in communities. Its mission is achieved through the application of health promotion and disease prevention and control efforts designed to improve health and enhance quality of life.[1-4]

Public health services incorporate the roles of a myriad of public health professionals in various sectors and from diverse disciplines that form the public health workforce in the United States.[4,5] Public health professionals belong to many professional disciplines including oral health, nursing, nutrition, social work, health promotion, laboratory science, environmental health, administration, and epidemiology. Public health professionals have expertise in diverse public health practices.[5] Education and training guidelines have been developed to extend capacity and to ensure that current and future public health professionals have expertise in key public health services.[4,5]

Successful provision of public health services requires collaboration among private and public partners within a given community and across various levels of government.[4] To fulfill these goals, partnerships must have broad-based representation of constituency and stakeholder groups including private, voluntary, nonprofit, and public agencies or organizations involved in health, mental health, substance abuse, environmental health protection, and public health.[6] Examples of organizations and agencies that can be engaged in coalitions and collaborative partnerships to improve health in communities are presented in Appendix C.

ASSESSMENT: A CORE PUBLIC HEALTH FUNCTION

The contemporary principles of public health practice and science have been highlighted in several national reports.[3-5] These reports, published by the Institute of Medicine (IOM), detail past contributions and identify future challenges to public health. They outline recommendations to improve the nation's public health system and to ensure universal access to necessary public health services.

The Future of Public Health report specified three core public health functions that shape the basic practice of public health at the state and local level.[3] State health agencies and local health departments must perform these functions to protect and promote health, wellness, and quality of life and to prevent disease, injury, disability, and death. These functions (as noted in Chapter 1) are (1) assessment,

(2) policy development, and (3) assurance.[3] This chapter emphasizes the core public health function of assessment in the community.

The IOM report called for public health agencies to promote, to facilitate, and—when necessary and appropriate—to perform community health assessments and to monitor change in key measures to evaluate performance. **Assessment** is defined as the regular and systematic collection, assemblage, analysis, and communication on the health of the community.[3] The IOM report stated that assessment includes statistics on health status, community health needs, and epidemiologic and other studies of health problems.[3]

ROLES OF PUBLIC HEALTH PROFESSIONALS IN ASSESSMENT

The effective use of information in the twenty-first century is crucial to ensure that healthy children and adults are living in healthy communities. New technologies influence the capacity and ability to generate and collect a vast amount of information.[1,2] In addition, evidence-based decision making is shaping the development of public health policies, programs, and practices.[4] Therefore it is essential for public health practitioners to have skills in collecting, analyzing, disseminating, and effectively using data and information.[5] Public health professionals must have the knowledge, skills, and values to[5,7]:

- Work with communities to form partnerships
- Gather health-related data
- Identify health issues and resources
- Determine priority health concerns
- Implement solutions to address community health problems
- Use data and evaluate outcomes of public health policies and interventions[8]

Future public health dental hygienists are likely to become more involved in community oral health assessments.[9,10] As agencies and organizations take on greater

GUIDING PRINCIPLES

Essential Public Health Services for Oral Health Related to Assessment[9]

- Assessment of oral health status and needs so that problems can be identified and addressed
- Analysis of determinants of identified oral health needs, including resources
- Assessment of the fluoridation status of water systems and other sources of fluoride
- Implementation of an oral health surveillance system to identify, investigate, and monitor oral health problems and health hazards
- Evaluation of effectiveness, accessibility, and quality of population-based and personal oral health services

responsibility in conducting periodic assessments, public health dental hygienists are expected to evaluate assets, needs, problems, and resources of the populations they serve in the community. Dental public health professionals within local and state health agencies are likely to be responsible for community oral health assessment.[9] Essential public health services for oral health were developed to describe community oral health assessment (see Chapter 6 and "Guiding Principles").

Dental hygienists working within the public, private, or nonprofit sectors must have skills to assess community health problems and evaluate outcomes of community health solutions. Dental hygienists working in community settings generally participate in a variety of assessment and evaluation activities. Examples of some of these roles and potential activities are shown in Box 3-1.

Box 3-1   Examples of roles of public health dental hygienists in assessment

- Oral health program director evaluates the attainment of goals, objectives, and performance measures set out in the oral health improvement plan for the state.
- Oral health policy analyst determines the number and geographic distribution of dentists statewide who participate in the Medicaid and state Children's Health Insurance Program (S-CHIP) programs and provide oral health care to young children under 5 years of age.
- Oral health program administrator with a city health department assesses the oral health assets, needs, and resources of a metropolitan area.
- Oral health educator assesses the knowledge, attitudes, and opinions of a community about community water fluoridation to develop an oral health promotion campaign.
- Public health dental hygienist from a county health department assesses dental sealants in third-grade children in schools throughout the county.
- Oral health program manager evaluates the quality and outcomes of clinical preventive services in a school-based oral health program.
- Oral health service provider monitors oral health indicators in the neighborhood surrounding a community health center.
- Private practice dental hygienist, appointed to a state oral health advisory committee, evaluates the oral health indicators in the state and the annual performance of the state oral health program.

OVERVIEW OF EPIDEMIOLOGY: POPULATION-BASED STUDY OF HEALTH

Public health dental hygienists involved in assessment and evaluation should become well versed in the basic concepts of epidemiology, which is a core science of community health. This section provides a basic overview of epidemiology. Table 3-1 provides the definitions of terms used in epidemiology and community health assessments.

Table 3-1   **Common terms used in epidemiology**

Term	Definition
Acute	Referring to a health effect, brief exposure of high intensity
Case	Epidemiologic study that compares persons with a disease or condition ("cases") with another group of people from the same population without the disease or condition ("controls"). The study is used to identify risks and trends, suggest some possible causes for disease, or for particular outcomes.
Chronic	Referring to a health-related state, lasting a long time
Cohort study	The method of epidemiologic study in which subsets of a defined population can be identified and observed for a sufficient number of person-years to generate reliable incidence or mortality rates in the population subsets; usually a large population, study for a prolonged period (years), or both (Synonym: concurrent, follow-up, incidence, longitudinal, prospective study)
Cross-sectional study	A study that examines the relationship between diseases (or other health-related characteristics) and other variables of interest as they exist in a defined population at one particular time
Dichotomous scale	A measurement scale that arranges items into either of two mutually exclusive categories
Ecoepidemiology	Conceptual approach that unifies molecular, social, and population-based epidemiology in a multilevel application of methods aimed at identifying causes, categorizing risks, and controlling public health problems
Ecologic study	Epidemiologic study in which the units of analysis are populations or groups of people rather than individuals
Endemic disease	The constant presence of a disease or infectious agent within a given geographic area or population group
Epidemic	From Greek epi (upon), demos (people); occurrence in a community or region of cases of an illness, specific health-related behavior, or other health-related events clearly in excess of normal expectancy
Eradication (of disease)	Termination of all transmission of infection by extermination of the infectious agent through surveillance and containment
Etiology	Literally, the science of causes, causality; in common use, cause
Incidence	(Synonym: incident number); the number of instances of illness commencing, or of persons falling ill, during a given period in a specified population; more generally, the number of new events (e.g., new cases of a disease in a defined population) within a specified period of time
Index	In epidemiology and related sciences, usually referring to a rating scale or a set of numbers derived from a series of observations of specified variables (e.g., health status index, scoring systems for severity or stage of cancer, heart murmurs, mental retardation)

Adapted from Last JM (ed): A Dictionary of Epidemiology, 4th ed. New York, Oxford University Press, 2001.

Table 3-1   Common terms used in epidemiology—cont'd

Term	*Definition*
Monitoring	Intermittent performance and analysis of routine measurements aimed at detecting changes in the environment or health status of populations; not to be confused with surveillance, which is a continuous process
Morbidity	Any departure, subjective or objective, from a state of physiologic or psychologic well-being; in this sense, sickness, illness, and morbid condition are similarly defined and synonymous
Mortality	Related to death
Multifactorial etiology	Referring to the concept that a given disease or other outcome may have more than one cause; a combination of causes or alternative combinations of causes may be required to produce the effect
Occurrence	In epidemiology, a general term describing the frequency of a disease or other attribute or event in a population without distinguishing between incidence and prevalence
Pandemic	An epidemic occurring over a very wide area and usually affecting a large proportion of the population
Prevalence	Number of instances of a given disease or other condition in a given population at a designated time; when used without qualification, term usually refers to the situation at a specified point in time (point prevalence)
Prospective	A research design used that looks forward
Retrospective	A research design that uses a review of past events
Sensitivity	(of a screening test); proportion of truly diseased persons as identified by the screening test; is the measure of the probability of a correct diagnosis or the probability that any given case will be identified by the test (synonym: true-positive rate)
Specificity	Proportion of truly nondiseased persons identified by the screening test; a measure of the probability of correctly identifying a nondiseased person with a screening test (synonym: true-negative rate)
Surveillance	Ongoing systematic collection, analysis, interpretation of health data essential to planning, implementation, and evaluation of public health practice. Generally using methods distinguished by their practicability, uniformity, and rapidity. Closely integrated with the timely dissemination of health information to responsible parties. Application of data in public health decision making and use of data to prevent and control diseases and conditions. Surveillance is the essential feature of epidemiology
Surveillance system	Functional capacity for data collection, analysis, and dissemination linked to public health programs
Trend	A long-term movement in an ordered series (e.g., a time series); an essential feature is that the movement, while possibly irregular in the short term, shows movement consistently in the same direction over a long term

Epidemiology is the study of the distribution and determinants of health-related states and events in specified populations and the application of this study to the prevention and control of health problems.[11] Epidemiologists consider the interactions and relationships among the multiple factors that influence health status and health problems.[12] Methods used in epidemiology and research are combined to focus on comparisons between groups or defined populations. Epidemiologists make comparisons by examining the occurrences of the health events, locations, times, and variations to assess the distribution and determinants of health events.[13] The principal factors analyzed in epidemiology are as follows:

- Distribution
- Population dynamics
- Occurrences
- Affected population
- Place characteristics
- Time
- Determinants

Epidemiology is based on a multifactorial perspective, with consideration given to the interacting relationships among host factors, agent factors, and environmental factors.[12,14]

Host Factors

The host may be a person, an animal, or plant. **Host factors** relate primarily to susceptibility and resistance to disease through biologic immunity, knowledge and cognition, behavior modification, screening, and personal power. Age, gender, socioeconomic status, race, ethnicity, culture, genetic endowment, behavior, physiologic and nutritional state, previous exposure, and other factors influence susceptibility and resistance.

Agent Factors

Agent factors are the biologic or mechanical means of causing disease, illness, injury, or disability, such as microbial, parasitic, viral, or bacterial pathogens or vectors; physical or mechanical irritants; chemicals; drugs; trauma; and radiation. Biology, marketing, engineering, regulations, and legislation can influence agent factors.

Environmental Factors

Environmental factors include physical, sociocultural, sociopolitical, and economic components. The media, beliefs, occupation, food sources, geography, climate, housing, social roles, technology, and other factors can influence the environmental conditions.

The "epidemiologic triangle" depicts disease as the outcome of the interactions among host, agent, and environmental factors.[12] For example, the development and

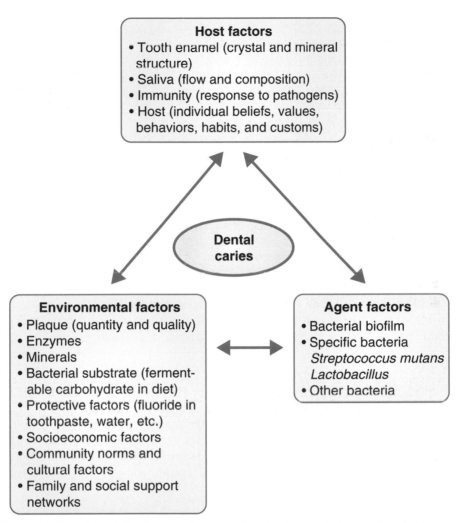

Figure 3-1 Epidemiologic triangle: Dental caries is a multifactorial oral disease.

progression of dental caries is attributed to multiple factors.[15,16] Figure 3-1 portrays the epidemiologic triangle, with dental caries shown as a multifactorial disease influenced by host, agent, and environmental factors.

Uses of Epidemiology

Health represents a general balance among host, agent, and environmental factors; health problems occur when the balance is threatened by changes in host, agent, or environment.[14] Prevention is concerned with maintaining or initiating a balance of these factors. Disease or health status depends on multiple factors such as

Box 3-2   USES OF EPIDEMIOLOGY

- Describe patterns among groups.
- Describe normal biologic processes.
- Elucidate mechanisms of disease transmission.
- Describe the natural histories of acute and chronic diseases.
- Test hypotheses for prevention and control of diseases, injuries, disabilities, and deaths through special studies in populations.
- Evaluate services (e.g., community preventive services, population-based health promotion services, and clinical health services).
- Study nondisease health and social problems such as occurrences of intentional and unintentional injuries.
- Measure the distribution of health status, diseases, injuries, disabilities, births, and deaths in populations.
- Identify determinants (e.g., protective and risk factors) for death or acquiring diseases, injuries, and disabilities.
- Evaluate interventions and strategies to prevent and control diseases, disabilities, injuries, and deaths.
- Predict trends of diseases, disabilities, injuries, and deaths.
- Identify health assets, gaps, needs, problems, resources, solutions, and partnerships within the context of a community assessment.

exposure to a specific agent, strength of the agent, susceptibility of the host, and environmental conditions.[12]

Epidemiology can be used to provide many pieces of data and information.[17] Epidemiologists in public health agencies are responsible for surveillance, investigation, analysis, and evaluation.[12,14] The various uses of epidemiology are illustrated in Box 3-2. The three classifications of epidemiologic studies are outlined in the Guiding Principles feature shown next.

GUIDING PRINCIPLES

Classification of Studies in Epidemiology
- *Descriptive studies.* Involve description, documentation, analysis, and interpretation of data to evaluate a current event or situation
- *Analytic studies.* Identify the cause of diseases, disabilities, injuries, and deaths; determine that a causal relationship exists between a factor and a disease or condition
- *Experimental studies.* Are used when the etiologic mechanism of the disease is established and the investigator determines the effectiveness of altering factors; applying or withholding the supposed cause of a condition and observing the results

Box 3-3   Trends shaping the perceptions of health in the twentieth century

- Changes in social conditions and mores, professional ethos, and social institutions
- Shifts in views of civil and human rights
- Population growth and demographic change
- Recognition of environmental health and ecology
- Technologic changes influencing work, home, and life in communities (e.g., transportation, telecommunications, computing)
- Advancements in the biologic, physical, quantitative, social, and behavioral sciences
- Acknowledgement of the impact of globalization on population health

CHANGING PERSPECTIVES OF HEALTH

During the twentieth century, major transformations took place in the concepts of health and the understanding of the determinants of diseases, disabilities, and injuries. Many historic developments contributed to these expanded visions and had a profound effect on the health of individuals and populations.[1,2,18] These developments contributed to changes in clinical health care and public health practice. Box 3-3 outlines broad trends that influenced the conceptions of health in the twentieth century.

There was a broadening of the concepts of health promotion and disease prevention from an individual focus toward a human ecologic perspective.[17] Health promotion theory has moved toward a complex, holistic, interactive approach, with a systems orientation focused on healthy people living in healthy communities.[19] Health promotion approaches have begun to embrace the principles of population health, social ecology, and community participation.[17,19,20,21] These transformations about the meanings of health, wellness, and quality of life as well as health problems within communities are continuing to evolve in the twenty-first century.

CONCEPTUAL MODELS OF THE DETERMINANTS OF HEALTH

Many models describing the multiple factors that influence the broader dimensions of health in individuals and populations were developed in the second half of the twentieth century.[4] Multicausal perspectives of health and disease began to take precedence over monocausal models.[12] The epidemiologic triangle model waned as the emphasis on infectious diseases diminished in the later part of the century. The concept of a "web of causation" emerged as multifactorial perspectives grew, with attention focused on the various determinants of chronic diseases, disabilities, and injuries.

Hancock, proposing a comprehensive framework to better understand the **determinants of health,** described the **mandala of health,**[22] a model of the human ecosystem (Figure 3-2). Its circular pattern symbolizes symmetry and wholeness. The confluent circles represent the multiple determinants of health. The center illustrates an individual whose total health and well-being are represented by the integration of mind, body, and spirit but not in isolation from other conditions. Within the global community of the biosphere, the individual is presented as only an element interdependent upon larger systems. These larger systems include the family and the community within society. All domains depicted in the model are surrounded and affected by ubiquitous cultural influences.

Also incorporated into the model are four groups of factors that influence the health of individuals, families, and communities:
- The psychosocioeconomic environment
- The physical environment

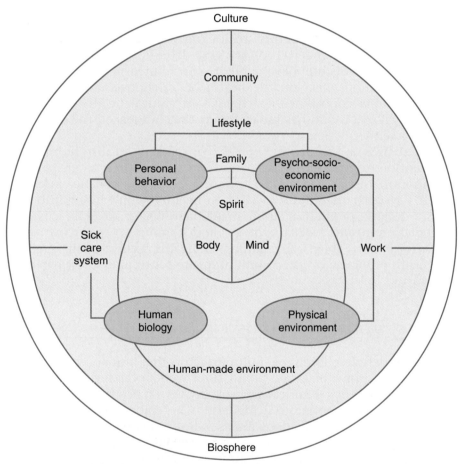

Figure 3-2 Mandala of health. *(From Hancock T: The mandala of health: A model of the human ecosystem. Fam Commun Health 8:1, 1985.)*

- Human biology
- Personal behavior

In the United States, a multidimensional perspective of health has shaped the development of the national health goals and objectives for *Healthy People 2010.* The decade-long strategy is based on a conceptual framework, the **systematic approach to health improvement.** This framework is grounded in the Force Field Model (Figure 3-3).[4,23] The Systematic Approach to Health Improvement framework describes the interrelated determinants of health. It includes the goals

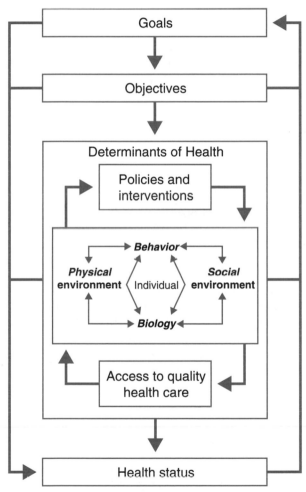

Figure 3-3 Conceptual framework from *Healthy People 2010* for a systematic approach to health improvement. *(From U.S. Department of Health and Human Services, 2000.)*

and objectives necessary to improve health. The determinants of health, according to this model, are classified as:

- Individual biology
- Individual behavior
- Physical environment
- Social environment
- Policies and interventions
- Access to quality health care

See Chapter 4 for further discussion of the national health objectives and *Healthy People 2010.*

DETERMINANTS OF HEALTH IN INDIVIDUALS AND POPULATIONS

The determinants of health have a profound effect on the health status of individuals, families, communities, nations, and thus the world.[6,23,24] The determinants of health are the factors that interact to create circumstances and produce specific health conditions; they can be classified as[1]:

- Physical (environmental)
- Biologic
- Behavioral
- Social
- Cultural
- Spiritual

These determinants may also be classified as follows[14]:

1. *Inherited* determinants are factors that are inborn or genetically determined.
2. *Acquired* determinants, which influence health and are obtained after birth and throughout life, include multiple factors such as infections, trauma, cultural characteristics, and spiritual values.

Many determinants of health influence the health of individuals and populations.[4,20-23,25-30] Multiple determinants of oral health have been described in the literature.[16,31] The boundaries between the specific categories of determinants are indistinct because they interact and influence each other continuously.[1,14] During different stages of human development, the multiple determinants act synergistically, rather than separately, to affect health. No single determinant of health is the most important because multiple factors work in combination. Thus causation is often described as multifactorial; that is, multiple factors determine health conditions, including diseases, disabilities, and injuries among individuals living in communities.

Several factors[14,23,32,33] are generally recognized as broader determinants of health (e.g., employment; education; environment; income; shelter; food; social justice and equity; family, friends, and social supports; peace and safety; culture and race relations).[22,24,32,33] Other factors (e.g., language, learning, meaningful work, recreation, self-esteem, personal control) are considered contributors to well-being.

A contemporary movement in public health called "Healthy Cities/Healthy Communities" has accepted a broader multidimensional perspective of health.[19,32] The World Health Organization has promoted this concept, which focuses on the root determinants of health.[19,15,31,34] Nations and communities around the world have adopted community health approaches based on this perspective.[19,35] Healthy Communities groups ascribe to key principles.

Healthy Communities: Perspective of Health[19]
- Broad definition of health
- Broad definition of community
- Shared vision from community values
- Quality of life addressed for everyone
- Diverse citizen participation and widespread community ownership
- "Systems change" emphasized
- Capacity built with the use of local assets and resources
- Progress and outcomes benchmarked and measured

The next topic is an overview of assessment as a key component within a comprehensive process that communities can adopt to improve health.

THE PLANNING CYCLE

The **planning cycle** is a model commonly used in public health practice; it provides a basic flowchart of steps in a process to (1) **assess,** (2) **plan,** (3) **implement,** and (4) **evaluate.** Figure 3-4 shows a basic planning cycle. The planning cycle is continuous[2]; each stage can be further subdivided into detailed steps for a long-term health improvement process in the community. The Community Health Improvement Process has been described as a comprehensive approach for communities to achieve sustained improvements in community health.[23]

Embedded into the basic planning cycle is a framework for a **community oral health improvement process** (Figure 3-5). Because of dynamics in community health, it is important to understand the necessity of flexibility in public health plans. If new circumstances arise, activities outlined initially in a plan may not be followed as sequentially ordered, and work would need to be adjusted. However, it is important to include all of the steps for a community oral health improvement process.

Following such a planning cycle allows a systematic approach of assessing different factors, considering options for action, planning and implementing policies

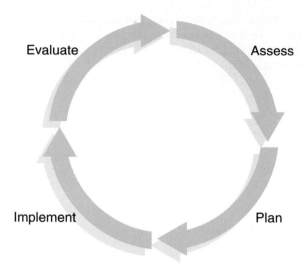

Figure 3-4 Planning cycle.

or programs, and evaluating their outcomes. This process can allow for coordinated community efforts in assessment, planning, implementation, and evaluation. When these efforts are institutionalized over time into the community fabric, long-term oral health benefits are likely to be achieved by the community.

ASSESSMENT OF ORAL HEALTH IN COMMUNITIES

This section reviews community oral health assessment, one component of a community oral health improvement process. It describes the steps undertaken and the indicators that can be included in an assessment.

A **community oral health assessment** is a multifaceted process that is community-oriented and community-directed. It focuses on population health, and it can concentrate on the entire population or a specific segment of the population in a community.

An oral health assessment considers assets, gaps, needs, problems, resources, solutions, and partnerships within the context of the community. Its purpose is to identify factors that affect the oral health of a population and to determine the availability of resources and interventions that affect these factors. Communities are better served and improved outcomes are more sustainable when assets-oriented assessment methods are used, in contrast to deficiency-based approaches that focus on needs and problems. By engaging and fostering the community in a community-building process, one can gain insight about the specific factors in the community that influence health. Through a participatory framework for action and capacity

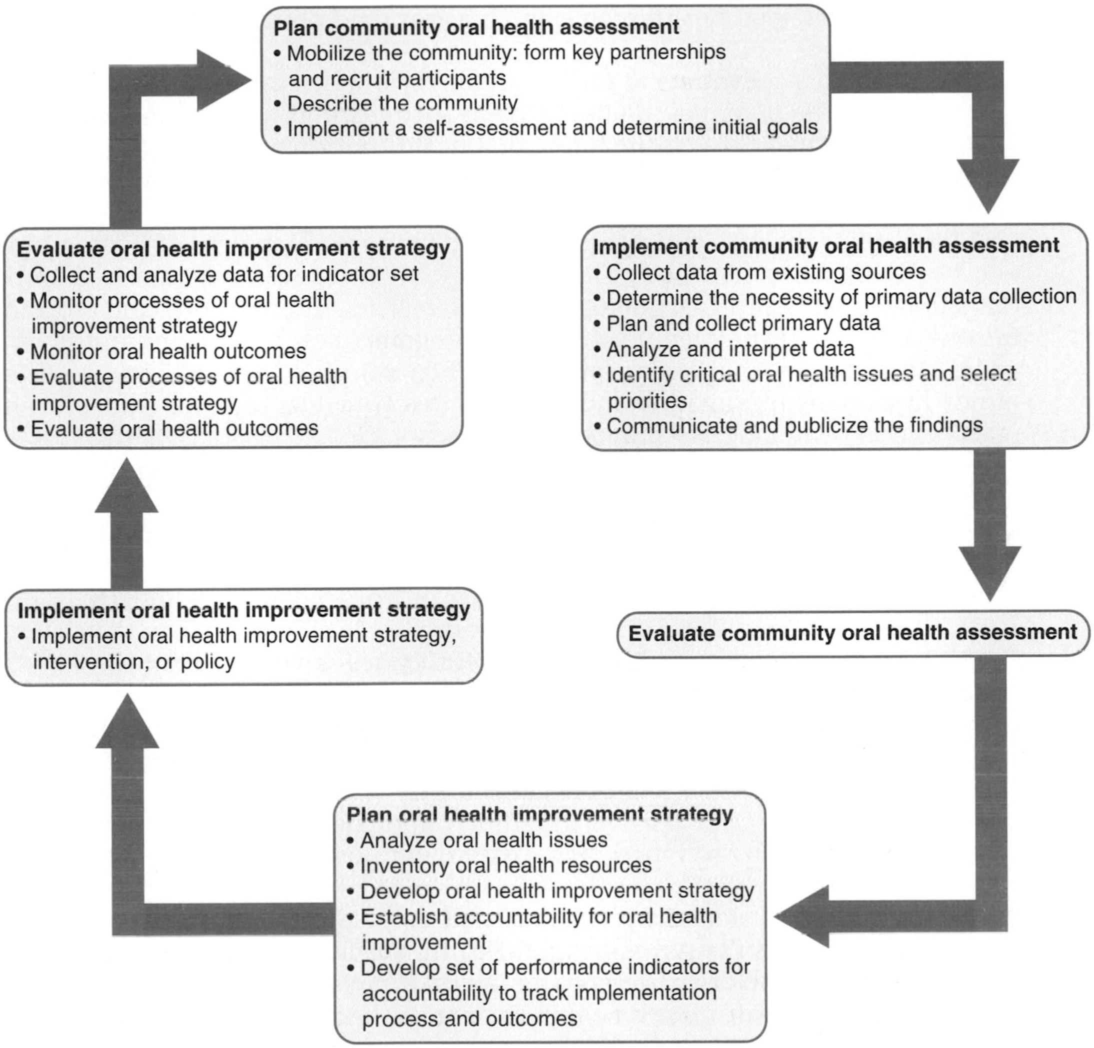

Figure 3-5 Community oral health improvement process.

development, a better understanding of opportunities for health enhancements can emerge over time.

With information gleaned from a broad-based assessment process, a community can begin to answer these questions about oral health:

- What community strengths, assets, and resources influence oral health in the community?
- What capacities, resources, and interventions are available within the community to promote oral health?

- What are the oral health problems, concerns, and obstacles faced by the community?
- What factors contribute to these community oral health gaps and needs?
- What are the potential solutions? What partnerships in the community can support strategies to ensure future oral health improvements?

Answers to these questions assist in final determination of critical oral health issues and priorities.

Assessment is the first, and an essential, step in the development of a community oral health improvement plan. The findings from the assessment can lead to the formation of oral health goals, objectives, plans, policies, interventions, and programs to solve oral health problems. Oral health programs best serve communities and address community oral health problems when priorities and actions are determined by current information and are grounded in evidence-based public health practices and contemporary principles.

Several models are available to guide collaborative health planning in communities. These models include:

- The MAPP: Mobilizing for Action through Planning and Partnerships developed by the National Association of County and City Health Officials in collaboration with the Centers for Disease Control and Prevention (CDC)[4]
- PATCH: the Planned Approach to Community Health developed by the CDC[4]
- CHIP: the Community Health Improvement Process reviewed in an IOM Report[23]

Many ways exist to collect information that can be used to evaluate the determinants of health for a population and a community. Numerous resources are available to describe methods and to offer guidance for community health assessments. Use of these resources can assist in a methodic approach to the assessment process in communities (see References and Assessment Resources at the end of this chapter).

One resource, developed by the Association of State and Territorial Dental Directors (ASTDD), is the Assessing Oral Health Needs: ASTDD Seven-Step Model. This publication provides a step-by-step guide for planning, implementing, and evaluating an oral health assessment.[10] The comprehensive guidebook outlines the main steps of a systematic and effective oral health assessment and reviews a broad array of alternatives that can be adapted for an oral health assessment.

The Division of Oral Health, CDC has also developed a resource, Oral Health Infrastructure Development Tools. This manual is a "how to" guide for planning and implementing evaluation activities. It focuses on the priorities of the CDC for program planning, monitoring, and evaluation and uses Logic Models for guidance. The purpose of this manual is to assist programs in planning, designing, implementation, and use of practical and increasingly comprehensive evaluation of oral health promotion and disease prevention efforts. The manual is a resource for dental public health professionals responsible for program planning and evaluation activities to demonstrate accountability to diverse stakeholders (see References and Assessment Resources at the end of this chapter).

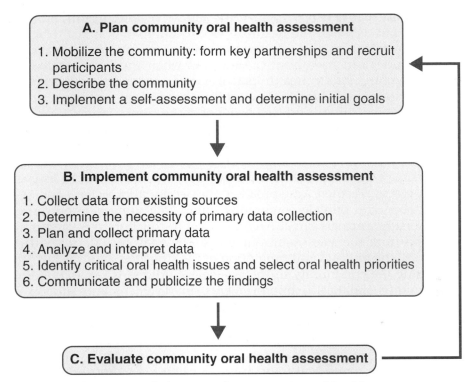

Figure 3-6 Essential elements of a community oral health assessment.

No single formula exists for conducting a community oral health assessment. However, the ASTDD outlines a useful model. A community oral health assessment should be developed on the basis of the specific aims and available resources, special circumstances, and expertise in the community. The essential components should be included in all community oral health assessments (Figure 3-6). The essential elements are reviewed in more detail in the following section.

Planning a Community Oral Health Assessment

The first step in any assessment process is the planning stage. During this stage it is important to methodically consider the overall purpose, potential partners, resources, and alternatives for conducting a community oral health assessment.

Mobilizing the Community: Forming Key Partnerships and Recruiting Participants

Community involvement is crucial in identifying oral health concerns and actions to resolve oral health problems. Collaborative partnerships and community coalitions are prominent strategies for community health improvement.[4,35-37] Mobilization of community partnerships to identify and solve oral health problems has been identified as a key public health service to improve oral health in communities.[9] Community action and community-building efforts that engage and empower communities can have positive outcomes when they are sustained over time.[7,35] Contemporary public health practices and principles encourage multisectorial collaboration and broad community engagement to improve health-related conditions, outcomes, and well-being of entire communities.[4,23,24,30]

At the beginning and throughout a community assessment process, it is essential to involve diverse partnering agencies, organizations, associations, and individuals to collaborate in partnerships.[38] Looking to the public, private, and nonprofit sectors may offer opportunities for potential champions of the assessment mission and process. Partners can broaden the scope, approaches, and perspectives in the process and provide community input, data sources, resources, expertise, and sponsorship. Partners can also lend support to collaborative community efforts that develop from the assessment outcomes. This may include support for communication of the findings and promotion of the strategies identified by the assessment. Engaging the community in the assessment process is key to building support for community oral health improvements. Involvement and support of partnering agencies and organizations throughout the assessment process can have a positive influence on the attainment of mutual missions and goals.

Potential partners should include a cross-section of the community such as technical staff, program managers, and leaders from business, media, religious, civic, philanthropic, community, and political realms.[27,39,40] Appendix C outlines partners that can be supportive in community-based efforts, including an assessment. The partners should represent a broad spectrum of the community and involve a wide variety of constituents and stakeholders from health and social service groups, organizations, and associations, governmental agencies and programs, community organizations, education-related groups (schools, colleges, universities), advocacy organizations, nonprofit, charitable and services groups, media, and business organizations.[27,38-40] The partners involved in an assessment may vary according to the overall focus of the assessment process.[38]

Mechanisms for community participation, input, and dialog must be incorporated throughout the assessment process.[38] It is imperative to a successful community oral health assessment that the community be mobilized and actively involved throughout the process.[7] Broad-based community partnerships should be engaged and participants enlisted to reflect the cultural, racial, ethnic, gender, economic, and linguistic diversities of the community.[38] Procedures should be in place to ensure opportunities for communication with and feedback to the community, sustaining support throughout the process, and evaluation of the assessment.

It is important to consider ways of identifying and recruiting partners in the development of an inclusive and empowering process. Resource materials can be helpful by offering innovative ideas about building effective collaborative partnerships and community coalitions.[35] Many of these resources discuss in-depth ways to initiate and sustain vitality of collaborative relationships. Specific factors and conditions that are conducive to effective collaborative partnerships should be supported and nurtured for measurable and lasting results (see References and Assessment Resources at the end of the chapter).

Describing the Community

An important task of the assessment is to provide a description of the community, which must be clearly defined.[13,27] Communities are a collection of peoples, places, and systems that define how people and places interact.[4,7] The Guiding Principles below can be used to provide an understanding and a description of a community.

Initially, the description can include a general overview of the community but not detailed statistics at this point. More comprehensive, detailed community data should be compiled during the data collection phase. This information should be incorporated into the **community profile,** a comprehensive description of the community.[13,20,27] Examples of information in a community profile are presented in Appendix D.

GUIDING PRINCIPLES

Factors to Use in Understanding and Describing a Community[7]
- People (socioeconomics and demographics, health status, risk profiles, cultural and ethnic characteristics)
- Location (geographic boundaries)
- Connectors (shared values, interests, motivating factors)
- Power relationships (communication patterns, social and political networks, formal and informal lines of authority and influence, stakeholder relationships, resource flows)

Implementing a Self-Assessment and Determining Initial Goals

During the initiation of an oral health assessment process, it is worthwhile to conduct a self-assessment.[10] At this step of self-reflection, it is useful to conduct an internal assessment to evaluate your organization and to consider its role. It is important to make an external assessment by exploring the missions and roles of other organizations in the community. Organizational capacity, power structures, strategic plans, commitment, and resources should be considered during this phase.

The next step is to determine the goals of the assessment. The goals should come from the self-assessment and through a group consensus process among the partnering organizations. Before embarking on an oral health assessment process, partners must understand why the community is conducting an assessment and what the community hopes to achieve from it. It is important to clarify the scope and size of the assessment. The objectives and activities undertaken to achieve the goals of the assessment must be refined continually as information is collected and in light of available resources.

Implementing a Community Oral Health Assessment

Collecting Data from Existing Sources

Data collection is the gathering of information that the community can use to make decisions and to set priorities. Different types, sources, and levels of information are needed for a comprehensive assessment.[41-49] For a community health assessment, it is vital to collect information and evaluate data related to the current status of assets, gaps, needs, problems, resources, solutions, and partnerships in the community.[47-49]

A standard element of an assessment is the compilation and synthesis of existing data and information from secondary sources.[10] After existing information is assessed, a decision should be made about the collection of new information from primary sources.

Which data sources are available?

Multiple resources of information are widely available to the general public. The sources of data used in an oral health assessment should be diverse to ensure a broad portrayal of the factors influencing oral health in the community.[10,16,40-44] A variety of data resources should be tapped to compile and review information during the data collection process.[46-49] Government agencies and private and non-profit organizations produce and compile excellent reports on the various determinants of health and oral health. Sources of local information include local reports, literature reviews, magazines, newspapers, newsletters, maps, and marketing data. It is also important to review previous assessments that have been conducted in the community. Table 3-2 outlines examples of various sources of information for community health assessments. Examples of government resources for health data are provided in Appendix D.

During data collection it is important to systematically conduct a broad search of available information and to organize an inventory of this information. It is essential to carefully compile the information from secondary sources and to establish a system to record, process, and organize the data and information.

What types of information should be included?

Different types of information are necessary to ensure that a complete assessment accurately describes the factors influencing health in the community.[7,12,14,46] Community health assessment efforts can accomplish the following[46]:
1. Evaluate determinants of health.
2. Assess needs and assets.

Table **3-2**   **Sources of information**

Potential Source	Example
Federal, state, and local government agencies (see Appendix D)	Health department, human services department, and social services department; department of aging; department of disabilities and special needs; highway safety department; police departments (documents, reports, surveys, statistics)
	Population surveys
	National, state, and local health surveys
	Surveillance system; reports and records
	Population-based registries
	Health agency records and reports of participants enrolled in programs
	Agency records and reports of health professionals; health professional shortage areas; community health centers
	State or local child protection agency records
	Environmental agency records and reports
Private and public (community) health, health care (clinical or personal health care), social, and human service programs	Hospitals; health plans (health insurance claims data); health care systems (health charts and dental records, pathology reports); professional associations; trade groups; community advisory committees; community collaborative groups and coalitions (community surveys); health and social service groups; organizations; societies; associations (documents; reports, surveys, statistics)
Philanthropic, nonprofit, and charitable organizations	Religious organizations and groups; voluntary agencies; civic organizations; service and voluntary groups; community organizations; advocacy groups (documents, reports, surveys, and statistics, local information and referral service inventories)
Schools and colleges	School districts; school boards; school campuses; colleges; universities (student statistics, school health reports, school entry records)
Businesses, employers, and business organizations	Major employers or chambers of commerce; marketing data and survey data (e.g., Claritas, AC Nielsen); economic statistics and financial records; corporate annual reports (e.g., sales of drugs, foods, tobacco)
Media	Media sources (television, radio, Internet, newspapers, magazines, newsletters)

3. Quantify disparities among population groups.
4. Measure preventable disease, injury, disability, and death.

Two main classes of data are used to describe a community and to characterize dimensions of health within the community:

1. **Quantitative data** refer to information that is objective and measurable. The data can be expressed in a quantity or amount (e.g., the percentage of children with dental sealants or the percentage of young children with dental caries).[6,10,16,41] These data numerically represent the size of a problem and determine its statistical significance. Data may include demographic information and vital statistics such as numbers of births or deaths, incidence or prevalence rates of disease, number of schools in a county, and employment statistics.

2. **Qualitative data** refer to information that reflects the quality or nature of things that cannot be numerically measured or analyzed.[43] Qualitative data add meaning to the numbers and help to answer the question of why a problem exists in a community. Data may include information gleaned from personal interviews, descriptions of traditions and the history of a community, and information gathered from participant observations or focus groups.[10,16,27,40,42-45,47]

The types of data collected and the selection of a data collection method and instrument used depend on the aims of an assessment and the resources available for the assessment.[10,13] Various data collection methods and instruments are indicated for specific types of assessments. Each method has advantages and limitations.[10,43] Appendix D summarizes the diverse data collection methods, instruments, and applications used in community assessments.

A spectrum of health indicators can be used to profile the health of a community.[46] Data collected for a "snapshot" in a community health assessment can describe:

- Population characteristics
- Summary measures of health status in the community
- Leading causes of death
- Measures of birth and death
- Measures of disease, injury, and disability
- Vulnerable populations
- Environmental health
- Use of community preventive services and personal health services
- Protective factors and risk factors for disease, injury, disability, and death
- Access to public health (e.g., community preventive services), personal health care, and social service system in the community

A new tool to assess national health, the Leading Health Indicators, was unveiled along with *Healthy People 2010*, the health goals for the decade in the United States.[6] These first-ever Leading Health Indicators include 10 focus areas, based upon the *Healthy People 2010* objectives. These measures allow Americans to easily assess the overall health of the nation and their communities to make comparisons and improvements over time. The 10 Leading Health Indicators cover the following[6]:

- Physical activity
- Overweight and obesity
- Tobacco use
- Substance abuse
- Mental health
- Injury and violence
- Environmental quality
- Immunizations
- Responsible sexual behavior
- Access to personal health care

The Leading Health Indicators are supported by 21 specific measurable objectives that reflect the influence of behavioral and environmental factors and community health interventions. These objectives can be assessed by states and communities to assess their current health status and to monitor changes over time. Examples of information for a community health assessment are presented in Appendix D.

Chapter 4 reviews specific measures that can be used in an assessment of oral health in a community and details the *Healthy People 2010* initiative.

Determining the Necessity of Primary Data Collection

A key step in the assessment process is determining the need for additional data and information.[10] This decision should be made based on:

1. A reevaluation and possible refinement of the assessment goals.
2. An analysis of the findings from the existing data sources.
3. Available resources to support future assessment activities.

The partners determine and prioritize information needs and evaluate alternative methods of data collection. One option might be the integration of specific measures into ongoing surveys and assessments. Sometimes it may be necessary to collect original data.

During this phase it is crucial to study the many alternative ways by which data can be collected for community health assessments. It is essential to consider both the advantages and disadvantages of the data collection options that are available to the group. After this analysis the group strategically determines the final goals according to identified priorities and resources.

Planning and Collecting Primary Data

When it is necessary to collect original data, the partners develop a work plan that outlines the objectives, activities, roles, responsibilities, budget, and timetable.[10] Once the scope of the assessment is determined, methods can be selected and criteria defined in preparation for the primary data collection phase. Examples of tasks that should be considered for conducting primary data collection are listed in Appendix D.

Analyzing and Interpreting Data

Analysis and interpretation of data often require knowledge and experience, and this is where the backgrounds and experience of community members, representatives of partnering organizations, and professionals in the community are invaluable. Partners can call upon local community members to enlist their expertise and assistance in validating impressions and interpretations of the data examined for the assessment.

To analyze and interpret both primary and secondary data, numerous steps are necessary. The initial step is to synthesize the information and summarize the findings. Data collected must be analyzed to determine meaning and significance.[10] A critique of each data source is required to assess its trustworthiness. The partners must consider the limitations of the data and data sources by checking for potential errors or biases. It is important to consider the sampling technique such as type of sample, sample size, participation of population segments, and generalization of findings to population groups based on the sample.

Because potential errors can be made in collecting, recording, and analyzing data, it is essential to review the data collection process to check that protocols have been followed to ensure standardization and to reduce the potential of bias or variation. The partners should evaluate that methods and techniques were in place to collect information consistently, record and compile information accurately, and analyze data completely and appropriately. Information should be reviewed carefully to consider the possibility of misinterpretation, errors in coding and groupings, erroneous instructions, or typographic errors.

When the data have been determined to be reasonably free of errors, they should be compared with other data. The partners ensure that the data being compared are alike as possible. Data of a community can be compared with those of surrounding communities, other counties, the region, the state, or the nation. It may be worthwhile to compare data with those of a baseline source such as the *Healthy People 2010* objectives (see Chapter 5). Analysis of trends can be included by comparison of new data in one time period with data from previous years. This comparison may show changes in the community over a specific time period. Also, data showing changes among communities over time can be very useful for planning purposes.

The group determines whether there are opportunities to analyze existing data sets further. If existing data sets are available and additional analysis will generate new information, this alternative may result in more insight. In addition, the group might add or integrate the collection of new types of data into ongoing data collection efforts.

The group assesses the significance of the data collected; the term significance means that the information truly reflects a problem existing in a community.

Studying the data for significance means that possible misleading findings are identified before conclusions are drawn from the findings. An abundance of data combining different data types allows for an easier determination of the significance of the findings.

Numeric calculations are made through statistical analysis for data collected by means of quantitative methods. A mathematical method is used to calculate relationships among quantitative variables to determine statistical significance. The calculations show whether the observed relationships among the variables happened by chance or not by chance (see Chapter 7 for an explanation of data analysis in research).

The relationships among data collected by qualitative methods are not calculated through statistical analysis. Textual data collected from transcripts of interviews or focus groups or field notes of observations are explored with the use of contextual analysis.[43] Steps in qualitative data analysis include familiarization, identifying a thematic framework, indexing, charting, mapping, and interpreting.[45] With the use of specific methods, data in contextual form are indexed to assess common or unique themes and to generate analytic categories and theoretic explanations.

The following questions are answered:
• Does this information reflect relationships?
• Does this information describe a pattern of key themes and explain a social phenomena?

The partners with expertise and experience can provide feedback on the findings. Partners can consider the implications of the data by evaluating the meaning of the data within the context and expectations of the community.

The findings from quantitative and qualitative data can provide direction for future actions to build on community assets. With potential strategies indicated, this step may move the assessment phase toward the planning stage of a community oral health improvement process. At the same time, additional questions may arise that may direct the process toward the need for more information and supplementary assessment activities.

Identifying Critical Oral Health Issues and Selecting Priorities

In conjunction with the community, it is essential to identify critical oral health issues. During this stage it is important to consider the identified assets, gaps, needs, problems, resources, solutions, and partnerships in the community. During the assessment process, community partners should evaluate the community's assets and resources to create a shared vision of change.[47] This encourages greater creativity when community partners begin to address problems and obstacles.

Community partners should be actively involved in all aspects of determining and prioritizing the critical issues. Based on all the evidence, it is crucial to analyze the situation and to determine the priority of oral health problems to be addressed in the future. Through a deliberative process, the community partners must reach a consensus about long-term and short-term solutions to address the identified oral health problems.

Key steps to determine and prioritize community oral health issues include the following:

1. Develop a prioritization process. Community input is vital in this process.
2. Ensure clear determination of oral health priorities in conjunction with the community.
3. Determine the community's capacity to address oral health priorities. Consider the assets and resources that were identified during the assessment process. How can the wide array of community assets and resources be expanded and maximized to address the oral health issues?
4. Consider how amenable each oral health priority is to change. What realistic degree of change can the community achieve in a specific time period?
5. Assess the economic, social, and political issues that influence the community's ability to address the priority oral health issues. When formulating oral health improvement strategies to address public health priorities, be cognizant of economic, social, and political factors that can affect plans and strategies.
6. Identify community programs currently addressing oral health priorities that were identified through the assessment efforts. Consider expanding partnerships and building upon effective strategies. This may allow for more effective and efficient use of limited resources.
7. Identify best practices to determine effective approaches to guide future planning, development, implementation, and evaluation of policies and programs.

Communicating and Publicizing the Findings

It is essential to establish a plan to communicate and disseminate the findings. The partners present the findings from the data collection and analysis and share information about the overall assessment quest. These findings should be publicized and distributed widely to various community members with the use of the diverse channels of communication available such as public forums, news conferences, and publications. Components of a report can include a statement of the purpose, materials and methods used, results, a discussion, conclusions, a summary, and an abstract. An executive summary and a full report may be useful to communicate the findings.

The outcomes should be communicated in a straightforward manner. It is important to summarize the findings by highlighting key findings and by including the outcomes of the inventory of community assets and resources to emphasize the availability of resources and to note the limitations of existing resources in the community. It is helpful to illustrate the findings through charts, graphs, and tables. In addition, partners can provide the audience with a frame of reference to show

how the community data compare with similar data from other local, state, or national figures. It is vital to explain the limitations of the data.

Chapter 8 describes contemporary strategies for promoting community oral health and communicating oral health findings.

Evaluating the Assessment Process

As with any process, it is important to incorporate evaluation. Throughout the oral health assessment process, the collaborating partners should, on a systematic basis, step back and evaluate the process.[10] Allowing time for evaluation along the way can provide opportunity to implement changes and to improve the process. Recording a critique of the assessment at the end of the process can allow a feedback loop in which lessons can be learned for future health assessments in the community.[10]

NEXT STEPS: DEVELOPING AND IMPLEMENTING AN IMPROVEMENT PLAN

With the published report of the assessment disseminated and the priorities identified, it is time to move to the next phase of the community oral health improvement process. At this stage oral health improvement strategies can be developed to address the prioritized oral health issues outlined in the oral health assessment. Concrete goals, objectives, policies, and programs can be planned and implemented based on the findings, evidence, best practices, and priorities from the oral health assessment.

A community oral health assessment is virtually useless unless the information is used to develop and implement evidence-based oral health strategies. *Healthy People 2010* (see Chapter 4) can provide guidance in the development of an oral health improvement plan.

SUMMARY

Assessment is a core public health function, and dental hygienists involved in public health practice must be proficient in the various aspects of oral health assessment. Assessment is an integral component of a community oral health improvement process. Information gained from a community assessment can be used to plan, implement, and evaluate oral health improvement strategies.

Community health assessment efforts are applied to evaluate assets, gaps, problems, resources, solutions, and partnerships in the community. This allows a community to assess the determinants of health, evaluate needs, quantify disparities among population groups, and measure preventable disease, injury, disability, and death. A systematic approach is crucial to accomplish a comprehensive community oral health assessment. This chapter has reviewed the key elements necessary when a community undertakes an assessment. Data collection methods and instruments are varied, and their application depends on the overall aims of the assessment in the community.

The chapter has reviewed how epidemiology involves a multifactorial perspective to analyze the interacting relationships among host factors, agent factors, and environmental factors that contribute to health in populations. As the concepts of health broaden and the information age grows, it will be essential that dental public health professionals be skilled in working with communities to assess the determinants of oral health.

Acknowledgment

The author wishes to acknowledge the contribution of S.E. Cunningham, MS, RD/LD, CDE, Assistant Professor, Department of Community Dentistry, Dental School, University of Texas Health Science Center at San Antonio for her insights and review of the chapter.

Applying **Your Knowledge**

---

1. Illustrate the determinants of oral health for the following groups and situations:
   a. Oral cancer among older adults in a county
   b. Early childhood caries among preschool children in a state
   c. Periodontal disease among disabled young adults in a region of a state
   d. Dental caries among adolescents in a city without fluoridated drinking water
   e. Adults without access to annual dental visits in a rural county
   f. Dental injuries among schoolchildren in a neighborhood
2. Group discussion: Read over the following situations and discuss your answers within small groups.
   A: The social worker from the County Agency on Aging calls you to discuss the dental problems of the senior citizens attending local nutrition sites near your community health center. The state health department has recently distributed the State Oral Health Improvement Plan, which notes a high rate of oral cancer among older men and a low rate of dental attendance for older edentulous adults. How would you maximize these "windows of opportunity" to initiate a community oral health assessment? Whom would you contact? What steps would you take? Do you think these efforts could advance the development and implementation of a community oral health improvement plan?
   B: At a local child care conference, a prominent speaker describes the high rate of early childhood caries among preschool children attending Head Start programs in the city. Also, during the conference, the new Director for the Supplemental Food Program for Women, Infants, and Children (WIC) from the local health department highlights the need to improve the

nutrition, health, and dental education for families enrolled in WIC. After the conference, the Community Coalition for Healthy Children (CCHC) asks you to join as a representative of the local component of the American Dental Hygienists Association. How would you maximize this opportunity to focus on oral health and young children? Whom would you contact? What steps would you take to initiate a community oral health assessment? How might the CCHC evaluate the assets, gaps, needs, problems, resources, solutions, and partnerships within the context of your community? How might this assessment promote the development and implementation of a community oral health improvement plan?

DENTAL HYGIENE COMPETENCIES

Reading the material in this chapter and participating in the activities of Applying Your Knowledge will contribute to the student's ability to demonstrate the following competencies:

Community involvement

CM.1 Assess the oral health needs of the community and quality and availability of resources and services.

CM.6 Evaluate the outcomes of community-based programs and plan for future activities.

Health promotion and disease prevention

HP.4 Identify individual and population risk factors and develop strategies that promote health-related quality of life.

HP.5 Evaluate factors that can be used to promote patient adherence to disease prevention and health maintenance strategies.

Community Case

You are a dental hygienist serving on a health team at a community health center. The Executive Director has called a meeting about the need to plan a community health assessment in the surrounding neighborhood served by the community health center. This community health assessment is an essential component of the center's application to receive continued funding. Your role as a member of the planning committee is to provide input on the components of the community health assessment.

   1. What would be the first step the committee should take for the community health assessment?
     a. Collect data from existing resources
     b. Identify critical health issues and select health priorities

    c. Mobilize the community by forming key partnerships and recruiting participants to collaborate in the community health assessment

    d. Plan and collect primary health data in the community

    e. Evaluate the community health assessment process

2. During the data collection phase of the community health assessment, all of the following are government resources for health data that the committee could use except one. Which one is not a government resource?

    a. Population surveys from the Bureau of the Census

    b. State health surveys

    c. Health and dental records from a private hospital

    d. CDC Cancer Registry

    e. National Health Interview Survey

3. The initial description and general overview of the community is called

    a. Community asset map

    b. Community profile

    c. Primary data collection

    d. Plan for the community assessment

    e. Inventory of community health resources

4. The data collection method that would be the most costly and time-consuming would be which of the following?

    a. Windshield tour

    b. Mailed survey

    c. Person-to-person interview

    d. Telephone interview

    e. Document study

5. Both qualitative and quantitative data can be used to describe the health status of the community. Qualitative data are expressed in a quantity or amount.

    a. The first statement is true and the second statement is false

    b. The second statement is true and the first statement is false

    c. Both statements are true

    d. Both statements are false

Assessment Resources

American Public Health Association
    http://www.apha.org
Association for Community Health Improvement
    http://www.communityhlth.org/
Association of State and Territorial Dental Directors
Assessing Oral Health Needs: ASTDD Seven-Step Model
Basic Screening Survey
Proven and Promising Best Practices for State and Community Oral Health Programs
    http://www.astdd.org

Community Toolbox
        http://ctb.ukans.edu
International Healthy Cities Foundation
        http://www.healthycities.org
National Association of County and City Health Officials: Mobilizing for Action through Planning and Partnerships (MAPP) (Part of the Assessment Protocol for Excellence in Public Health [APEXPH] project
        http://www.naccho.org
        http://mapp.naccho.org/MAPP_Home.asp
National Institute of Dental and Craniofacial Research
Healthy People 2010 Oral Health Toolkit
        http://www.nidr.nih.gov/hp2010/
National Maternal and Child Oral Health Resource Center
        http://www.mchoralhealth.org/
Office of Disease Prevention and Health Promotion, DHHS
Public Health Foundation
Healthy People 2010 Toolkit: A Field Guide to Health Planning
        http://www.healthypeople.gov/state/toolkit/default.htm
State *Healthy People 2010* Tool Library
        http://www.phf.org/HPtools/state.htm
U.S. Department of Health and Human Services, *Healthy People 2010*
        http://www.health.gov/healthypeople
Healthy People Publications
        http://www.healthypeople.gov/Publications/
Healthy People in Healthy Communities: A Community Planning Guide *Using Healthy People 2010*
        http://www.healthypeople.gov/Publications/HealthyCommunities2001/default
Healthy People 2010 Companion Websites and Documents
        http://www.healthypeople.gov/Implementation/compdocs.htm
State *Healthy People 2010* Plans
        http://www.healthypeople2010.gov/implementation/stateplans.htm
Tracking *Healthy People 2010*
        http://www.healthypeople.gov/Document/tableofcontents.htm#tracking
U.S. Department of Health and Human Services, Centers for Disease Control and Prevention (CDC)
CDC, Data 2010: The *Healthy People 2010* Database
        http://wonder.cdc.gov/data2010
CDC, Division of Oral Health and Association of State and Territorial Dental Directors
National Oral Health Surveillance Systems (NOHSS)
        http://www.cdc.gov/nohss/
CDC, Division of Oral Health
Oral Health Infrastructure Development Tools and State Oral Health Plans
        http://www.cdc.gov/OralHealth/state_reports/index.htm
        http://www.cdc.gov/OralHealth/library/infrastructure.htm
        http://www.cdc.gov/OralHealth/data_systems/index.htm

CDC, National Center for Chronic Disease, Prevention and Health Promotion (NCCDPHP) Planned Approach to Community Health (PATCH)
    http://www.cdc.gov/nccdphp/patch/
CDC, Public Health Practice Program Office (PHPPO), National Public Health Performance Standards Program (NPHPSP)
    http://www.phppo.cdc.gov/nphpsp/index.asp
World Health Organization (WHO), Oral Health
    http://www.who.int/oral_health/en/
WHO Oral Health Country and Area Profile Programme
    http://www.whocollab.od.mah.se/

REFERENCES

1. Scutchfield FD, Keck CW: Principles of Public Health Practice. Albany, NY: Delmar, 1997.
2. Turnock BJ: Public Health: What It Is and How It Works. Gaithersburg, Md, Aspen, 1997.
3. Institute of Medicine, Committee for the Study of the Future of Public Health: The Future of Public Health. Washington, DC, National Academy Press, 1988.
4. Institute of Medicine, Committee on Assuring the Health of the Public in the 21st Century: The Future of the Public's Health in the 21st Century. Washington, DC, National Academy Press, 2003.
5. Institute of Medicine, Committee on Educating Public Health Professionals for the 21st Century: Who Will Keep the Public Healthy? Educating Public Health Professionals in the 21st Century. Washington, DC, National Academy Press, 2003.
6. U.S. Department of Health and Human Services: Healthy People 2010: Understanding and Improving Health (2nd ed). Washington, DC, U.S. Government Printing Office, 2000.
7. Centers for Disease Control and Prevention: Principles of Community Engagement. Atlanta, Public Health Practice Program, 1997.
8. Centers for Disease Control and Prevention: Framework for program evaluation in public health. MMWR Morb Mortal Wkly Rep 48(RR11)1, 1999.
9. Association of State and Territorial Dental Directors: Guidelines for State and Territorial Oral Health Programs. Jefferson City, Mo, 2001.
10. Kuthy RA, Siegal MA, Phipps K: Assessing Oral Health Needs: ASTDD Seven-Step Model. Association of State and Territorial Dental Directors, Jefferson City, Mo, 2003.
11. Last JM (ed): A Dictionary of Epidemiology, 4th ed. New York, Oxford University Press, 2001.
12. Timmreck TC: An Introduction to Epidemiology, 2nd ed. Boston, Jones & Bartlett, 1998.
13. Abramson JH, Abramson ZH: Survey Methods in Community Medicine, 5th ed. New York, Churchill Livingstone, 1999.
14. Last JM: Public Health and Human Ecology, 2nd ed. Stamford, Conn, Appleton & Lange, 1998.
15. Nikiforuk G: Understanding Dental Caries: Etiology and Mechanisms. New York, Karger, 1985.
16. Cohen LK, Gift HC (eds): Disease Prevention and Oral Health Promotion: Socio-dental Sciences in Action. Copenhagen, Munksgaard, 1995.
17. Green LW, Ottoson JM: Community and Population Health, 8th ed. Boston, McGraw-Hill, 1999.
18. Starr P: The Social Transformation of American Medicine. New York, Basic Books, 1982.
19. Lee PR: Focus on healthy communities: Healthy communities—a young movement that can revolutionize public health. Public Health Rep 115:114, 2000.
20. Huff RM, Kline MV: Promoting Health in Multicultural Populations: A Handbook for Practitioners. Thousand Oaks, Calif, Sage Publications, 1999.
21. Airhihenbuwa CO: Health and Culture: Beyond the Western Paradigm. Thousand Oaks, Calif, Sage Publications, 1995.
22. Hancock T: The mandala of health: A model of the human ecosystem. Fam Commun Health 8:1, 1985.
23. Institute of Medicine: Improving Health in the Community. Washington, DC, National Academy Press, 1997.

24. Institute of Medicine: Healthy Communities: New Partnerships for the Future of Public Health. Washington, DC, National Academy Press, 1996.
25. Spector RE: Cultural Diversity in Health and Illness, 5th ed. Upper Saddle River, NJ, Prentice Hall, 2000.
26. Hahn RA: Anthropology in Public Health: Bridging Differences in Culture and Society. New York, Oxford University Press, 1999.
27. Aspen Reference Group: Community Health Education and Promotion: A Guide to Program Design and Evaluation. Gaithersburg, Md, Aspen, 1997.
28. Waxler-Morrison N, Anderson J, Richardson E: Cross-cultural Caring. Vancouver, BC, University of British Columbia Press, 1990.
29. Mechanic D: Medical Sociology, 2nd ed. New York, The Free Press, 1978.
30. Amick BC, Levine S, Tarlow AL, Walsh DC (eds): Society and Health. New York, Oxford University Press, 1995.
31. U.S. Department of Health and Human Services (DHHS): Oral Health in America: A Report of the Surgeon General. Rockville, Md, DHHS, National Institute of Dental and Craniofacial Research, National Institutes of Health, 2000.
32. Flynn BC: Healthy cities: Toward worldwide health promotion. Annu Rev Public Health 17:299, 1996.
33. Roseland M (ed): Eco-City Dimensions: Healthy Cities, Healthy Planet. Gabriola Island, BC, New Society Publishers, 1997.
34. Duhl L, Hancock T, Twiss JM: A dialogue on healthy communities: Past, present, and future. Natl Civic Rev 87:283, 1998.
35. Roussos ST, Fawcett SB: A review of collaborative partnerships as a strategy for improving community health. Annu Rev Public Health 21:369, 2000.
36. Berkowitz W, Wolff T: The Spirit of the Coalition. Washington, DC, American Public Health Association, 1999.
37. Kaye G, Wolff T: From the Ground Up (companion workbook to The Spirit of Coalition). Washington, DC, American Public Health Association, 1995.
38. Community Roots for Oral Health: Guidelines for Successful Coalitions. Olympia, Wash, Washington Department of Health, Community and Family Health, 2000.
39. Kretzmann JP, McKnight JL: Building Communities from the Inside Out. Chicago, ACTA Publications, 1993.
40. McKnight JL, Pandak CA: New Community Tools for Improving Child Health: A Pediatrician's Guide to Local Associations. National CATCH Meeting, American Academy of Pediatrics, Community Access to Child Health (CATCH) Program and Asset-Based Community Development Institute, Institute for Policy Research, Northwestern University, CATCH 2000, Elk Grove Village, Ill, April 15-16, 1999.
41. Weintraub JA, Douglass CW, Gillings DB: Biostats: Data Analysis for Dental Health Care Professionals. Chapel Hill, NC, CAVCO, 1984.
42. Blinkhorn AS: Qualitative research: Does it have a place in dental public health? J Public Health Dent 60:3, 2000.
43. Bailey KD: Methods of Social Research, 4th ed. New York, The Free Press, 1994.
44. Marshall C, Rossman GB: Designing Qualitative Research, 2nd ed. Thousand Oaks, Calif, Sage Publications, 1995.
45. Pope C, Mays N. Qualitative Research in Health Care, 2nd ed. London, BMJ Books, 1999
46. Health Resources and Services Administration (HRSA), Community Health Status Indicators Project (CHSI): Community Health Status Report: Data Sources, Definitions, and Notes. Washington, DC, U.S. Department of Health and Human Services, 2000.
47. Sharpe PA, Greaney ML, Lee PR, Royce SW. Assets-oriented community assessment. Public Health Rep 115:114, 2000.
48. Minkler M: Community Organizing and Community Building for Health. New Brunswick, NJ: Rutgers University Press, 1998.
49. Anderson E, McFarlane J: Community as Partner: Theory and Practice in Nursing, 2nd ed. Philadelphia, JB Lippincott, 1996.

4

Measuring Progress in Oral Health

Jane E.M. Steffensen, RDH, BS, MPH, CHES

Objectives

Upon completion of this chapter, the student will be able to:

- Discuss the health goals and health objectives of *Healthy People 2010*
- Describe the oral health objectives of *Healthy People 2010*
- Discuss measures used to assess oral health
- Compare and contrast the procedures and methods used in oral health surveys

Key Terms

Healthy People 2010
Quality of Life
Disparities
Index
Decayed, missing, and filled teeth (DMFT)
Decayed, missing, and filled surfaces (DMFS)
Association of State and Territorial Dental Directors

(ASTDD) Basic Screening Survey
National Health and Nutrition Examination Survey (NHANES)
World Health Organization (WHO) Basic Methods for Oral Health Surveys
Community Periodontal Index (CPI)

Behavioral Risk Factor Surveillance Survey (BRFSS)
National Health Interview Survey (NHIS)
Water Fluoridation Reporting System (WFRS)
Medical Expenditure Panel Survey (MEPS)

OPENING STATEMENT

National 2010 Objectives for Leading Health Indicators

- Increase access to health insurance
  - 100% of children and adults (under 65 years) have health insurance

- Increase access to personal health care
  - 96% of children and adults have a source of ongoing primary health care

- Increase access to prenatal care
  - 90% of pregnant women receive prenatal care during the first trimester

- Immunizations
  - 80% of young children (aged 19 to 35 months) are fully immunized

- Increase physical activity
  - 50% of adults are physically active on a regular basis

- Decrease obesity
  - 15% of adults are obese

- Decrease tobacco use
  - 12% of adults smoke cigarettes

- Decrease substance abuse
  - 89% of adolescents do not use alcohol or illicit drugs during the past month

- Increase access to mental health services
  - 50% of adults with recognized depression receive treatment

- Reduce deaths caused by motor vehicle crashes
  - 9.2 deaths per 100,000 population due to motor vehicle crashes

- Improve environmental quality
  - 0% of Americans are exposed to harmful air pollutants

- Increase responsible sexual behavior
  - 0.7 deaths per 100,000 population due to HIV/AIDS*

From Data 2010: The Healthy People 2010 Database. Centers for Disease Control and Prevention, National Center for Health Statistics, DHHS, http://wonder.cdc.gov/data2010/ (accessed July 2004).
*HIV, Human immunodeficiency virus; AIDS, acquired immunodeficiency syndrome.

ORAL HEALTH ASSESSMENT: ESSENTIAL IN MONITORING COMMUNITY HEALTH

To ensure that a comprehensive profile of a community's health is depicted, oral health should be included in a community health assessment. When the health of a community is assessed, oral health is often found to be an important concern for both children and adults.[1,2] Common oral and craniofacial diseases and conditions that can be assessed include:

- Dental caries
- Periodontal diseases
- Edentulism (complete tooth loss)
- Oral and pharyngeal cancer
- Soft tissue lesions
- Craniofacial anomalies, including cleft lip and palate
- Malocclusion
- Orofacial injuries
- Temporomandibular dysfunction (TMD)

Multiple determinants influence oral health in populations.[3] The etiology and pathogenesis of diseases and disorders affecting craniofacial structures are multi-factorial and complex. They involve the interplay among social, cultural, behavioral, environmental, and biologic dimensions.[1] These factors contribute to the development and progression of oral diseases, conditions, and injuries.[1] In addition, various factors affect the access of population groups to community preventive services (e.g., community water fluoridation) and clinical dental services. These measures can prevent and control oral problems. In a community oral health assessment, it is worthwhile to evaluate key determinants that influence oral health status and access to services. Appendix E outlines oral conditions and factors influencing oral health that have been assessed in oral health surveys. The national health objectives outlined in *Healthy People 2010* provide an important framework for the development of an oral health assessment at the state or local level.

HEALTHY PEOPLE 2010: NATIONAL OBJECTIVES FOR IMPROVING HEALTH

Health promotion and disease prevention are important concepts in the United States. Therefore the nation has developed a plan for the prevention of diseases and the promotion of health, embodied in the publication called ***Healthy People 2010***.[4] These national health objectives shape the health agenda in the United States and guide health improvements. The *Healthy People* initiative has been the nation's blueprint for disease prevention and health promotion beginning in the 1980s. *Healthy People 2000 (HP 2000)* set measurable national targets to be achieved by the year 2000.[5] *Healthy People 2010 (HP 2010)*, the third generation of national benchmarks, was launched in 2000 and established national objectives to be reached by the year 2010.[4] The initiative originated in a 1979 report by the U.S. Surgeon General that established the precedent for setting national health objectives and monitoring progress over an interval of a decade.[6]

Healthy People 2010 was developed through an extensive goal-setting, consultation process that involved the Healthy People Consortium, a public-private alliance of more than 350 national membership organizations and 270 state, territorial, and tribal public health, mental health, substance abuse, and environmental agencies.[4] This national effort brought together national, state, and local agencies; nonprofit, voluntary, and professional organizations; businesses; communities; and individuals to focus on improvements in the health of all Americans.

The national objectives have served as a basis for the development of state and community plans to improve health for two decades. In the early 2000s, many states and localities used the *Healthy People 2010* framework to guide the development of health improvement plans and performance standards. Several resources based on the national health objectives outlined in *Healthy People 2010* have been developed to guide these planning initiatives. (See Resources and Assessment Resources at the end of Chapter 3).

The *Healthy People 2010* framework is built on a systematic approach to health improvement[4] (see Chapter 3 and Figure 3-3). The goals outlined in *Healthy People 2010* provide a general focus and direction and serve as a guide for the development of a set of objectives that will measure progress in population health within a specified time period. The objectives focus on the determinants of health, which encompass the combined effects of individual and community physical and social environments. Also, the objectives consider policies and interventions used to promote health; prevent diseases, injuries, and disabilities; and ensure access to effective personal and public health services. The ultimate measure of success in any health improvement effort is the health status of the target population.

The *Healthy People 2010* initiative has a vision of healthy people in healthy communities. It aims to promote healthy behaviors, promote healthy and safe communities, improve systems for personal health and public health, and prevent diseases, injuries, disabilities, and disorders. *Healthy People 2010* provides a mechanism for monitoring and tracking health status, health risks, protective factors, and use of services.

Healthy People 2010 includes two overarching goals[4]:
1. To increase quality and years of healthy life by ensuring that people of all ages enjoy increased life expectancy and improved **quality of life.**
2. To eliminate **disparities** in health among different segments of the population, whether the disparities are related to age, gender, race and ethnicity, education level, income, disability, sexual orientation, or geographic location.

Ten Leading Health Indicators have been designated in *Healthy People 2010* as key measures for national report cards on population health.[4] *Healthy People 2010* contains 467 objectives, grouped in 28 focus areas; each focus area has a specific overall goal (Box 4-1).

HEALTHY PEOPLE 2010: NATIONAL ORAL HEALTH OBJECTIVES

The national oral health objectives have defined the nation's oral health agenda and served as a road map for national benchmarks since the early 1980s. Oral health

Box 4-1   HEALTHY PEOPLE 2010 SUMMARY

Goals

Goal 1: Increase quality and years of healthy life.

To help individuals of all ages increase life expectancy and improve their quality of life.

Goal 2: Eliminate health disparities among different segments of the population.

These health disparities include differences that occur by age, gender, race, ethnicity, education, income, disability, geographic location, or sexual orientation.

Focus Areas

Each focus area has a specific goal and multiple objectives.

Chapter	Focus Area
1	Access to quality health services*
2	Arthritis, osteoporosis, and chronic back conditions*
3	Cancer*
4	Chronic kidney disease
5	Diabetes*
6	Disability and secondary conditions*
7	Educational and community-based programs*
8	Environmental health*
9	Family planning
10	Food safety
11	Health communication*
12	Heart disease and stroke*
13	Human immunodeficiency virus infection
14	Immunization and infectious diseases*
15	Injury and violence prevention*
16	Maternal, infant, and child health*
17	Medical product safety*
18	Mental health and mental disorders*
19	Nutrition and overweight*
20	Occupational safety and health*
21	Oral health*
22	Physical activity and fitness*
23	Public health infrastructure*
24	Respiratory diseases
25	Sexually transmitted diseases*
26	Substance abuse*
27	Tobacco use*
28	Vision and hearing

Adapted from Healthy People 2010: Understanding and Improving Health, 2nd ed. Washington, DC, U.S. Department of Health and Human Services, 2000.[4]

*Oral Health Related Objective included in Focus Area according to National Institute of Dental and Craniofacial Research. Healthy People 2010 Oral Health Toolkit <http://www.nidr.nih.gov/hp2010/> Accessed July 2004.

is a specific focus area in *Healthy People 2010*.[4] Oral health is integrated into many of the other 27 focus areas in the *Healthy People 2010* objectives for the nation. Table 4-1 outlines the key topics of the *Healthy People 2010* national oral health objectives. Table 4-2 describes selected other health objectives related to oral health. The *Healthy People 2010* Oral Health Objectives are based on the latest research and scientific evidence related to oral health. They combine current information with contemporary public health principles to benefit the largest number of people in the United States.

Table **4-1**   *Healthy People 2010:* **Oral health objectives**

Oral health goal: To prevent and control oral and craniofacial diseases, conditions, and injuries and improve access to related services	
Number	*Topic of Objective*	*Measure to Monitor Objective*
21-1*	Dental caries experience	% of persons with ≥1 dft or DMFT
21-2	Untreated dental decay	% of persons with ≥1 dt or DT
21-3	No permanent tooth loss	% of persons with 28 teeth, no teeth extracted
21-4	Complete tooth loss	% of persons with all teeth extracted, edentulous
21-5	Reduce periodontal disease Gingivitis	% of persons with ≥1 bleeding site
	Destructive periodontal disease	% of persons with ≥4 mm LOA in at least 1 site
21-6	Early detection of oral and pharyngeal cancers	% of individuals with oral and pharyngeal cancer diagnosed at earliest stage
21-7	Annual examinations for oral and pharyngeal cancer	% of individuals with recent oral and pharyngeal examination past year
21-8	Dental sealants	% of persons with ≥1 sealant on permanent molars
21-9	Community water fluoridation	% of people served by community water systems with optimal levels of fluoride
21-10	Use of oral health care system	% of individuals with annual dental visit
21-11	Use of oral health care system by residents in long-term care facilities	% of nursing home residents with dental service within past year
21-12	Dental services for low-income children	% of low-income children and adolescents with preventive dental service within past year

Adapted from Healthy People 2010: Understanding and Improving Health, 2nd ed. Washington, DC, U.S. Department of Health and Human Services, 2000.[4]
Numbers refer to the chapter and objective as referenced in Healthy People 2010. For example, 21-1 is Chapter 21, Objective 1.
DT, Decayed permanent teeth; DMFT, decayed, missing, and filled permanent teeth; dft, decayed and filled primary teeth; dt, decayed primary teeth; LOA, loss of attachment.

Table **4-1**   *Healthy People 2010:* **Oral health objectives—cont'd**

	Oral health goal: To prevent and control oral and craniofacial diseases, conditions, and injuries and improve access to related services	
Number	*Topic of Objective*	*Measure to Monitor Objective*
21-13	School-based health centers with oral health component	% of school-based health centers with an oral health component
21-14	Health centers with oral health component	% of local health departments and community-based health centers with oral health component
21-15	Referral for cleft lip or palate	% of states with system for recording and referring orofacial clefts
21-16	State-based surveillance system	% of states with an oral health surveillance system
21-17	Tribal, state, and local dental programs	% of state, tribal, territorial, and local health agencies with an effective public dental health program (directed by a dental professional with public health training)

Table **4-2**   *Healthy People 2010:* **Selected health objectives related to oral health**

Number	*Topic of Objective*	*Measure to Monitor Objective*
01-8*	Racial and ethnic representation in dental education programs	% of dental degrees (DDS and DMD) awarded to members of underrepresented racial and ethnic groups
03-6	Oropharyngeal cancer deaths	Number of oral cancer deaths per 100,000 population
03-10	Health provider counseling about cancer prevention and tobacco cessation	% of dentists who have counseled their at-risk patients about tobacco cessation
05-15	Annual dental examination for persons with diabetes	% of persons with diabetes who have had an annual dental examination
07-11	Local health departments established culturally appropriate and linguistically competent community health promotion and disease prevention programs	% of local health departments that have provided culturally appropriate and linguistically competent community oral health promotion and disease prevention programs to their jurisdiction in the past year

Adapted from Healthy People 2010: Understanding and Improving Health, 2nd ed. Washington, DC, U.S. Department of Health and Human Services, 2000.[4]
*Numbers refer to the chapter and objective as referenced in Healthy People 2010. For example, 18 is Chapter 1, Objective 8.

The oral health objectives inform decision making and resource allocation by driving action at national, state, and local levels toward the achievement of common oral health improvement goals. States, territories, tribes, and localities can use the framework to guide health plans for oral health improvements. The oral health objectives can shape the development and implementation of policies, interventions, programs, and practices tailored to specific population groups. The objectives identify significant opportunities to improve oral health for all Americans by providing a focus for efforts in the public, private, and nonprofit sectors. These objectives provide a framework for measuring oral health indicators and progress toward achievement of targets.

ORAL HEALTH SURVEILLANCE SYSTEMS

A comprehensive public health surveillance system integrates oral health and is essential for programmatic activities to improve oral health. Several agencies and national organizations have stressed the importance of oral health surveillance systems to routinely collect data on oral health outcomes, risk factors, and intervention strategies for the whole population or representative samples of the population.[7,8] Oral health surveillance systems are not only oral health data collection systems but also involve timely communication of oral health findings to responsible parties and to the public and the use of oral health data to initiate and evaluate public health measures to prevent and control oral diseases and conditions.[7,8] An oral health surveillance system should contain, at a minimum, a core set of oral health measures that describe the status of important oral health conditions to serve as benchmarks for assessing progress in achieving oral health.

Steps have been taken in the United States at the national and state levels to formulate a systematic approach for oral health data collection and reporting. The focus of these collaborative efforts among organizations and agencies was to promote oral health assessment and monitoring that could be applied in a wide range of environments. These efforts also stressed the importance of oral health program evaluation in light of contemporary public health principles. An important aim of these efforts has been the dissemination of procedures for collecting comparable data to assess oral health. A long-term goal includes an approach for continuous monitoring of oral health at the community level and expansion of indicators in oral health surveillance systems. Results of these endeavors included the development of standard ways to monitor the national oral health objectives, an oral health needs assessment model, and documentation of methods to measure community oral health.[4,5,9-13] Several resources have been developed to provide guidance to state, territorial, tribal, and local oral health programs in planning and implementing oral health surveillance systems.

The National Oral Health Surveillance System (NOHSS) is an important oral health data system. NOHSS is a collaborative effort between the Center of Disease Control and Prevention (CDC), Division of Oral Health and the Association of

State and Territorial Dental Directors. It is designed to help public health programs monitor the burden of oral disease, use of the oral health care delivery system, and status of community water fluoridation on both a state and a national level. NOHSS includes indicators of oral health from national and state data sources, information on state oral health programs, and links to sources of oral health information. NOHSS has been developed to track eight basic oral health indicators based on *Healthy People 2010* (see Guiding Principles).[7] NOHSS includes a minimal set of standard oral health indicators, to be expanded in the future, based on data sources and surveillance capacity available to most states.

GUIDING PRINCIPLES

Oral Health Indicators
- Dental visits
- Teeth cleaning
- Complete tooth loss
- Fluoridation status
- Dental caries experience
- Untreated dental caries (tooth decay)
- Dental sealants
- Cancer of the oral cavity and pharynx

The Dental, Oral, and Craniofacial Data Resource Center (DRC) is an important source of information for oral health surveillance and oral health assessments. The DRC is co-sponsored by the National Institute for Dental and Craniofacial Research (NIDCR), National Institutes for Health (NIH), and the Division of Oral Health, CDC. The DRC serves as a resource on dental, oral, and craniofacial data for the oral health educators, researchers, clinical practitioners, public health planners, policy makers, advocates, and the general public. Key resources related to oral health assessment are available from the DRC and include: (a) *Catalog of Oral Health Surveys and Archive of Procedures Related to Oral Health* and (b) *Oral Health Survey Questions: A Compilation of Dental and Oral Health Questions Included on National Health Surveys.* See Appendix D for additional information about the NOHSS, DRC, and other Oral Health Data Systems and Data Sources.

MEASURING ORAL HEALTH AND ITS DETERMINANTS IN POPULATIONS

This chapter focuses on measurements of oral health used in population-based oral health surveillance systems and oral health surveys. The text highlights common measures used to assess population oral health, specifies oral health indicators included in *Healthy People 2010,* and provides an overview of clinical and non-clinical data collection methods related to oral health assessment. Measures and methods used for assessment of individual patients in clinical settings or in clinical studies (including clinical trials) are not emphasized in this chapter. Other books review clinical evaluation techniques or clinical research methods.[14]

Selection of a data collection method for a community oral health assessment should be based on:

1. Information of interest (e.g., types of conditions and factors to be assessed).
2. Social and demographics of the population and community.
3. Purpose of the assessment (e.g., how the data collected are to be used after the assessment).

Common nonclinical measures include face-to-face personal interviews, telephone interviews, a self-administered questionnaire, and a computer-assisted personal interview, although other nonclinical methods can be used to assess different factors influencing oral health.[11] The topics of oral health questions that can be used in oral health surveys are outlined in Appendix E.

Clinical methods include basic screenings and epidemiologic examinations.[9,11,12,15,16]

Basic screenings involve the use of direct observation techniques established for visual detection and identification of gross dental and oral lesions in the oral cavity with a tongue blade, a dental mirror, and appropriate lighting. Epidemiologic examinations entail the use of detailed visual-tactile assessment of the oral cavity with dental instruments and a light source in an oral health survey.

Basic screenings and epidemiologic examinations do not constitute a thorough clinical examination[9,11]; they do not involve making a clinical diagnosis that would result in a treatment plan. Surveys are cross-sectional when they look at a population at a point in time. Surveys are descriptive, as they allow for oral health determinants to be ascertained and oral health status to be estimated for a defined population.

Common dental indexes are used for clinical measures in oral health surveys. A dental **index** is an abbreviated measurement of the amount or condition of oral disease in a population. An index is based on a graduated numeric scale with defined upper and lower limits. It is an aid in data collection, allowing for comparisons among population groups that are classified by the same criteria and methods (see Guiding Principles).

GUIDING PRINCIPLES

Attributes of a Good Index[17]
- Valid
- Reliable
- Clear, simple, and objective
- Sensitive to shifts in disease
- Acceptable to the participants involved
- Amenable to statistical analysis

TYPES OF MEASUREMENTS

Measurements of Dental Caries

Permanent Dentition

Dental caries (tooth decay) is an infectious disease that results in demineralization and, ultimately, cavitation of the tooth surface if the process is not controlled or if the tooth is not remineralized. This bacterial infection is influenced by a variety of factors in the host, agent, and environment. Unless dental caries is arrested early, the process is irreversible.

Dental caries can occur in primary or permanent teeth. General types of tooth decay include coronal (occurring on the crowns of teeth) and root surface (occurring on the roots of teeth). Coronal and root surface caries can be assessed by a systematic evaluation of teeth through epidemiologic examination or screening procedures. The status of **decayed, missing, and filled teeth (DMFT)** or **decayed, missing, and filled surfaces (DMFS)** is commonly recorded by a basic screening or oral epidemiologic examination.[9,12,15,16]

The conventional DMF indexes are used to count coronal caries of permanent teeth (DMFT) or surfaces (DMFS). Although the DMF Index has been used extensively in oral health surveys and has been a standard measurement in many countries, it is limited in its ability to measure thoroughly the characteristics of dental caries.[15,16] As patterns of dental caries change, technology develops, and the goals of oral health surveys shift toward more situational analyses in communities, different approaches for the measurement of dental caries may emerge in the future.[9,11]

For the DMF Index, each tooth space is scored as to whether it is sound or is diseased and whether there is evidence of treated or untreated clinical caries.[18,19] In surveys of populations, the DMF Index can be based on 28 or 32 permanent teeth. If ever diseased, the tooth must show one of three conditions:

1. Untreated, frank cavitation (decayed = D).
2. Evidence of restorative treatment resulting from caries (filled = F).
3. Evidence of a lost tooth caused by caries or periodontal disease (missing = M).

The DMF Index for an individual is the sum of either teeth (DMFT) or surfaces (DMFS) having these three conditions. The DMF Index is considered irreversible, as it indicates cumulative, lifetime caries experience and is used to measure past and present caries experience.

The **Association of State and Territorial Dental Directors (ASTDD)** has developed the **Basic Screening Survey**. It assesses untreated dental caries and dental caries experience on a per-person basis.[9] Dichotomous measures (e.g., yes or no) are used during the screening of each individual to record the absence or presence of untreated dental caries and experience of dental caries (at least one decayed tooth, restored tooth, or missing tooth). Population measures are formulated to indicate the percentage of the population with untreated dental caries and dental caries experience. See Table 4-1 for a summary of the ways in which dental caries will be monitored for *Healthy People 2010.*

In oral health surveys, the terms *caries-free* and *caries experience* are commonly used to describe the status of population groups. When the DMFT score is equal to or more than 1, the person is considered to have experienced dental caries (at present, D; at some time in the past, M or F). When the DMFT equals 0, the person is considered to be caries-free. Population measures are used to indicate the percentage of the population with dental caries experience and, its complementary measurement, the percentage of the population that is caries-free. For example, a survey can show that 52% of children in the population have experienced dental caries and the other 48% are caries-free.

In the United States, oral health surveys typically have used a dichotomous scale for the diagnosis of coronal caries. Dental caries is scored by the presence or absence of a cavitated lesion based on established diagnostic criteria. According to the ASTDD Basic Screening Survey methods, untreated dental caries is detected and recorded by the screener on the basis of observation of the following two criteria[9]:

- A loss of at least 0.5 mm of tooth structure at the enamel surface
- Brown or dark brown discoloration of the walls of the cavity

It has been suggested that protocols to assess coronal dental caries in the future may extend the diagnostic criteria and definitions to evaluate specific stages of dental caries progression by including enamel carious lesions and dentinal carious lesions at the cavitated and noncavitated levels. Findings from such assessments would be helpful in targeting prevention programs at the earliest stages of dental caries progression.

Intraoral epidemiologic examinations can be used to assess the occurrence of root surface caries in oral health surveys.[19] Assessments of each tooth (and surface) present can be evaluated by scoring:

- Sound root
- Decayed root
- Filled root but with decay
- Filled root without decay
- Unexposed root (no gingival recession beyond the cementoenamel junction [CEJ])
- Bridge abutment/implant

The measurement of root surface caries in populations is generally based on the number of exposed root surfaces decayed or filled, with consideration given to the number of surfaces present in the mouth and at risk for dental caries.

Other surveys have used intraoral epidemiologic examinations and used a dichotomous scale for assessing root caries.[18] The examiner scores the status of the survey participant's whole mouth for the following variables:

- Root caries detected/root caries not detected
- Root restoration detected/root restoration not detected

Additional measurements of dental caries have been developed to reflect treatment needs and to provide a broader profile of the impact of dental caries in population groups.[15] A measure of selected restoration and tooth conditions was developed to supplement the DMF Index and to characterize the prevalence and severity of physical and biologic conditions that result from dental caries. The Restorations and Tooth Conditions Assessment (RTCA) was measured in the third **National Health and Nutrition Examination Survey (NHANES III)**.[20] The RTCA was used to evaluate permanent teeth or tooth spaces of adults (18 to 74 years of age). For the RTCA, evaluations were recorded on the basis of the following criteria[20]:

- Soundness
- Defective intracoronal restorations, crowns, or bridges
- Gross loss of tooth structure associated with a restoration
- Pulpal involvement
- Retained roots

Scoring of teeth and tooth conditions for the RTCA is based on a hierarchical approach to measure severity by recording the worst condition.

Primary Dentition

The DMF Index can be modified for primary teeth in children.[18,21] Indexes commonly used for assessing the primary dentition include the df index or dmf index. The df index is the sum of decayed (d) and filled (f) primary tooth surfaces (dfs) or teeth (dft). It does not include missing teeth because of the difficulty in distinguishing primary tooth loss as a result of dental caries from those lost by natural exfoliation.

Note: Upper case letters (e.g., DMFT) signify *permanent* teeth; lower case letters (e.g., dft) signify *primary* teeth.

For use in children before the age of exfoliation (<5 years), the dmf index can indicate the number of teeth or surfaces with history of decay: d denotes decayed teeth, m denotes missing teeth resulting from caries, and f denotes teeth that had been previously filled.

For preschool-age children the assessment of early childhood caries has been used in population-based surveys. To assess the early childhood caries pattern, an examiner evaluates a young child's six maxillary anterior teeth and determines whether one or more of the teeth are decayed, filled, or missing because of dental caries.[9] Missing front teeth for preschool children are most likely a result of caries or traumatic injury. Therefore the cause of missing anterior teeth must be identified by questioning the parent or guardian, if present, during the screening or must include a question on the consent form. The ASTDD Basic Screening Survey methods outline assessment of early childhood caries for young children. As more attention is focused on the prevention of early childhood caries, discussions will emerge in the future about case definitions, diagnostic criteria, and stages of progression related to dental caries in the primary dentition.

Measurement of Dental Treatment Need

The **World Health Organization (WHO)** has established **Basic Methods for Oral Health Surveys** in its "Pathfinder" approach.[16] WHO includes the assessment of treatment needs. During the epidemiologic examination, the examiner records a treatment need for each tooth separately, and the treatment needs can be tabulated for population groups. Treatment categories include[16]:

- No treatment
- Preventive or caries-arresting care
- Sealant
- Restoration(s) (one or two or more surfaces)
- Crown for any reason
- Veneer or laminate
- Pulp care and restoration
- Indication for extraction
- Other treatment

For each person examined, the current status of a prosthesis and need for a prosthesis can be recorded by assessing the type of prosthesis needed and the arch in need.[15,16] It is also common to assess need for dental care and referral.

The assessment of treatment needs may be a problem because it is difficult to standardize clinical judgments for the most appropriate treatment required based on the treatment needs of the average person in the community. Findings of treatment needs can be useful for planning and monitoring purposes. They can be helpful in estimating personnel and service requirements, with demand levels for these services taken into consideration.

Summary assessments that record overall need for dental care (e.g., treatment urgency) are also used in oral health surveys. The ASTDD Basic Screening Survey methods use the following three categories measured during a screening to assess need and referral for dental care[9]:

1. *None*—no obvious oral health problem; routine dental care (next regular checkup) recommended.
2. *Early*—observable oral health problem (dental caries without accompanying signs or symptoms, spontaneous bleeding of the gums, white or red soft tissue areas suggestive of a problem or ill-fitting denture); early dental care (within several weeks) recommended.
3. *Urgent*—signs or symptoms that include pain, infection, swelling, soft tissue ulceration of more than 2 weeks of duration (determined by questioning), emergency dental care (within 24 hours) recommended.

Measurement of Dental Sealants

Dental sealants are traditionally assessed in populations through a basic screening or epidemiologic examination procedure.[9,22] Tooth surfaces and teeth can be evaluated for the presence or absence of dental sealants in the pits and fissures of erupted primary or permanent teeth. Sometimes oral health survey protocols limit measurements for dental sealants to selected tooth surfaces or teeth (e.g., permanent molars).[9] The screener can assess for the presence of dental sealants on a per-person basis with the use of the ASTDD Basic Screening Survey methods.[9] This screening protocol focuses on the eight permanent molar teeth. During the screening a dichotomous measure is used to assess for the presence or absence of dental sealants.

When a tooth is scored for treatment need in an oral health survey, the examiner can record the need for sealant or other preventive and caries-arresting care.[16] This measurement is included in the WHO Pathfinder methodology. This measure can be a problem, because criteria for dental sealant need and caries-arresting care have not been standardized for oral epidemiologic surveys.

See Table 4-1 for a summary of how dental sealants will be monitored for *Healthy People 2010*.

Measurement of Periodontal Disease

Gingivitis is characterized by localized inflammation, swelling, and bleeding of the soft tissues surrounding a tooth without loss of connective tissue or bone support. The condition results in swelling and bleeding of the gums. Gingivitis usually is reversible with proper daily oral hygiene, and its presence or absence serves as a crude measure of a person's self-care practices (e.g., toothbrushing).[23] Although not all occurrences of gingivitis progress to periodontal disease, all periodontal disease starts as gingivitis.[17] Destructive periodontal disease is manifested by the loss of the connective tissue and bone that support the teeth.[23] Destructive periodontal disease places a person at risk for eventual tooth loss unless appropriate treatment commences.

Contemporary indexes to assess the health of periodontal tissues in population-based surveys reflect current theories of the pathogenesis of periodontal diseases. A disaggregated approach is taken to evaluate and record clinical signs of disease. Each measure usually is scored separately. Typical clinical signs that can be measured to assess periodontal status include[24]:

- Gingival bleeding
- Loss of supporting structure as a measure of past disease (recession or loss of periodontal attachment)
- Pocket formation
- Calculus as a contributing risk factor

For the oral epidemiologic examination procedures in NHANES, explicit protocols and criteria were outlined for assessments of periodontal status.[18,25] In the epidemiologic examination the examiner measured gingivitis with the use of the gingival bleeding index by "walking" the probe inside the gingival sulcus to determine the number of sites of gingival bleeding. In addition, periodontal pocket depth on probing, calculus (supragingival or subgingival), and furcations were assessed in the epidemiologic examination. The measurements allowed for the calculation of recession and loss of attachment. The loss of clinical periodontal attachment is defined as the distance in millimeters between the CEJ and the bottom of the sulcus (e.g., periodontal depth minus the distance from the CEJ to the free gingival margin). The extent and severity of destructive periodontal disease are often measured by loss of periodontal attachment, pocket-probing depth, and furcation involvement. The periodontal assessments for NHANES 1999-2002 include measures to determine loss of attachment and to identify bleeding on probing.[18]

See Table 4-1 for a summary of how periodontal disease will be monitored for *Healthy People 2010.*

The presence of at least one bleeding site has been used to define gingivitis in populations and is used to measure progress in *Healthy People 2010.* The occurrence of destructive periodontal disease is often measured by loss of periodontal attachment. The presence of one or more sites with loss of periodontal attachment of 4 mm or greater has been used to delineate destructive periodontal disease in a population. This measure has been used to monitor achievement of targets for the national oral health objectives, and it has allowed the monitoring of changes in destructive periodontal disease over time, distinguishing the status of one population from that of another.

A method of assessing periodontal health status, the **Community Periodontal Index (CPI),** has been developed by WHO and is included in the WHO basic methods for oral health surveys.[16] It is a modification of the Community Periodontal Index of Treatment Needs (CPITN). The CPI allows for a rapid assessment of periodontal status of a population according to various grades of periodontal health.

The CPI divides the teeth into sextants for measurement. The severest measurement of the sextant is scored during an epidemiologic examination. The CPI provides a measurement of:

- Healthy gingival
- Presence or absence of gingival bleeding
- Supragingival or subgingival calculus
- Periodontal pockets (shallow, 4 to 5 mm, and deep, 6 mm or more)

Loss of periodontal attachment is measured, and the highest score is recorded by sextant.

The treatment need codes for observed conditions were eliminated from the original CPITN because they did not reflect contemporary theories of periodontal diseases. The CPI calls for a specially designed lightweight probe with a 0.5-mm ball at its tip and bearing specific millimeter markings. In the United States a modified version of the CPI, the Periodontal Screening Record (PSR), is used for screening in the clinical setting.[14]

Sometimes, to increase efficiency, to lower cost, and to decrease time spent on the epidemiologic examination, partial-mouth periodontal measurements are made to assess periodontal health. Historically, the Periodontal Disease Index (PDI) included specific index teeth to be measured, dubbed the "Ramfjord teeth."[17] The CPI identifies specific index teeth for different age groups.[16] Two quadrants (one maxillary and one mandibular) were randomly selected, and specific tooth sites were measured for the periodontal examination in the NHANES.[18,24] This method, used in NHANES, allowed comparison with the periodontal findings from other NHANES surveys and the National Survey of Oral Health in U.S. Employed Adults and Seniors, 1985-1986, conducted by the National Institute for Dental Research (NIDR) of the NIH.

Retention and Loss of Teeth

"No tooth loss" is equivalent to "tooth retention." "Complete tooth loss" reflects no remaining teeth regardless of the cause of the loss.[9,26] Lack of any natural teeth is defined as edentulousness or edentulism. An individual with at least one natural tooth is considered dentate. Tooth retention and tooth loss can be measured in oral health surveys.[9,16,26]

The ASTTD Basic Screening Survey methods assess edentulousness on a per-person basis.[9] A dichotomous measure is used during the screening of each individual to record the absence of all natural teeth or the presence of all natural teeth.

In an epidemiologic examination each tooth space can be assessed and scored to evaluate retention or loss of natural teeth.[16,26] Data collected about the presence or absence of each tooth are used as indicators of tooth retention and tooth loss at the tooth level, arch level, or individual level for population studies.

Missing teeth can be assessed by tooth type and are scored by cause of loss (e.g., caries, periodontal disease, trauma, congenital absence, or orthodontia). However, determining the exact cause of tooth loss is difficult and can be a problem for a dental examiner. Assessment of tooth retention and loss can be made in the primary or permanent dentition. The missing primary tooth score should be used only in an age group in which normal exfoliation would not sufficiently explain tooth absence.

Self-reported dentition status can be provided in a face-to-face interview or in a telephone interview. Tooth loss was assessed in 2004 through the **Behavioral Risk Factor Surveillance System (BRFSS)** by asking survey participants the following question in a telephone interview:
- How many of your permanent teeth have been removed because of tooth decay or gum disease? Do not include teeth lost for other reasons, such as injury or orthodontics. (Note: if third molars [wisdom teeth] are removed because of tooth decay or gum disease, they should be included in the count for lost teeth. Include teeth lost as a result of "infection.")
  1. 1 to 5
  2. 6 or more but not all
  3. All
  4. Don't know/Not sure
  5. None
  6. Refused

In addition, complete tooth loss can be tracked through personal interviews, and this method constitutes the basis of the measure used for *Healthy People 2010.* Two questions from the **National Health Interview Survey (NHIS),** used in 1997, ask for edentulous status of each arch, and responses of "yes" to both questions determined complete tooth loss.[27] The questions are:

- Have you lost all of your upper natural (permanent) teeth? Yes No
- Have you lost all of your lower natural (permanent) teeth? Yes No

The NHIS in 2004 used the following single question to assess edentulism:

- Have you lost all of your upper and lower natural permanent teeth? Yes No

See Table 4-1 for a summary of the ways in which tooth loss will be monitored for *Healthy People 2010.*

Measurement of Oral and Pharyngeal Cancer

Data to measure the number of deaths resulting from cancer of the oral cavity or pharynx are obtained from death certificates collected through the National Vital Statistics System, within the National Center for Health Statistics (NCHS) of the CDC; such data are available at the state and local levels.[4,13] This measure is based on the number of deaths resulting from oropharyngeal cancer per 100,000 people attributed to cancers classified in coded categories 140 to 149 of the tenth edition of the *International Classification of Diseases (ICD-10).* The original baseline statistic for *Healthy People 2010* was based on codes 140-149 of the ICD-9. Oral and pharyngeal cancers include cancers of the lip, tongue, buccal mucosa, floor of the mouth, and pharynx.

A second measure tracked is the proportion of oral and pharyngeal cancer lesions diagnosed at the earliest stage (e.g., stage 1, localized).[4] This measure is collected through state cancer registries and the Surveillance, Epidemiology, and End Results (SEER) of the National Cancer Institute (NCI) of the NIH. Specific factors related to population groups (e.g., age, gender, race, ethnicity) are often identified in assessments of oral and pharyngeal cancers in populations.

Another measure related to oral and pharyngeal cancer is the receipt of an examination to detect oral and pharyngeal cancer. The National Health Interview Survey, used in 1998, assessed this action through self-reports.[27] The face-to-face interview included the following two questions:

- Have you ever had a test for oral cancer in which the doctor or dentist pulls on your tongue, sometimes with gauze wrapped around it, and feels under the tongue and inside the cheeks? Yes No
- When did you have your most recent oral cancer examination? Was it a year ago or less? More than 1 year but not more than 2 years? More than 2 years but not more than 3 years? More than 3 years but not more than 5 years? Over 5 years?

See Table 4-1 for a summary of how oral and pharyngeal cancers will be monitored for *Healthy People 2010.*

Measurement of Other Oral and Craniofacial Diseases, Conditions, and Injuries

Malocclusion and Craniofacial Anomalies

Malocclusion through evaluation of occlusal characteristics can be assessed during a population-based oral health survey. Some measurements focus on clinical measures of function, whereas other measurements are used to assess aesthetics.

The evaluation of occlusal traits was included in the epidemiologic examination protocol for persons aged 8 to 50 years for NHANES III.[28] It included measurements of incisor alignment, overjet, overbite, presence or absence of a posterior cross-bite, and presence or absence of a maxillary midline diastema. In addition, two questions were included in the face-to-face interview to ascertain the receipt of orthodontic treatment and age at initiation of orthodontic treatment.

WHO incorporates the Dental Aesthetics Index (DAI) in its epidemiologic examination protocol for a basic oral health survey.[16] The DAI considers an individual's social and psychologic well-being as the main benefit of orthodontic treatment. It includes objective measurements of aesthetic acceptability according to social norms.[25] Clinical assessments of missing incisors, canines, or premolars are recorded along with the following evaluations:

- Crowding and spacing in the incisal segments of both arches
- Diastema
- Largest anterior maxillary and mandibular irregularities (rotations or displacements from normal alignment)
- Anterior maxillary and mandibular overjet
- Vertical anterior open bite
- Anteroposterior molar relation

In the United States craniofacial anomalies (including cleft lip and palate) are usually expressed as a proportion or rate based on recordings of congenital anomalies in birth certificates.[29] Recordings of craniofacial anomalies and oral clefts on birth certificates may not be universal.

Orofacial Injuries

Tooth trauma can be assessed through oral epidemiologic examination procedures to evaluate clinical evidence of tooth injury and treatment received for the injury.[30] Incisor trauma has been assessed in NHANES, and the NIDR Trauma Index was used in NHANES III among persons of specific ages to assess, retrospectively, the outcomes of injuries to anterior teeth. The index was developed at the National Institute for Dental Research, the predecessor agency to NIDCR. The index tracks the status of the tooth, from sound (no evidence of trauma) through a missing tooth due to trauma, and reflects selected sequelae of trauma.[18,30] The classification scheme measures soundness or six levels of tooth trauma and is applied to each of the incisor teeth or tooth spaces. A history of trauma is obtained by questioning individuals in the sample, and assessments are recorded for the eight permanent incisors in specific aged children and adults.

Orofacial Pain and Temporomandibular Dysfunction

A temporomandibular joint (TMJ) assessment is included in the WHO basic oral health survey guide.[15] The guide suggests evaluation of signs such as the occurrence of clicking, tenderness on palpation, and reduced jaw mobility on opening greater than 30 mm during an epidemiologic examination. Brief interview questions are added to ascertain symptoms and include self-report of clicking, pain, or difficulties in opening or closing the jaw once or more within a week.

An Orofacial Pain Assessment has been added to the NHANES 1999-2002 with the use of the Orofacial Pain Questionnaire and Orofacial Pain Examination.[18] The Orofacial Pain Questionnaire assesses the frequency of experiences in the past 30 days with specific types of orofacial pain including toothache, sores or irritations, pain in the jaw joint, dull, aching pain across the face, and burning sensations in the mouth. Positive responses to questions about orofacial pain lead to quality of life questions assessing worry or concerns about the pain sensations and days lost to usual activities of daily life (e.g., work, school, self-care, recreation) because of orofacial pain. In addition, an extraoral examination is conducted to assess orofacial pain by measuring the maximal incisal opening in millimeters and palpating the muscles of mastication and the TMJ region for tenderness.

Dental Fluorosis

Dean's Fluorosis Index is the conventional index used to assess for dental fluorosis.[16] This index is one of the most universally accepted classifications for dental fluorosis. Each tooth present in an individual's mouth is rated according to these classifications: normal, questionable, very mild, mild, moderate, and severe. The classifications are based on specific criteria describing the enamel. The individual's fluorosis score is based on the severest form of fluorosis recorded for two or more teeth. The criteria for classifying and scoring dental fluorosis have been slightly modified from the system originally described by Dean for the NHANES 1999-2002.[18]

Dean's Fluorosis Index is included in the WHO basic oral health survey methods.[16] Dental fluorosis has been classified in a number of other ways including the Tooth Surface Index of Fluorosis, the Thylstrup-Fejerskov Index, and the Fluorosis Risk Index.[14,17]

Access to Oral Health Services

Access to Community Prevention: Water Fluoridation

Community water fluoridation, a community preventive service, is measured by the percentage of persons served by public water systems containing optimally fluoridated water.[31] Optimal levels of fluoridation are achieved by adjusting fluoride to obtain a concentration between 0.7 and 1.2 parts per million (ppm). The optimal fluoride concentration is determined by geographic areas based on mean daily temperature; thus states have different levels of optimal concentration of fluoride in water.

To characterize a community as optimally fluoridated, it is necessary to compare tap water or water samples from water treatment plants with the level determined by the state to be optimal for that community. National information related to public water systems and community water fluoridation is obtained from the **Water Fluoridation Reporting System (WFRS),** an interactive Web-based monitoring and surveillance program available for use by state and tribal fluoridation managers. WFRS is one of the first CDC surveillance systems to collect and edit data over the Internet in "real time" (information entered instantaneously updates data records). The application was developed by CDC in collaboration with the ASTDD to monitor fluoridation at the local and state levels in the United States.

WFRS allows state and tribal fluoridation managers to update basic water system information such as populations served, fluoridation status, communities and counties served, and contact information for more than 56,000 community water systems directly over the Internet. WFRS maintains the relationships among water systems that buy and sell water to each other, allowing the fluoride content of a water system to be found, whether it produces its own water or purchases water from another system.

Although knowing which systems are fluoridated is important, WFRS was also designed as a tool to assist states and tribes in monitoring the quality of fluoridation. Users can enter monthly data such as high, low, and average fluoride concentrations and split-sample analysis and can indicate whether the water system met the daily testing requirements. Using criteria supplied by the state or tribe, WFRS evaluates the data entered to determine whether the water system provided "optimally" (e.g., the fluoride concentration is within the desired range) fluoridated water for the month. Numerous reports provide fluoridation managers with the tools they need to improve the quality of fluoridation. This voluntary reporting system compiles information on the number of people served by the fluoridated water system, the number of counties and cities served by the fluoridated water system, and the quality of the fluoridated water system. These quality measures will include the number of months the system is operating with optimal fluoride concentration. Data from WFRS is used to update the water fluoridation information and maps on the NOHSS. CDC produces an annual report from the WFRS database. See Table 4-1 for a summary of the ways in which community water fluoridation will be monitored for *Healthy People 2010*.

Access to the Oral Health Care System

Access to the oral health system consists of many facets including availability, accessibility, accommodation, affordability, and acceptability.[32] Multiple factors have been assessed to explain the use of clinical oral health services. These factors have been summarized as epidemiologic, social, demographic, personal, and psychologic, as well as characteristic of the oral health care system.[3]

A common measure of access to and use of the oral health care system is having an annual dental visit. This measure is assessed by determining the length of time since the last visit to a dentist or dental clinic. See Table 4-1 for a summary of the ways in which use of the oral health care system will be monitored for *Healthy People 2010.*

Responses to interview questions have been used to measure the percentage of persons who have had a dental visit in the past year. The **Medical Expenditure Panel Survey (MEPS),** which uses a face-to-face interview to assess dental visits, is used to measure progress of the *Healthy People 2010* objectives regarding dental attendance. Other national surveys such as NHANES and NHIS use face-to-face interviews with structured questionnaires to evaluate dental visits. Specific questions about dental visits are included in these questionnaires.

The CDC, through its state-specific BRFSS, conducts telephone interviews to assess dental attendance. In addition, self-administered questionnaires have been used by states and localities to determine access to dental care. The questionnaire may be completed by adult participants in surveys or by parents of children participating in school-based oral health surveys. The National Nursing Home Survey, conducted by the National Center for Health Statistics, CDC in 1997 and 1999, measured the receipt of dental care services by nursing home residents.

Other important measures associated with access to oral care include the following:

- Dental attendance for routine checkups or cleanings
- Assessment of dental insurance coverage
- Usual source of dental care
- Reason for not having a dental visit in the past year
- Difficulty in obtaining needed dental care
- Purpose of last dental visit

Box 4-2 outlines examples of questions about access to care that are included with the Basic Screening Survey methods developed by the ASTTD.[9] These questions can be included in a self-administered questionnaire or can be asked during a telephone or face-to-face interview.

Measurement of Oral Health, Well-Being, and Quality of Life

A better understanding of cultural, social, behavioral, psychologic, and economic factors related to oral conditions and treatments can contribute to oral health efforts at the community level.[33,34] During an assessment it is also important to consider the belief systems and cultural values, customs, traditions, and institutions related to the oral health of individuals and groups.[3] Measurements of knowledge, attitudes, beliefs, and behaviors traditionally have been used to evaluate personal oral health practices and use of the oral health care system.[1,3]

BOX 4-2   QUESTIONS TO EVALUATE THE USE OF THE ORAL HEALTH CARE SYSTEM

1. During the past 6 months, did {you/your child} have a toothache more than once, when biting or chewing? [Source: National Health Interview Survey, 1989]
   1. Yes
   2. No
   3. Don't know/don't remember

2. About how long has it been since {you/your child} last visited a dentist? Include all types of dentists, such as orthodontists, oral surgeons, and all other dental specialists, as well as dental hygienists. [Source: National Health Interview Survey, 1997]
   1. 6 months or less
   2. More than 6 months, but not more than 1 year ago
   3. More than 1 year ago, but not more than 3 years ago
   4. More than 3 years ago
   5. Never have been
   6. Don't know/don't remember

3. What was the main reason that {you/your child} last visited a dentist? (Please check one.) [Source: National Health Interview Survey, 1986]
   1. Went in on own for checkup, examination, or cleaning
   2. Was called in by the dentist for checkup, examination, or cleaning
   3. Something was wrong, bothering, or hurting
   4. Went for treatment of a condition that dentist discovered at earlier checkup or examination
   5. Other
   6. Don't know/don't remember

4. During the past 12 months, was there a time when {you/your child} needed dental care but could not get it at that time? [Source: National Health Interview Survey, 1994]
   1. Yes
   2. No
   3. Don't know/don't remember

5. The last time {you/your child} could not get the dental care {you/he/she} needed, what was the main reason {you/he/she} couldn't get care? (Please check one.) [Source: National Health Interview Survey, 1994]
   1. Could not afford it
   2. No insurance
   3. Dentist did not accept Medicaid/insurance
   4. Not serious enough
   5. Wait too long in clinic/office
   6. Difficulty in getting appointment
   7. Don't like/trust/believe in dentists

Continued

BOX 4-2   QUESTIONS TO EVALUATE THE USE OF THE ORAL HEALTH CARE SYSTEM—cont'd

    8. No dentist available
    9. Didn't know where to go
   10. No way to get there
   11. Hours not convenient
   12. Speak a different language
   13. Health of another family member
   14. Other reason
   15. Don't know/don't remember

6. Do you have any kind of insurance that pays for some or all of {you/your child's} medical or surgical care? Include health insurance obtained through employment or purchased directly as well as government program like Medicaid.
    1. Yes
    2. No
    3. Don't know/don't remember

7. Do you have any kind of insurance that pays for some or all of {your/your child's} dental care? Include health insurance obtained through employment or purchased directly as well as government programs like Medicaid.
    1. Yes
    2. No
    3. Don't know/don't remember

Additional questions for survey planners to consider:

8. During the past 12 months, was there a time when you felt that {you/your child} needed medical care or surgery but could not get it at that time? [Source: Modified from National Health Interview Survey, 1994]
    1. Yes
    2. No
    3. Don't know/don't remember

9. The last time {you/your child} could not get the medical care or surgery {you/he/she} needed, what was the main reason {you/he/she} couldn't get care? [Source: National Health Interview Survey, 1994]
    1. Could not afford it
    2. No insurance
    3. Doctor did not accept Medicaid/insurance
    4. Not serious enough
    5. Wait too long in clinic/office
    6. Difficulty in getting appointment
    7. Don't like/trust/believe in doctors
    8. No doctor available
    9. Didn't know where to go

Box 4-2   Questions to evaluate the use of the Oral Health Care System—cont'd

> 10. No way to get there
> 11. Hours not convenient
> 12. Speak a different language
> 13. Health of another family member
> 14. Other reason
> 15. Don't know/don't remember

Adapted from Association of State and Territorial Dental Directors: Basic Screening Surveys: An Approach to Monitoring Community Oral Health, 2003.[9]
For all questions, refused/no response is a coding option but is not listed as a choice on the questionnaire. For one-digit variables, 9 is coded. For two-digit variables, the refused/no response code is 99.

Data collection methods have been developed to assess oral health knowledge, attitudes, beliefs, and behaviors. Multiple measurements have been designed to evaluate diverse factors as they relate to oral health care–seeking behaviors, oral hygiene and home care practices, dietary practices, use of tobacco and alcohol, age-appropriate safety measures, and use of protective gear.[1]

The development of sociodental indicators has been advocated to assess the non-clinical aspects of oral diseases.[3] Measures have been recommended to document the full impact of oral disorders and treatment within populations. Different measures have been used to evaluate economic impact and social and psychologic consequences of oral diseases, conditions, and injuries. These measures have been developed to assess outcomes at the individual and societal levels. The term *oral health-related quality of life* has been adopted as a construct that considers multiple dimensions of oral health.[35]

Perceived health status and general assessment of oral health are common measurements used in population-based oral health surveys. These questions were included in the International Collaborative Study of Oral Health Outcomes, sponsored by WHO.[36] The questions use a basic Likert measurement scale to assess self-perceived health status. The NHANES 2001-2002 included the following questions:[18]

- Would you say your health in general is excellent, very good, good, fair, or poor?
- How would you describe the condition of your teeth and gums? Is it excellent, very good, good, fair, poor, or very poor?

Satisfaction with oral health status is another measurement used in surveys. Assessment instruments such as the Geriatric Oral Health Assessment Instrument (GOHAI) and the Oral Health Impact Profile (OHIP) have been developed to evaluate oral health–related quality of life.[1,35]

The psychosocial and functional dimensions of oral health have been used in studies of population groups.[1,34] These dimensions consider the crucial sensory, communicative, gustatory, and psychosocial functions of the structures related to the teeth, mouth, and face, such as social function, and the impact of oral disorders on intimacy, personal contact, social integration, and social roles.[1]

The functional dimensions of oral health have been assessed and include measurements of self-perceived oral functional status and well-being including self-reported evaluations of tooth loss, oral pain, eating ability, and ability to sleep. The impact of oral symptoms and pain can also be included in assessments.

Self-reported evaluations can assess presence or absence of pain in the teeth or soft tissues of the mouth from acute or chronic oral pain, dental pain, and facial pain. In addition, studies have considered social response to facial appearance by assessing social and psychologic outcomes of malocclusion, craniofacial anomalies, and oral cancer. Such assessments can include measurements of self-concept, psychosocial development, and social perceptions.

Economic dimensions include indirect and direct economic impacts of oral health problems and their treatments.[1] A measurement of indirect economic impacts is self-reported reductions in normal activities related to dental conditions and dental attendance.[1] Answers to questions in a structured questionnaire can evaluate work-loss days, school-loss days, reduced activity days, and bed days resulting from acute dental conditions and dental visits. This measure has been included in the National Health Interview Survey. Years of life lost can be calculated on the basis of premature deaths from oral and pharyngeal cancer.[1]

Direct economic impacts include direct costs related to dental and oral problems for society and individuals. In addition, analyses of cost benefit and cost-effectiveness can be made for preventive and therapeutic treatments to evaluate direct economic impacts of oral health problems and their treatments.

Measures of oral health, well-being, and quality of life can be used to demonstrate the significance of oral health conditions for individuals and for society as a whole. It helps to ensure that treatments provided result in health gains that enhance not only the individual's clinical status but also his or her psychologic well-being. Assessing social, psychologic, and economic impacts can be used to identify population subgroups and oral diseases that need to be targeted for health promotion and disease prevention efforts.[1]

Measurement of Infrastructure, Capacity, and Resources

Infrastructure, capacity, and resources are key elements by which states and localities can effectively address oral health problems.[7]

Infrastructure consists of systems, people, relationships, and resources that enable states and localities to perform public health functions and address oral health problems. Within a public health agency, infrastructure includes assessment, surveillance, information systems, planning, policy development, applied research, training, standards development, quality management, coordination, and systems of care.

Capacity enables the development of expertise and competence and the implementation of strategies.

Resources include personnel, financial capital, and available time. The public health and personal health workforce must have the necessary capacity and expertise to effectively address oral health problems and issues in jurisdictions and states.[10]

See Table 4-1 for a summary of the ways in which infrastructure and capacity of the oral health system will be monitored for *Healthy People 2010.*

To ensure achievement of the *Healthy People 2010* oral health objectives, it is necessary that instruments and methods be developed to assess the current status, best practices, and future development of infrastructure, capacity, and resources necessary to improve oral health at state and local levels. States and localities that can evaluate and develop these key elements will be better prepared to maintain fully effective essential public health services for oral health and to achieve the oral health objectives.

FUTURE DIRECTIONS

A core foundation of successful planning in dental public health is information collected though oral health surveillance systems about the epidemiology of oral diseases and factors that could be targets for prevention. Assessment of key oral health indicators is crucial to effective public health planning that tailors oral health policies, programs, and practices based on oral health status and the progression of oral diseases among population groups. Oral health assessment methods should evolve as oral disease patterns and population demographics change. These changes will demand new techniques and the development of skills by dental professionals working in public health.

SUMMARY

This chapter presented the goals and health objectives of *Healthy People 2010;* these benchmarks provide an important framework for the assessment of health in the United States in the coming decade. It focused on oral health surveillance as the ongoing and systematic collection, analysis, and interpretation of oral health indicators for use in planning, implementing, and evaluating dental public health practice. The chapter described how assessments are important to monitor changes in:

- Oral health and disease patterns
- Use of services
- Social, demographic, and economic factors influencing oral health
- Workforce and service system capacity within the public, private, and nonprofit sectors

Specific measures used in assessing oral health in populations were discussed in the chapter. The chapter highlighted examples of oral health surveys and discussed the importance of using standardized measurements to assess oral health trends.

Applying **Your Knowledge**

1. Apply your knowledge about community assessment and oral health surveys.
   a. Select three oral health objectives from *Healthy People 2010*.
   b. For each objective, describe how you would assess it in the coming year in the following situations:
      Objective 1—in an urban inner-city community
      Objective 2—in a suburban community
      Objective 3—in a rural county
2. Read over the following situations and questions. Discuss your ideas and answers in small groups.
   a. The chair of the Healthy Communities Task Force contacts you at the State Health Department. The number 1 priority issue for the Task Force is fluoridation of the municipal water supply. The Task Force is interested in your technical assistance in developing this local initiative and would like your suggestions about assessments in the community that are necessary to get this initiative implemented in the coming year. What assessment issues might the Task Force need to address? Whom should they contact? What steps may it need to take? How could this community process instigate the development and implementation of a community oral health improvement plan?
   b. ARC, a community-based organization that provides vocational opportunities for disabled adults, has become concerned about its clients' dental status and lack of access to dental care. A legislator from this rural area takes up this issue and is interested in improving access to dental care for adults. She asks her legislative aide to evaluate the dental access problems and to study the options in the Medicaid program to provide dental coverage for low-income adults, especially adults with disabilities. Representatives from a State Disability Coalition meet with you at the State Health Department to discuss your insights. The next day, the Executive Director of the State Association of Community Health Centers calls you and asks you to describe some of the barriers to dental care that adults face in rural counties across the state. How would you capitalize on these unique circumstances to develop a state oral health assessment? Whom would you contact? What steps would you take? How could these activities contribute to the development and implementation of a state oral health improvement plan?

DENTAL HYGIENE COMPETENCIES

Reading the material in this chapter and participating in the activities of Applying Your Knowledge will contribute to the student's ability to demonstrate the following competencies:

Health promotion and disease prevention

HP.4 Identify individual and population risk factors and develop strategies that promote health-related quality of life.

Community involvement

CM.1 Assess the oral health needs of the community and the quality and availability of resources and services.

Patient/client care

PC.1 Systematically collect, analyze, and record data on the general, oral, and psychosocial health status of a variety of patients or clients using methods consistent with medicolegal principles.

PC.2 Use critical decision making skills to reach conclusions about the patient's or client's dental hygiene needs based on all available assessment data.

PC.5A Determine the outcomes of dental hygiene interventions using indexes, instruments, examination techniques, and the patient's or client's self-report.

Community Case

In your position as the State Dental Director, the State Health Officer for the State Department of Public Health has requested that the State Health Surveillance System be reorganized and changed based on the *Healthy People 2010* Health Objectives. You are asked to develop a plan to integrate an updated oral health component for this State Health Surveillance System.

1. All of the following resources should be reviewed during the early planning of the oral health component for the State Health Surveillance System except:
   a. National *Healthy People 2010* Oral Health Objectives
   b. National Oral Health Surveillance System
   c. Reports from the Behavioral Risk Factor Surveillance Survey
   d. The Dental, Oral, and Craniofacial Data Resource Center
   e. The Oral Health Impact Profile
2. What measure would be used to assess untreated tooth decay?
   a. Percentage of persons with ≥1 bleeding site
   b. Percentage of nursing home residents having a dental visit in the past year
   c. Percentage of persons with ≥1 dft or DMFT
   d. Percentage of persons with ≥1 dt or DT
   e. Percentage of persons with all teeth extracted, edentulous
3. In conducting a survey to evaluate access to dental care, the following information is most often collected with the use of a questionnaire except?
   a. Dental insurance coverage
   b. Oral cancer experience

     c. Usual source of dental care

     d. Annual dental visit

     e. Reason for not having a dental visit in the past year

4. Which survey method would you select to replicate in the state to assess the presence of dental sealants among third-grade students?

     a. National Nursing Home Survey

     b. National Health Interview Survey

     c. Association for State and Territorial Dental Directors (ASTDD) Basic Screening Survey

     d. Behavioral Risk Factor Surveillance Survey

     e. National Vital Statistics System

5. An important goal of an Oral Health Surveillance System is to assess disparities among different segments of a population. All of the following factors are important to include in a State Oral Health Surveillance System to track oral health disparities except?

     a. Geographic location

     b. Age

     c. Income

     d. Social class based on occupational ranking

     e. Racial and ethnic background

REFERENCES

1. Oral Health in America: A Report of the Surgeon General. Rockville, Md, U.S. Department of Health and Human Services, National Institute of Dental and Craniofacial Research, National Institutes of Health, 2000.
2. U.S. Department of Health and Human Services: A National Call to Action to Promote Oral Health. Rockville, Md, U.S. Department of Health and Human Services, Public Health Service, Centers for Disease Control and Prevention, National Institutes of Health, National Institute of Dental and Craniofacial Research, May 2003.
3. Cohen LK, Gift HC (eds): Disease Prevention and Oral Health Promotion: Socio-dental Sciences in Action. Copenhagen, Munksgaard, 1995.
4. Healthy People 2010: Understanding and Improving Health, 2nd ed. Washington, DC, U.S. Department of Health and Human Services, 2000.
5. Healthy People 2000: National Health Promotion and Disease Prevention Objectives. Washington, DC, U.S. Department of Health and Human Services, 1990.
6. Healthy People: Surgeon General's Report on Health Promotion and Disease Prevention. Washington, DC, U.S. Department of Health, Education, and Welfare, 1979.
7. Beltran-Aquilar ED, Malvitz DM, Lockwood SA, et al: Oral health surveillance: Past, present, and future challenges. J Public Health Dent 63:141, 2003.
8. Association of State and Territorial Dental Directors: Best Practice Approaches for State and Community Oral Health Programs: State-Based Oral Health Surveillance System. Jefferson City, Mo: Association of State and Territorial Dental Directors, 2003.
9. Association of State and Territorial Dental Directors. Basic Screening Surveys: An Approach to Monitoring Community Oral Health. Columbus, Ohio: Association of State and Territorial Dental Directors, 2003.
10. Association of State and Territorial Dental Directors: Guidelines for State and Territorial Oral Health Programs. Jefferson City, Mo, 2001.
11. Kuthy RA, Siegal MA, Phipps K: Assessing Oral Health Needs: ASTDD Seven-Step Model. Association of State and Territorial Dental Directors, Jefferson City, Mo, 2003.

12. Carnahan BW: Oral Health Examination Survey Manual (companion document to 1997 version of Assessing Oral Health Needs: ASTDD Seven-Step Model). Arlington, Va, National Center for Education in Maternal and Child Health, 1997.

13. U.S. Department of Health and Human Services: Tracking Healthy People 2010. Washington, DC, U.S. Government Printing Office, November 2000. *http://www.healthypeople.gov/Document/tableofcontents.htm#tracking*

14. Wilkins EM: Clinical Practice of the Dental Hygienist, 9th ed. Philadelphia, Lippincott Williams & Wilkins, 2004.

15. Drury TF, Winn DM, Snowden CB, et al: An overview of the oral health component of the 1988-1991 National Health and Nutrition Examination Survey (NHANES III, Phase 1) (special issue). J Dent Res 75:620, 1996.

16. Oral Health Surveys: Basic Methods, 4th ed. Geneva, World Health Organization, 1997.

17. Burt BA, Eklund SA: Dentistry, Dental Practice, and the Community, 5th ed. Philadelphia, WB Saunders, 1999.

18. Centers for Disease Control and Prevention, National Center for Health Statistics: National Health and Nutrition Examination Survey: Dental Examiners Procedures Manual. Hyattsville, Md, National Center for Health Statistics, CDC, DHHS, 2001.

19. Winn DM, Brunelle JA, Selwitz RJ, et al: Coronal and root caries in the dentition of adults in the United States, 1988-1999 (special issue). J Dent Res 75:642, 1996.

20. White BA, Albertini TF, Brown LJ, et al: Selected restoration and tooth conditions: United States, 1988–1991 (special issue). J Dent Res 75:661, 1996.

21. Lewitt EM, Kerrebrock N: Child indicators: Dental health. Future Child 8:133, 1998.

22. Selwitz RH, Winn DM, Kingman A, Zion GR: The prevalence of dental sealants in the US population: Findings from NHANES III, 1988-1991 (special issue). J Dent Res 75:652, 1996.

23. American Academy of Periodontology: Consensus report on periodontal diseases: Epidemiology and diagnosis. Ann Periodontol 1:216, 1996.

24. Brown LJ, Brunelle JA, Kingman A: Periodontal status in the United States, 1988–1991: Prevalence, extent, and demographic variation (special issue). J Dent Res 75:672, 1996.

25. Cons NC, Jenny J, Kohout FJ: DAI: The Dental Aesthetic Index. Iowa City, University of Iowa College of Dentistry, 1986.

26. Drury TF, Brown LJ, Zion GR: Tooth retention and tooth loss in the permanent dentition of adults: United States, 1988-1991 (special issue). J Dent Res 75:684, 1996.

27. Centers for Disease Control and Prevention: National Health Interview Survey 1998 Questionnaire: Adult Prevention Module. Hyattsville, Md, National Center for Health Statistics, Centers for Disease Control and Prevention, June 27, 2000.

28. Brunelle JA, Bhat M, Lipton JA: Prevalence and distribution of selected occlusal characteristics in the U.S. population, 1988-1991 (special issue). J Dent Res 75:706, 1996.

29. Tolarova MM, Cervenka J: Classification and prevalence of orofacial clefts. Am J Med Genet 75:126, 1998.

30. Kaste LM, Gift HC, Bhat M, Swango PA: Prevalence of incisor trauma in persons 6 to 50 years of age: United States, 1988-1991 (special issue). J Dent Res 75:696, 1996.

31. Centers for Disease Control and Prevention, National Center for Health Statistics: Healthy People 2000 Review, 1999–2000. Hyattsville, Md, Public Health Service, 1999.

32. Warren RC: Oral Health for All: Policy for Available, Accessible, and Acceptable Care. Washington, DC, Center for Policy Alternatives, September 1999.

33. Schou L, Blinkhorn AS: Oral Health Promotion. New York, Oxford University Press, 1993.

34. Weintraub JA: Uses of oral health–related quality of life measures in public health. Community Dent Health 15:8, 1998.

35. Inglehart MR, Bagramian R: Oral Health-Related Quality of Life. Chicago, Quintessence Publishing, 2002.

36. Chen M, Andersen RM, Barmes DE, et al: Comparing Oral Health Care Systems: A Second International Collaborative Study. Geneva, World Health Organization, 1997.

5

Oral Health Status and Trends

Jane E.M. Steffensen, RDH, BS, MPH, CHES

Objectives

Upon completion of this chapter, the student will be able to:

- Describe the current status of oral health in the United States
- Discuss oral health trends in the United States
- Compare the indicators for oral health included in the national oral health objectives for *Healthy People 2000* and *2010*
- Identify oral health disparities among population groups
- Discuss the factors that influence oral health in populations

Key Terms

Oral Health Disparities
Healthy People 2000
Healthy People 2010
Status
Trend
Behavioral Risk Factor
  Surveillance Survey (BRFSS)

National Health and
  Nutrition Examination
  Survey (NHANES)
National Health Interview
  Survey (NHIS)
Medical Expenditure Panel
  Survey (MEPS)

National Oral Health
  Surveillance System
Dental Health
  Professional Shortage
  Area (Dental HPSA)

OPENING STATEMENT

The Burden of Oral Diseases in the United States[1,5,6,16]

- Of young children 2 to 4 years of age, 23% have already experienced dental caries.

- Fifty percent of children 6 to 8 years of age and 59% of 15-year-old adolescents are affected by dental caries.

- Approximately 162 million persons, or 66% of the population served by public water systems, received optimally fluoridated water and the benefits for prevention of dental caries.

- Only 28% of children (8 years of age) and 14% of adolescents (14 years of age) have received dental sealants.

- Of adults (35 to 44 years of age), 20% have destructive periodontal disease.

- Oral diseases continue to burden older adults, and 25% of seniors (65 to 74 years of age) are edentulous and no longer have their natural teeth because of dental caries or periodontal disease.

- Nearly 30,000 Americans are found to have oral and pharyngeal cancer, and approximately 7800 people die of these cancers each year.

- More than 100 million Americans lack dental insurance.

- Nearly two thirds (57%) of children (>2 years of age) and adults have not had a dental visit in the past year.

- Only 23% of edentate adults 18 years and older had an annual dental visit in the preceding year.

- Adults miss more than 164 million hours of work each year because of dental concerns.

- Approximately $40 billion have been saved in reduced oral health care expenditures in the United States over the past 40 years as a result of public water fluoridation.

ORAL HEALTH IN THE UNITED STATES

In the United States, progress has been made in reducing the extent and severity of common oral diseases.[1] Over the past 50 years, major improvements in oral health have been seen nationally for many Americans, yet oral diseases remain common and widespread in the United States.[2-5] Oral diseases and conditions still afflict most people at some time throughout their life span.[1,6] Safe and effective measures of preventing oral diseases exist but are underused.[7-11] Effective preventive measures include (1) community water fluoridation, (2) application of dental sealants, (3) regular dental care, and (4) tobacco cessation.[8-11] Preventive measures need to be adopted and applied by communities, individuals, and professionals to ensure marked improvements of the nation's oral health in the future.[1,6]

SOCIAL IMPACT OF ORAL DISEASES

Oral diseases are progressive and cumulative and become more complex over time.[1,6] They can jeopardize physical growth, development, self-concept, and the capacity to learn. They influence eating and communicating. Oral diseases affect economic productivity and compromise a person's ability to work at home or on the job or to concentrate in school.[5]

The social impact of oral disease in children is substantial. More than 51 million school hours are lost each year as a result of dental problems.[1,5] Poor children experience nearly 12 times more restricted activity days than do their counterparts from higher-income families. Among those who lost school time, youngsters from low-income families, members of minority communities, and families without insurance missed more hours.[12] Children with early childhood caries—oftentimes a severe and painful form of dental caries—can demonstrate failure to thrive and be underweight.[13] Serious lifetime functional, aesthetic, and social consequences can be outcomes for children and adults with severe developmental and acquired oral and facial conditions.[1] The Centers for Disease Control and Prevention (CDC) estimated that 16.2 years of life were lost per person who died prematurely of oral and pharyngeal cancer.[1] This figure exceeds the average 15.4 years lost for all cancer sites.

Dental diseases in adults affect their economic productivity and compromise their ability to get jobs. Employed American adults lose more than 164 million hours of work each year because of dental disease or dental visits.[1,5] Among those who miss work, women, African Americans, low wage earners, employees with less education, and the uninsured miss the greatest number of hours. Employees of service industries lose from 2 to 3.5 times more hours of work than executives or professional workers.[12]

Oral and dental diseases influence an individual's ability to eat, communicate, and interact in society. For example, a study supported by the World Health Organization (WHO) found that among Navajo schoolchildren living in parts of the Navajo reservation in Arizona and New Mexico, 25% avoided laughing or smiling and 20% avoided meeting other people because of the way their teeth looked. Because of dental pain, almost 25% of Navajo adults were unable to chew hard foods, and nearly 20% reported difficulty sleeping.[14]

BURDEN OF ORAL DISEASES AND CONDITIONS

Despite improvements in oral health status, profound **oral health disparities** remain in specific population groups in the United States.[5,15-16] For some oral diseases and conditions, the magnitude of the differences in oral health status among population groups is striking.[1,16] Oral health disparities are defined as differences in oral health status among population groups. Many different demographic and social characteristics are associated with oral health disparities. These factors include income, education, race/ethnicity, culture, geography (urban/rural), age, sex, disability status, behavioral lifestyles, and other factors. These factors reflect the diversity of the U.S. population. Oral health disparities can be due to lack of information or access to preventive measures.

The burden of oral diseases is spread unevenly throughout the population.[1,6,16] People who experience the worst oral health are found among the poor of all ages, with poor children and poor older Americans particularly vulnerable. Members of racial and ethnic minorities experience a disproportionate level of oral health problems. People who are medically compromised or who have disabilities are at greater risk for oral disease; in turn, oral diseases further jeopardize their overall health and well-being. This burden of oral disease restricts activities in school, work, and home and often significantly diminishes quality of life.

ORAL HEALTH STATUS AND TRENDS

National benchmarks have been established to assess health in the United States through **Healthy People 2000** and **Healthy People 2010**.[2,4] Tracking systems have been developed and regular progress reports are used to monitor the attainment of the national oral health objectives.[3,5,15] Table 5-1 summarizes the progress in reaching the *Healthy People 2000* oral health objectives.[2,3] The national trends

Table **5-1**   **Progress in meeting *Healthy People 2000* oral health objectives**

Number	Oral Health Objective	Age (yr)	Baseline Data (%)	Healthy People 2000 Goal (%)	Final Data (%)	Summary
13.1	Reduce dental caries in children	6-8	54	35	52	Progress
	Reduce dental caries in adolescents	15	78	60	61	Progress
13.2	Reduce untreated dental decay in children	6-8	28	20	29	Reversed
	Reduce untreated dental decay in adolescents	15	24	15	20	Progress

Centers for Disease Control and Prevention, National Center for Health Statistics: Healthy People 2000 Review, 1998-1999. Hyattsville, Md, Public Health Service, 1999.

Table 5-1   **Progress in meeting *Healthy People 2000* oral health objectives—*cont'd***

Number	Oral Health Objective	Age (yr)	Baseline Data (%)	Healthy People 2000 Goal (%)	Final Data (%)	Summary
13.3	Increase adults who have never lost a permanent tooth	35-44	31	45	31	No change
13.4	Reduce adults who have lost all their teeth	65+	36	20	30	Progress
13.5	Reduce gingivitis among adults	35-44	41	30	48	Reversed
13.6	Reduce destructive periodontal disease among adults	35-44	25	15	22	Progress
13.7	Reduce oral and pharyngeal deaths in males	45-74	13.6	10.5	10.3	Met
	Reduce oral and pharyngeal deaths in females	45-74	4.8	4.1	3.5	Met
13.8	Increase dental sealants in children	8	11	50	23	Progress
	Increase dental sealants in adolescents	14	8	50	24	Progress
13.9	Increase persons on public water receiving fluoridated water		61	75	62	Progress
13.10	Increase topical/systemic fluorides among nonfluoridated		50	85	No data	No data
13.11	Increase caregivers using feeding practices that prevent early childhood caries		55	75	No data	No data
13.12	Increase oral health screening, referral, follow-up, first-time school attendee		66	90	75	Progress
13.13	For long-term care, oral examination and services provided within 90 days		No data	100	No data	No data
13.14	Increase use of oral health care system (adults)	35+	54	70	63	Progress
13.15	Increase states with system for recording and referring orofacial clefts		11 states	40 states	23 states	Progress
13.16	Extend use of protective head, face, eye, and mouth equipment		No data	No data	No data	No data
13.17	Reduce smokeless tobacco use among males	12-17	6.6	4	3.7	Met
		18-24	8.9	4	6.9	Progress

Table 5-2   Summary *Healthy People 2010:* oral health objectives

Number	Oral Health Objective	Baseline Age (yr)	Data (%)	Data 2000 (%)	Healthy People 2010 Goal (%)
21.1	Reduce dental caries experience in children				
	Young children (primary teeth)	2-4	18	23	11
	Children (primary or permanent teeth)	6-8	52	50	42
	Adolescents (permanent teeth)	15	61	59	51
21.2	Reduce untreated dental decay in children and adults				
	Young children (primary teeth)	2-4	16	20	9
	Children (primary or permanent teeth)	6-8	28	26	21
	Adolescents (permanent teeth)	15	20	16	15
	Adults (permanent teeth)	35-44	27	26	15
21.3	Increase adults with teeth who have never lost a tooth as a result of dental caries or periodontal disease	35-44	31	39	42
21.4	Reduce adults who have lost all their teeth	65-74	26(a)	25 (2002)	20
21.5a	Reduce gingivitis among adults	35-44	48	DNA	41
21.5b	Reduce destructive periodontal disease	35-44	21	20	14
21.6	Increase detection of stage 1 oral cancer lesions	All	36	35	50
21.7	Increase number of oral cancer examinations	40+	13	—	20
21.8	Increase dental sealants	8 (first molars)	23	28	50
		14 (first and second molars)	15	14	50
21.9	Increase persons on public water receiving fluoridated water	All	62	68 (2002)	75
21.10	Increase use of the oral health care system	2+	44	43	56
21.11	Increase use of dental services for those in long-term facilities (e.g., nursing homes)	All	19	—	25
21.12	Increase preventive services for low-income youth	2-17	20	31	57
21.13	Increase number of school-based health centers with oral health component	K-12	DNC	DNC	*
21.14	Increase number of community health centers and local health departments with oral health component	All	52	61 (2002)	75
21.15	Increase states with systems for recording and referring orofacial clefts	All	23	—	51 states
21.16	Increase number of states with state-based oral health surveillance systems	All	0	—	51 states
21.17	Increase the number of tribal, state, and local dental programs with public health trained directors	All	DNC	DNC	*

National Centers for Health Statistics, Centers for Disease Control and Prevention: Healthy People 2010 Progress Review: Briefing Book Materials–Data Summary Table for Focus Area 21—Oral Health, March 17, 2004.
DNA, *Data not analyzed;* DNC, *data for specific population are not collected.*
*Goal in developmental stage.

Table **5-3** **Summary *Healthy People 2010:* selected objectives related to oral health**

Number	Oral health objective	Age (yr)	Baseline data (%)	Data 2000 (%)	Healthy People 2010 Goal (%)
01-8	Increase racial and ethnic representation in dental education programs				
01-8m	American Indian or Alaska Native		0.5	0.7*	1.0
01-8n	Asian or Pacific Islander		19.5	20.8*	4.0
01-8o	Black or African American		5.1	5.7*	13.0
01-8p	Hispanic or Latino		4.7	5.7*	12.0
03-6	Decrease oropharyngeal cancer deaths		2.8	2.7	2.7
03-10 (c)	Increase the number of dentists counseling about cancer prevention and tobacco cessation		59	(2001) —	85
05-15	Increase annual dental examination for persons with diabetes	2 years and over	56	60	75
07-11 (t)	Increase the number of local health departments that have established culturally appropriate and linguistically competent community oral health promotion and disease prevention programs		25	—	50

Centers for Disease Control and Prevention, National Center for Health Statistics: Data 2010, Accessed September 1, 2004.
*1999-2000 data.

reveal progress for some oral health indicators. Other oral health indicators showed little or no improvement during the 1990s. Tables 5-2 and 5-3 review the national oral health targets established for 2010.[4,5] Also, Tables 5-2 and 5-3 describe the changes in the oral health indicators being tracked for *Healthy People 2010.*[4,5,15]

This chapter provides a broad overview of the status and trends associated with oral health. **Status** is the current state or condition, while a **trend** is the direction of a condition on a particular course over a period of time. National oral health indicators from the United States are included in international oral health surveillance systems. Selected oral health indicators are tracked by the 39 nations in the Americas and include those reported by the United States. The Pan American Health Organization (PAHO) serves as the World Health Organization Regional Office for the Americas (AMRO) and leads this regional oral health surveillance effort on an international level. In addition, selected U.S. oral health indicators are incorporated into the WHO Country-Area Profile, and these contribute to the Global Oral Health Data Bank that tracks oral health on an international level through the WHO Global Oral Health Program.

This chapter concentrates on the national oral health indicators for the United States and focuses on the indicators included in *Healthy People 2010.* Several surveys and data systems in the United States are used to track national oral health indicators.[15,16] The following national surveys monitor key oral health indicators in the United States:

- **Behavioral Risk Factor Surveillance Survey (BRFSS)**
- **National Health and Nutrition Examination Survey (NHANES)**
- **National Health Interview Survey (NHIS)**
- **Medical Expenditure Panel Survey (MEPS)**

The national oral indicators provide a framework for oral health assessments at the state and local levels. States and localities use several surveys and data collection systems to monitor oral health. State oral health indicators are included in state-based oral health surveillance systems and are integrated into the **National Oral Health Surveillance System.** Future progress in improving oral health will require diligent efforts to assess oral health, mobilize resources, and ensure that necessary oral policies, programs, and services are in place and are received by individuals and communities across the United States.[1,6,17,18]

Dental Caries

Children and Adolescents

Despite a tremendous decline in dental caries in children in the United States since the 1950s, tooth decay remains the single most common chronic disease of childhood.[1] It is five times more common than asthma and seven times more common than hay fever.[1]

Early childhood caries affects the primary teeth of infants and young children 1 to 5 years of age.[4] Sometimes referred to as baby bottle tooth decay or nursing caries, it can be a devastating condition, often requiring thousands of dollars and a hospital visit with general anesthesia during treatment.[19] Substantial pain, psychologic stress, health risks, and expense are associated with restorative care for children affected by early childhood caries.[20] Infant feeding practices, in which children are put to bed with formula or other sweetened drinks and fall asleep while feeding, have been associated with this condition.[20]

The average number of decayed and filled teeth (DFT) among 2- to 4-year-olds has remained unchanged over the past 25 years.[4] According to the NHANES, 23% of young children 2 to 4 years of age experienced dental caries in their primary dentition during the years 1999-2000.[5] Of these children, 20% had untreated caries in their primary teeth. Eighty percent of these children were free of dental caries.

The prevalence of dental caries in the permanent dentition of school-age children has been declining in the United States over the past two decades. This decline is the result of various preventive measures such as community water fluoridation and increased use of fluoride toothpastes and mouth rinses as well as the application of dental sealants.[1] Despite this reduction, one half (50%) of children aged 6 to 8 years experienced dental caries in their primary or permanent teeth in the years 1999-2000.[5] This proportion had decreased only slightly from 52% in the years 1988-1994.[5]

The proportion of untreated dental caries in school-aged children also has been declining overall. Twenty-six percent of 6- to 8-year-olds had untreated dental caries in 1999-2000, down from 28% in 1988-1994.[5] In the years 1988-1994, by the third grade, 60% of students had experienced tooth decay, and 33% of these third-graders had untreated dental caries.[5]

Caries experience is cumulative and thus is higher among adolescents than among young children.[5] By age 15 years, two thirds (59%) of teenagers had experienced dental caries in their permanent dentition, according to a national survey in 1999-2000.[5] Forty-one percent of these teens were caries-free. In comparison, 61% of adolescents during the period 1988-1994 had experienced dental caries.[5] In the years 1999-2000, 16% of teens 15 years of age had untreated tooth decay and were in need of treatment.[5] This proportion has decreased slightly from 20% of teens with untreated dental caries in the period 1988-1994.[5]

As with general health, oral health status in the United States tends to vary based on social and demographic factors. Dental caries, however, remains a significant problem in specific populations, particularly among poor children and adults from certain racial and ethnic groups.[1,5,21] Most tooth decay is experienced by only a few children. National data indicate that for those aged 2 to 5, 75% of dental caries in the primary dentition was found in 8% of the population.[22] Also, for those 6 years and older, 75% of dental caries in the permanent dentition was found in 33% of the population.[22]

Children from minority racial and ethnic groups (e.g., American Indian, Alaska Native, Asian or Pacific Islander, Mexican American, and black or African American) whose parents have less than a high school education or who have a low income are often markedly at increased risk for dental caries.[3-5,16,21] Minority children aged 2 to 4 years in the United States are more likely to experience dental caries than white children.[5] Also, preschool-age African American and Mexican American children have more untreated tooth decay compared with their white peers.[5] America's youngest and poorest young children, aged 2 to 4 years and living below the poverty level, have almost three times as much dental caries as children of higher-income families (>200% poverty).[3,21]

Also, the level of untreated dental caries among African American children aged 6 to 8 years (39%) and Mexican American children (42%) was greater than for white children (21%) in the United States in 1999-2000.[5] A statewide oral health survey in California found 69% of Asian or Pacific Islander children 6 to 8 years of age had dental caries in 1993-1994.[4] In 1999, the oral health survey of Native Americans reported that 71% of American Indian or Alaska Native children 6 to 8 years of age had untreated dental caries.[4] Oral health disparities for dental caries are also found among adolescents in the United States. Oral health disparities for dental caries among children and adolescents are shown in Figures 5-1 to 5-3.

Young and Older Adults

Of all adults 18 years of age and older, 85% have experienced dental caries.[1] In the United States, more than 37% of persons aged 65 years or older with teeth had

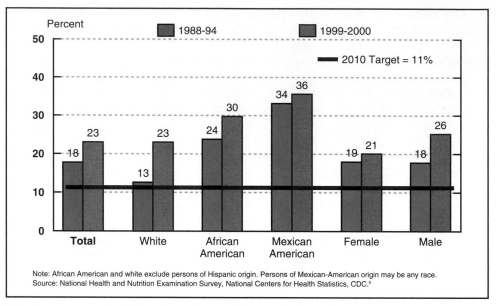

Figure 5-1 Percentage of children 2 to 4 years of age with dental caries experience in primary teeth, 1988-94 and 1999-2000.

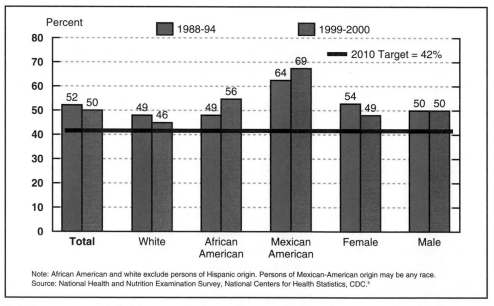

Figure 5-2 Percentage of children 6 to 8 years of age with dental caries experience in primary teeth or permanent teeth, 1988-1994 and 1999-2000.

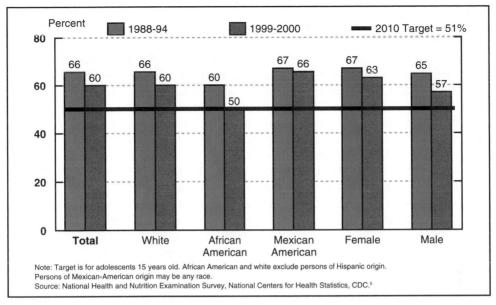

Figure 5-3 Percentage of adolescents 12 to 18 years of age with dental caries experience in permanent teeth, 1988-1994 and 1999-2000.

at least one decayed or filled root surface.[23] Also, 50% of people 75 years and older had root caries affecting at least one tooth.[1] Approximately 26% of adults 35 to 44 years of age had untreated dental caries in 1999-2000.[5] Findings from NHANES III 1988-1994 showed disparities in dental caries among adults, with 44% of African American and 41% of Mexican American adults 35 to 44 years of age with untreated tooth decay compared with 19% of white adults. In an earlier NHANES, 1988-1994, more than three times as many young adults (35 to 44 years of age) with less than a high school education (51%) had untreated dental caries than did adults with some college education (16%).[4] Untreated dental caries can lead to pain, abscesses, extensive dental treatment, extractions of teeth, and costly dental care. As the trends in aging continue, adults will lose fewer teeth as they age but will have more teeth that are at risk for dental caries throughout life.[5]

Preventive Interventions

Dental Sealants

Dental sealants can be very effective in preventing dental caries on the pit and fissure surfaces of teeth, but few children receive them. The percentage of school-age children with dental sealants has risen among specific groups in recent years as the public and private sectors increasingly use the procedure, dental insurance pays for dental sealants, and parents request sealants for their children.[24] Despite the effectiveness of dental sealants, only 28% of children aged 8 and 14% of adolescents aged 14 in the United States received dental sealants in 1999-2000.[5] Disparities in dental sealants have been shown among children based on race and ethnicity. In 1999-2000, 35% of white children 8 years of age had received sealants, and 23% of their African American peers had dental sealants. This same survey found 16% of white adolescents 14 years of age had a dental sealant compared with 14% of their African American counterparts. Also, disparities for dental sealants have been shown for family income and parental education.[4] As few as 3% of poor 8-year-old children had dental sealants, in contrast to 35% of children from families with higher income levels according to NHANES 1988-1994.[4] In 1990, the NHIS found that 23% of adults in the United States reported that dental sealants prevented dental caries.[25] Hispanic adults (12%), African American adults (12%), and adults with less than a high school education were less likely to know the purpose of dental sealants than white adults (25%).[25] Figure 5-4 illustrates disparities for dental sealants among children 6 to 11 years of age and adolescents 12 to 18 years of age.

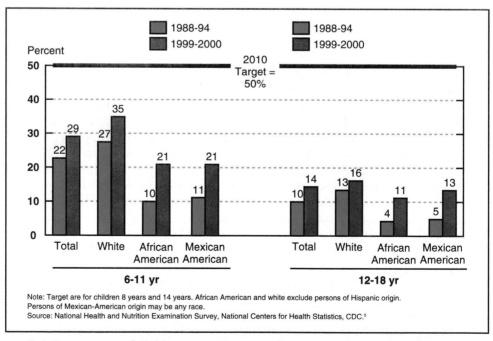

Figure 5-4 Percentage of children 6 to 11 years of age and adolescents 12 to 18 years of age with dental sealants, 1988-1994 and 1999-2000.

Community Water Fluoridation

Community water fluoridation is a cornerstone community preventive service in the United States. During the second half of the twentieth century, a major decline in the prevalence and severity of dental caries resulted from the use of fluorides as an effective method of preventing caries. Fluoridation of the public water supply is the most equitable, cost-effective, and cost-saving method of delivering fluoride to the community.[17] In the United States during 2000, approximately 162 million persons (66% of the population served by public water systems) received optimally fluoridated water compared with 144 million (62%) in 1992.[26] A key oral health objective outlined in *Healthy People 2010* calls for at least 75% of the population served by community water systems to receive optimal levels of fluoride.[4] To reach this goal, approximately 22.5 million more people must gain access to fluoridated water through public water systems.

According to a national survey of adults in 1998, 70% of respondents indicated that water supplies should be fluoridated in communities.[27] In 1990, only 62% of adults had recognized that the primary purpose of water fluoridation is to prevent dental caries. Persons with lower levels of education, Hispanic adults, and African American adults were less likely to know the purpose of water fluoridation.[28] When asked to identify the best method of preventing dental caries, only 7% of adults considered fluoride the correct answer, and 70% indicated toothbrushing and flossing to be the most effective.[25]

Periodontal Diseases

During the period 1988-1994, nearly half (48%) of adults aged 35 to 44 years had gingivitis (inflammation of the gums).[4] This figure represents an increase from the 41% of young adults with gingivitis in 1985-1986.[29] Gingivitis will probably remain a substantial problem and may increase as tooth loss from dental caries declines or may result from the use of some systemic medications.[4]

Destructive periodontal disease (defined as loss of attachment of 4 mm or greater) affected 20% of dentate adults 35 to 44 years of age in 1999-2000.[5] The incidence of this problem declined slightly among young adults from 21% in 1988-1994.[5] Severe periodontal disease (defined as 6 mm of loss of attachment) affected 14% of adults aged 45 to 54 years and 23% of adults aged 65 to 74 years in 1988-1994.[1] Destructive periodontal disease seems to increase with age.[1]

Gingivitis occurs frequently among American Indians, Alaska Natives, Mexican Americans, adults with low incomes, and adults with less than a high school education.[1] Among certain population groups, the prevalence of destructive periodontal disease is higher. In 1999-2000, 24% of African American, 17% of white, and 16% of Mexican American adults (35 to 44 years of age) had destructive periodontal disease. In addition, gender differences were found in the same survey, with 14% of female adults and 26% of male adults (35 to 44 years of age) with destructive periodontal disease. In addition, disparities for destructive periodontal disease have

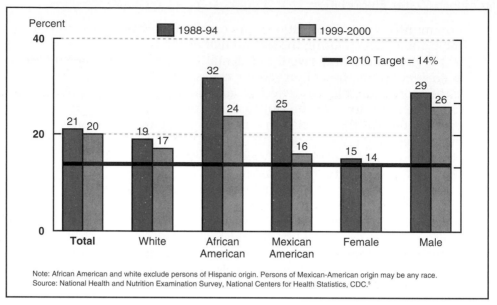

Figure 5-5 Percentage of adults with destructive periodontal disease, 1988-1994 and 1999-2000.

been shown among American Indian/Alaska Native adults, adults with low family incomes, and adults with less than a high school education.[4] At all ages more severe periodontal disease is seen among males and adults at the lowest income levels.[1] Figure 5-5 describes the disparities for destructive periodontal disease.

Tooth Loss

Fewer adults are undergoing tooth extraction because of dental caries or periodontal disease. The percentage of people who have lost all of their natural teeth has been declining over the past 50 years.[1] Of adults 35 to 44 years of age, 39% had never lost a permanent tooth during the period 1999-2000.[5] Differences were found by gender, as males (42%) were more apt to have permanent tooth loss than females (36%). White adults (43%) and Mexican American adults (38%) were less likely to have any loss of permanent teeth compared with African American (30%) adults (35 to 44 years of age) in 1999-2000.

Approximately 25% of the American population aged 65 to 74 years was edentulous (i.e., have lost all of their natural teeth) in 2002. Among persons aged 65 to 74 years in 2002, 43% of persons with less than a high school education were edentulous compared with 14% of persons with at least some college.[5] In this same age group, edentulousness was also higher among older African American (34%) than among Hispanic (20%) and white (23%) older adults.[5] Disparities related to tooth loss are shown in Figure 5-6.

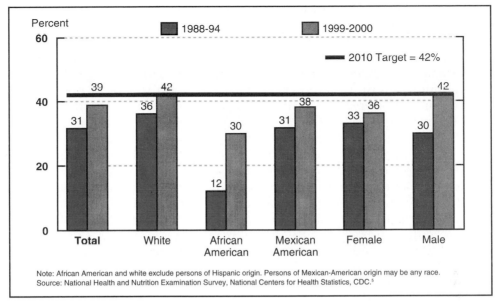

Figure 5-6 Percentage of adults 35 to 44 years of age without permanent tooth loss, 1988-1994 and 1999-2000.

Oral and Pharyngeal Cancer

Oral and pharyngeal cancers include different malignant tumors that affect the oral cavity and pharynx. Most of these tumors are squamous cell carcinomas.[30] These may include cancers of the lip, tongue, floor of the mouth, palate, gingival and alveolar mucosa, buccal mucosa, and oropharynx.[31] The American Cancer Society estimates that in 2004, 28,260 people will be found to have oral and pharyngeal cancers and 7230 persons will die of these cancers in the United States.[32] These cancers occur more frequently than leukemia, Hodgkin's disease, and cancers of the brain, cervix, ovary, liver, pancreas, bone, thyroid gland, testes, and stomach. Oral cancer accounts for 2% to 4% of all cancers diagnosed annually in the United States, but relative survival rates are among the lowest of major cancers.[16]

Oral cancer today occurs more often in males than in females.[16,33] For decades oral cancer has affected six men for every woman, but that ratio has now become two men to each woman. This increase in oral cancer occurrences among women may be due to lifestyle changes, primarily the increased number of women smoking over the last few decades.[31] Age is also a factor, with greater than 90% of oral cancers occurring among persons over the age of 45 and the average age at diagnosis about 60 years.[16]

Disparities related to oral and pharyngeal cancers have been shown in several reports. The occurrence of oral and pharyngeal cancers varies by race and ethnicity.[34]

African Americans and whites have 12.9 and 11.1 new cases of oral and pharyngeal cancers per 100,000 per year, respectively, whereas Asians or Pacific Islanders, American Indian/Alaska Natives, and Hispanics have 8.9, 7.6, and 6.8 new cases per year, respectively, according to Surveillance, Epidemiology, and End Results Program, 1992-2001.[35] In the United States oral and pharyngeal cancers constituted the fourth most common cancer among African American men, the eighth most common cancer among white men, and the fourteenth most common cancer among women in 2002.[36]

In addition, oral and pharyngeal cancer deaths (per 100,000) differ among population groups. Whereas in 2001, oropharyngeal cancer deaths for the overall population were 2.7 per 100,000, they were 4.1 for males and 1.6 for females.[33] Differences among racial and ethnic groups were shown in 2001, with 4.1 pharyngeal cancer deaths per 100,000 for African Americans, 2.6 for Asians/Pacific Islanders, 2.6 for American Indian/Alaska Natives, 2.5 for whites, and 1.6 for Hispanics/Latinos.[33] For adult men 50+ years, the mortality rate increased to 23.3 for African Americans and 13.0 for white males, according to Surveillance, Epidemiology, and End Results Program, 1969-2001.[35]

Only half the number of persons with the diagnosis of oral cancer are alive 5 years after the diagnosis. In contrast to other cancers (e.g., breast, colorectal, and prostate cancers) with longer survival rates, the 5-year survival rates for oral and pharyngeal cancers have remained unchanged since the early 1960s.[35] Survival rates for oral cancer in minorities have decreased. The survival rate is only 52%, and most of these cancers are diagnosed at late stages.[35] For only 35% of all individuals with oral and pharyngeal cancers is the diagnosis made at an early stage. The rate is 40% for females and 33% for males.

Disparities by race and ethnicity have been reported, with only 21% of African Americans and 24% of American Indian/Alaska Natives having their oral cancer detected at the earliest stage compared with 29% of Asians/Pacific Islanders, 35% of Hispanics/Latinos, and 37% of whites.[5] African American men have experienced increases in both death rates and new case rates, and their 5-year survival rate is much poorer than that for whites (36% vs. 60%).[34,35] African American men have the highest incidence of and the lowest survival rates from oral and pharyngeal cancers. At every stage of diagnosis, the survival rate for African Americans is lower than that for whites.[34]

The vast majority of oral cancers are attributed to the use of tobacco (smoked and smokeless tobacco) and alcohol use.[32] Those who chew tobacco are at high risk for oral lesions that can lead to oral cancer. In 2001, 23% of adults smoked cigarettes, 2.3% used smokeless ("spit") tobacco, 2.2% smoked cigars, 0.5 smoked pipes, and 0.09% smoked bidis.[37] Thirty-four percent of high school students reported using tobacco; of these students, 28% smoked cigarettes, 15% smoked cigars, and 8% used spit tobacco in 2001.[37] Alcohol consumption is another risk factor for oral cavity and pharyngeal cancers. Combinations of tobacco and alcohol represent substantially greater risk factors than either substance consumed alone. Other factors that can place a person at risk for these cancers are viral infections, immuno-deficiencies, poor nutrition, exposure to ultraviolet light (a major cause of cancer to the lips), and certain occupational exposures.[32] Consideration needs to be given to income levels, education, availability of proper health care, and use of tobacco and alcohol by different population groups when examining disparities related to oral cancer.

Overall, levels of knowledge about risk factors for oral cancer are low. There is extensive misinformation and a general lack of knowledge among American adults about the signs, symptoms, and risk factors for oral and pharyngeal cancers. According to the NHIS in 1990, this gap in knowledge was present across race, ethnic groups, and frequency of recent visits for dental and medical care. In 1990, only 25% of adults in the United States could identify one sign of oral cancer.[38] Tobacco use was the only risk factor most adults identified correctly. There was a lower level of knowledge of other risk factors across all racial and ethnic groups of American adults. Just one third (36%) of adults knew that excessive exposure to sunlight definitely increased the risk of lip cancer.

Only 13% of adults (40 years of age and older) in the United States reported ever having an oral cancer examination according to the NHIS in 1998.[5] Males (12%) were less likely to receive an annual oral cancer examination compared with females (12%).[5] Respondents more likely to have had an oral cancer examination included those with at least some college education (19%), whereas those with less than a high school education (5%) and high school graduates (10%) were less apt to report an examination for oral cancer.[5] Also, disparities for receipt of an annual oral cancer examination were noted for individuals based on race and ethnicity. Only 6% of Hispanic/Latinos and 7% of African Americans had an oral cancer examination, whereas 12% of Asians/Pacific Islanders and 14% of whites received an oral examination.[5] Figure 5-7 shows a comparison of the disparities related to early detection of oral and pharyngeal cancers based on race and ethnicity.

Other Oral Conditions

Cleft Lip and Cleft Palate

Cleft lip with or without cleft palate is one of the more common birth defects in the United States. The rate of cleft lip and/or cleft palate was 81.24 per 100,000 live births in the United States in 1998.[16] The cleft lip rate was highest for whites (96.1) followed by Hispanics (59.0) and African Americans (46.0).[16] The rate for whites was more than twice that for African Americans. States should have an efficient mechanism in place for identification, recording, referral, and follow-up of infants with oral clefts for treatment. Of 50 states plus the District of Columbia, 23 reported referral and reporting systems for persons with a cleft lip and/or palate.[4] Care by a multidisciplinary team has been shown to be an effective approach in providing services for people with craniofacial anomalies.

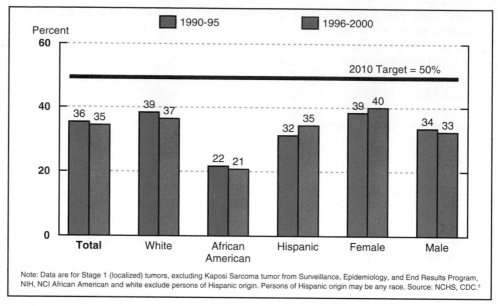

Figure 5-7 Percentage of individuals with early detection of oral and pharyngeal cancers, 1990-1995 and 1996-2000.

Malocclusion

In a national survey, it was found that 9% of persons 8 to 50 years of age had severe crowding of the anterior incisors and 25% had no crowding.[39] Approximately 9% of persons had a posterior crossbite; this condition was most common in whites. Severe overbite was found in 8%, and a similar percentage had a severe overjet. Fewer than 5% of whites had an open bite.

Craniofacial Injuries

Injuries to the head, face, and teeth are common. A national survey found that of all persons 6 to 50 years of age, 25% had sustained an injury that resulted in damage to one or more anterior teeth.[40] In 1991 more than 5.9 million injuries were treated in dental offices.[41] In 1999, 11% of the emergency room visits were due to craniofacial injuries.[16] Different rates of emergency department visits have been reported among demographic groups. Of the emergency department visits in 1999 for craniofacial injuries, 21% were for children less than 15 years of age, 12% for those 15 to 24 years of age, and 10% were for adults 75 years and older.[16] The leading causes of injuries to the head, face, and teeth are falls, assaults, sports-related activities, and bicycle and automobile collisions.[1,16] Community-based interventions, professional practices, and personal behaviors that increase the use of passenger restraints, air bags, helmets, protective gear, and mouth guards can prevent oral injuries in the future.

Dental Fluorosis

In a 1986-1987 national survey of American schoolchildren, dental fluorosis was present in 22% (grades 2 through 12) examined with Dean's Fluorosis Index.[41] The survey included children exposed to all sources of fluoride. The dental fluorosis by classification was:
- Very mild, 17%
- Mild, 4%
- Moderate, 1%
- Severe, 0.3%

Thus 78% of children were found not to have fluorosis.[41] The results of this survey can serve as a baseline for future national assessments of fluorosis in the United States.

ACCESS TO THE ORAL HEALTH CARE SYSTEM

Barriers to Dental Care

Many children and adults in the United States do not receive clinical dental care that is essential for their healthy growth, development, and well-being. Americans of all ages can gain improved oral health with increased access to appropriate, timely, and quality dental care. A host of barriers that prevent timely use of personal oral health services have been identified and include barriers related to patients, professionals, the health care system, and society. Some key barriers include the following[1]:
- Cost
- Lack of perceived need for regular dental care
- Lack of dental insurance
- Lack of dental providers
- Fear of dental visits

Vulnerable population groups, including low-income elderly people, homeless persons, migrant and seasonal farmworkers, disabled and medically compromised individuals, rural residents, and very young children, often lack access to dental care.[42]

Regular Dental Visits and Use of Dental Services

The percentage of people in the United States who have had at least one dental visit annually and the average number of visits vary among population groups. Regular dental attendance changes significantly according to social and demographic factors including age, gender, race and ethnicity, level of education, family income, family structure, place of residence (urban, rural, etc.), geographic location in the United States, health insurance status, disability, dentition status, current health status, and institutionalization.[4]

According to the MEPS in 2000, 43% of the total U.S. population over age 2 years had a dental visit in the past year.[5] Nearly half (48%) of children aged 2 to 17 years and 41% of adults 18 years and older reported an annual dental visit in 2000.[5] This survey found that females (39%) were less likely than males (46%) to have had a dental visit during the past year.[5]

Disparities in regular dental attendance for children and adults over age 2 were reported in the MEPS among racial and ethnic groups, with 46% white, 41% American Indian/Alaska Native, 36% Asian/Pacific Islander, 27% African American, and 27% Hispanic/Latino reporting an annual dental visit in 2000.[5] For persons aged 25 and older, differences were shown based on educational attainment. The percentage of persons with a dental visit in the last year increased with each successive level of education.[5] The MEPS found that adults with at least some college education (57%) and high school graduates (41%) were more likely to have an annual dental visit than adults with less than a high school education (24%) in 2000.[5] A greater percentage of persons (2+ years of age) living at or above the federal poverty level had a dental visit during the past year compared with those living below the federal poverty level according to NHANES 1988-1994.[16] Also, persons with disabilities (30%) were less likely to have regular dental visits than persons without disabilities (43%) in 2000, according to the MEPS.[5]

The percentage of people with an annual dental visit is lowest among children 2 to 4 years of age.[16] Children aged 2 to 4 years are less likely to have had an annual dental visit, whereas a much larger proportion of these children have had well-child visits and have received immunizations, health care, or anticipatory guidance for their parents.[43] NHANES 1988-1994 reported that only 36% of children aged 2 to 4 years had a dental visit in the past year.[16] According to the MEPS, 50% of children entering school (5 to 6 years) and 55% of third-grade children (8 to 9 years) had an annual dental visit in 2000.[5] This same survey reported that in 2000 a third (33%) of children, adolescents, and young adults aged 2 to 19 with a family income less than 200% of poverty level had a dental visit in the past year.[5] Only 31% of low-income youth received a preventive dental service in 2000 despite the promise of comprehensive coverage promised under Medicaid and the potential for coverage through the State Children's Health Insurance Program (SCHIP).[5,44] According to the 1997 survey 11% of children aged 2 to 17 years had a dental visit that was associated with pain in a 1-year period, and 20% of poor children had such a visit.[1] The MEPS found that low-income children experienced the highest disease prevalence, the most extensive disease, the most frequent bouts of dental pain, but the fewest dental visits in 1996.[44]

Older people are less likely to schedule dental visits on a regular basis. Of people 65 years of age and older, 40% reported a dental visit in 2000.[5] Among dentate adults, 44% had a dental visit in the past year; among edentulous adults, the rate

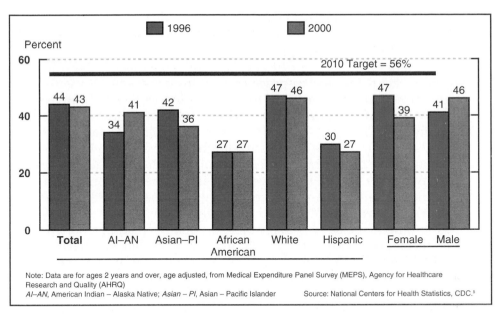

Figure 5-8 Percentage of population 2 years and over with annual dental visit by selected factors, 1996 and 2000.

was 23%.[5] In 1997 only 19% of residents in long-term care facilities received dental care during the last 30 days.[5] A greater percentage of younger residents in long-term care facilities received dental care compared with older residents. In addition, more males from long-term care facilities compared with females and African American compared with white residents received dental care. One in seven adults reported experiencing dental pain over a 6-month period.[1] According to NHANES 1988-1994, a third of poor adults 18 years and older had a dental visit in the past year compared with nearly two thirds of adults with middle-level or high-level incomes.[3] Disparities related to annual dental visits are shown in Figure 5-8.

Unmet Dental Needs

In 1994, 8% of the United States population wanted, but could not obtain, needed dental care.[45] Approximately 16% of individuals from households with low family incomes (e.g., poor and near-poor) reported unmet dental care needs.[45] More than 22% of persons who were uninsured reported unmet dental care needs.[45] Among children whose parents reported an unmet health care need, 73% of them had an unmet dental need, according to analysis of the NHIS, 1993-1996.[46] When communities assess their own health care needs, dental care is frequently cited as a primary unmet need.

Dental Care Coverage

Young and Older Adults

In 1999 more than 95% of dental expenditures were paid by private sources, either out-of-pocket (45.8%) or by private dental insurance (49.6%), with 4.6% by public sources of payment.[5] Spending for dental services in the United States has risen steadily but has remained fairly constant as a proportion of personal health care spending (~4.5%). Only 45% of persons in the United States have some form of private dental insurance (some with limited coverage and high co-payments), 9% have public dental insurance (Medicaid and Children's Health Insurance Program), 2% have other dental insurance, and 45% have no dental insurance.[1] Dental insurance coverage has not increased; approximately 108 million children and adult Americans have no form of dental insurance.[1]

According to the BRFSS, 56% of the U.S. adult population reported they had dental insurance and 44% of adults indicated that they did not have dental insurance in 1997.[16] Among the U.S. population, 86% of adults aged 18 years and older had medical insurance and 14% were without medical insurance in 1997.[16] Females reported less dental insurance (55%) and more medical insurance (97%) compared with males, with 57% with dental insurance and 85% with medical insurance.[16]

The percentage of the adult population with dental insurance was greatest among those 35 to 54 years of age (64%) and 18 to 34 years of age (58%) and least among the oldest age group, 55 years of age and older (42%) in 1997.[16] In comparison, medical insurance was highest among the oldest group (94%) and decreased for the middle-age adult group (86%) and the youngest age group (77%). Medicare does not provide reimbursement for routine dental services. Medicare dental benefits are not authorized, with the limited exception of special dental care associated with systemic diseases and their treatment (e.g., medical necessity related to selected transplants).

African American (61%) and white adults (56%) were most likely to have dental insurance in 1997. Hispanic adults (46%) were least likely to have dental insurance. Nearly ninety (89%) white adults, 82% of African American adults, and 69% of Hispanic adults reported coverage by medical insurance.[16] Coverage for dental and medical insurance increased as education levels increased among adults.[16] This same gradient was found in family income levels; as family income levels rose, so did dental and medical insurance rates among adults, according to the BRFSS in 1997.[16]

The out-of-pocket costs for dental care can be a significant burden on low-income Americans.[47,48] Often, dental care in the private sector is not accessible for many Americans, especially those from vulnerable groups.[47] Dental care coverage for adults is optional in Medicaid, and 2 million adults received dental services through Medicaid in 2000.[49] Eight states provided full coverage for adults, whereas 16 states provided partial coverage with limitations in 2003.[49] In 18 states emergency services were paid through adult Medicaid dental benefits, and nine states provided no dental benefits for adults in the Medicaid program in 2003.[49] Current fiscal demands in states have led some states to reduce or eliminate dental benefits for adults or

Medicaid beneficiaries with disabilities as cost-saving measures. These cuts leave millions of adults unable to access dental care in the face of pain and infection.

Children and Adolescents

Lack of insurance coverage can cause financial barriers that are a significant deterrent to obtaining timely medical and dental care, especially for children in families with low incomes. Overall, 14% of children were uninsured for medical care and 36% were uninsured for dental care according to the NHIS in 1995.[50] Thus 2.6 times as many children were uninsured for dental care than for medical care in 1995. Children from families with low incomes (100% to 199% federal poverty level defined as near-poor) and Hispanic children were most likely to be without medical or dental coverage. The near-poor children were more likely to be uninsured for dental care than for medical care (44% vs. 22%). Many more children are considered underinsured for dental care; they may receive only an oral examination and prophylaxis but not needed treatment of disease.

All states provide dental benefits for children under Medicaid and its Early Periodic Screening, Diagnostic, and Treatment (EPSDT) program according to the Centers for Medicare and Medicaid Services (CMS).[51] Quality dental coverage is essential to ensure access to dental services and improvement of oral health. The 29 million children in Medicaid and SCHIP are 1.5 times more likely to access dental care than uninsured children.[52] Children covered by Medicaid are 3.5 times less likely to have an unmet dental need than uninsured children.[53] In 1998, 20.2 million children were enrolled in Medicaid, and 19 million were considered beneficiaries because they had received at least a single health service.[54] In 2004, 26.6 million children were beneficiaries of the Medicaid EPSDT program, which mandates comprehensive dental care.

Nearly 4 million children received dental services through Medicaid in 2000.[49] Only 19% of children covered by Medicaid EPSDT received a preventive dental visit in fiscal year 1998.[48] Medicaid reports that 80% of children receive regular pediatric care, whereas fewer than 20% receive any preventive dental services.[55] Of children enrolled in Medicaid, 30% had a dental visit for any reason in fiscal year 1999.[48] Yet dental spending in Medicaid comprised only 1% of Medicaid expenditures in 2000.[49]

SCHIP provides important opportunities for improving access to dental care for children from low-income and modest-income families. Dental caries is increasingly a disease of such children—children covered by SCHIP. In many instances dental caries remains untreated.[21] Although dental benefits in SCHIP are optional, 54 of 56 states and territories include dental services in the approved benefit package for SCHIP.[49] Two states—Delaware and Texas—did not include dental benefits in SCHIP in 2003.[49] Unlike Medicaid's EPSDT benefit, which provides for comprehensive dental services, many SCHIP plans provide more limited benefits.[49] Because dental benefits in SCHIP are optional, state governments have the prerogative to include benefits in SCHIP programs.

Studies have shown that cost of dental care in Medicaid is disproportionate for a few, and most often young, preschool-aged children. These studies have found that a small percentage (~2% to 5%) of low-income children with devastating early childhood caries consume an overwhelmingly disproportionate share (25% to 45%) of Medicaid spending for dental care.[55-57] The cost to Medicaid for dental treatment of a very young child under general anesthesia for restorative dental care in the hospital was reported as $1500 to $2000 per episode.[56,57] Treatment of early childhood dental caries, a preventable disease, is expensive when the disease is not prevented, detected, or controlled early. Medicaid spends at least $100 million per year for operating room charges associated with early childhood caries in very young children.[54]

Early primary prevention and greater continuity of dental care for young children at highest risk for dental caries have been emphasized in recent reports.[56,57] This early intervention (EI) for early childhood caries holds promise for improving health and lowering public expenditures. It has been recognized that long-standing, complex barriers limit the potential of Medicaid to provide needed oral health services to children.[43] It is crucial that oral health programs within Medicaid and SCHIP be upgraded and improved based on identified best practices to ensure oral health outcomes.

Organizations and agencies at the national and state levels have begun to discuss and implement innovative ways to address dental care access problems for children.[58,59] Recently a compendium and a series of policy briefs were published by the American Dental Association (ADA) describing effective innovations that can be implemented to improve the Medicaid program and increase access for enrolled children.[60,61] It is essential that these discussions focusing on children be expanded to ensure access to dental services not only for children and adolescents but also for adults and seniors in communities across the United States.

ORAL HEALTH CARE SYSTEM

Changing demographics within the United States will have a long-term impact on the oral health care system in the future. These changes will affect patients and providers of oral health care services. A projected decline in the dentist workforce and the population's growing demand for dental services are likely to accelerate access problems for historically underserved segments of the U.S. population.[62]

Supply and Distribution of Dental Professionals

The oral health care system depends on the size, composition, characteristics, and distribution of the oral workforce.[63,64] Factors such as scope of practice, productivity, practice settings, and participation of providers have an impact on the capacity of the workforce to serve general and vulnerable populations.[62] Concerns have been raised about the adequacy of the number of dentists available to provide needed oral health services in the United States. Several factors have been implicated including the marked decline in the number of practicing dentists over the past two decades, the reduction of students graduating from dental schools, the number of dentists retiring, and the increase in the population of the United States. These factors are likely to influence the dynamics of the oral health care system in the next 20 years and could adversely affect access to oral health services for vulnerable population groups.

The ADA reported 141,396 U.S. dentists were in private practice in part-time or full-time positions in 1995.[65] A report indicates that the number of practicing dentists rose by 22% from 1982 to 1995; however, most of the increase was due to doubling of part-time dentists, with only an 8% increase in full-time dentists.[66] In comparison, the population in the United States increased by 13% during the same time period, with a 10% increase among children.[67] Since 1986, seven dental schools closed, three dental schools opened, and class sizes were reduced in the remaining dental schools.[62] The percentage of graduating dentists declined by 40% between 1986 and 2000.[64]

Even when the numbers of dentists may be adequate, the distribution of dentists remains a challenge. Of the nation's dentists, 90% provide dental care in the private sector of the oral health care system.[66] Most of these practitioners are in privately owned solo or two-person practices.[64,66] The employment status for dentists shows that 79% are sole proprietors, 13% are partners, 6% are nonowner dentists, and 2% are independent contractors.[62,64] Eighty percent of dentists are general dentists, and 20% are specialists.[68] This ratio of general dentists to specialists has remained stable, although owing to changes in public policies, it is projected that this ratio may decrease to 3 to 1.

The ratio of dentists to population increased in the 1980s and decreased in the 1990s as a result of the changing number of dentists entering and leaving the workforce.[69,70] In 1980 there were an estimated 53.6 dentists per 100,000 persons.[1] This ratio increased to 59.1 per 100,000 people in 1990 and decreased to 58.3 in 2000. By the year 2010 the ratio of dentists to population is expected to decrease to 57.2 and to decline even further, to 53.7 in 2020.[1] In contrast, the ratio of physicians to population has been increasing steadily since 1990.[1,16] Availability of dentists differs markedly among states—the dentist-to-population ratio ranges from 31.3 per 100,000 to 69 per 100,000, with the District of Columbia at 94.9 per 100,000.[16] The four states with the highest dentist to population ratio were New York, New Jersey, Connecticut, and Hawaii. The four states with the lowest dentist to population ratio were Mississippi, New Mexico, Nevada, and North Carolina.[16]

Dentists in the United States are distributed unevenly and are underrepresented in areas of high need. Privately owned dental practices tend to be disproportionately concentrated in suburban areas with high income and education levels, with dentists less available in inner cities or rural areas.[1] The distribution of dentists varies across regions in the United States and within each state.

A **Dental Health Professional Shortage Area (Dental HPSA)** is one of the three types of health professional shortage areas defined by the federal government.

Factors for identifying health professional shortage areas include primary care provider-to-population ratios, access to primary health care according to distance and time, incomes at poverty levels, and infant mortality and low birth-weight incidences. In addition to communities, special populations and institutions may be designated as shortage areas. Dental HPSAs have limited access to primary oral health care services because of financial, geographic, cultural, and language barriers. The federal government designates areas as having practitioner shortages if a minimum number of specified criteria are met. Dental HPSA is used to evaluate the eligibility of a given area or population for a number of federal and state programs to expand the oral health workforce.[71] These programs include the National Health Service Corps (NHSC), Federal and State Loan Repayment Programs, Community Health Center Programs, and several Title VII Health Professions Programs. The Health Resources and Services Administration (HRSA) reported that there were 1036 Dental HPSAs in 1998, which required 3984 dentists.[1] A total of 2477 Dental HPSAs were designated nationwide by the Shortage Designation Branch, National Center for Health Workforce Analysis, Bureau of Health Professions, HRSA in 2003.

Safety net facilities located in dental schools, community-based health centers, migrant and rural health clinics, school-based programs, and mobile van programs that target the underserved populations in primarily inner-city and rural areas are few in number.[63] HRSA reports only 61% of the federally supported community-based health centers include on-site dental services.[5] The "safety net" dental delivery system is under pressure and in short supply.[42] The nation's federally funded health centers are meeting a small part of the great need for dental care.[72] The distribution of the dental workforce is placing stress on the public, nonprofit, and private sectors that provide services in the oral health care system and is causing reductions in access to oral health services.[72-77]

Geographic maldistribution of dentists contributes to poor access to dental care in many communities, especially rural and urban centers and low-income and minority communities. African American dentists report that nearly 62% of their patients are African Americans, and approximately 45% of the patients of Hispanic dentists are Hispanic.[75] Minority dentists are more likely to provide care to minority populations, but minority dentists are a small portion of the dental workforce. The number of minorities in the dental professions is inadequate and underrepresented compared with the overall population.[78] In 1999, 89% of dentists were white, 5% were Asian/Pacific Islander, 2% were African American, 4% were Hispanic/Latino, and 0.1% were Native American/Alaska Native compared with the overall population of 72% white, 12% African American, 11% Hispanic/Latino, 4% Asian/Pacific Islander, and 0.9% Native American/Alaska Native. Representation by underrepresented minorities was low among undergraduate dental students enrolled in dental schools during 2003; the American Dental Education Association reported that 5.4% of dental students were African American, 5.9% were Hispanic/Latino, and 0.4% were Native American/Alaska Native in 2003.[79] This imbalance will become more exacerbated with the significant changes in racial and ethnic composition of the United States over the next 50 years. The greatest gains in dental school enrollment have been in increased representation of females. Female enrollees in dental schools in the United States increased from 5% in 1970 to 38% in 1999.[69]

There are approximately 100,000 dental hygienists, 200,000 dental assistants, and 70,000 dental laboratory technicians in the United States.[80] Two thirds of all dentists employ at least one dental hygienist, and most dentists work with dental assistants. In the United States there are 266 dental hygiene programs, 259 dental assisting programs, and 25 dental laboratory technology programs.[79] First-year enrollment has increased 9.5% in dental hygiene programs, decreased 7% in dental assisting programs, and declined 31% in dental laboratory technology programs from 1994-1995 to 1998-1999.[80] The current dental workforce is thought to have a reserve capacity largely through allied dental personnel. Table 5-4 summarizes the status of dental education programs and students in the dental professions as of 2003.

Innovative strategies are needed to recruit and retain dental professionals from specific racial and ethnic groups who will seek careers in oral health and public health, today and in the future.[62,74] Strategies must be implemented to ensure that the dental workforce is culturally competent to provide oral health services to increasingly diverse individuals and communities. As demands for oral health services increase both nationally and through programs for specific, vulnerable populations, groups, or communities, collaboration among state and local oral health programs and key stakeholders is essential to enhance development of the dental workforce.[62,74] Partnerships are necessary among state dental and dental hygienists' associations, dental and dental hygiene schools, state dental licensing boards, state primary care associations, community health centers, hospitals, and safety net oral health programs to increase the dental workforce, expand access to oral health services, and improve oral health outcomes.[62,74] With the current oral health disparities and expected population growth, creative measures are crucial to improve oral health, including developments in education, research, and health promotion and expansions of clinical care within the private, public, and nonprofit sectors.[62,74,81]

Public Health Infrastructure and Capacity

The proportion of dental care paid for with government revenues is small and declining. According to the Centers for Medicare and Medicaid Services, 6% of the

Table 5-4   Dental education programs and students in the dental professions, 2004.

	Schools and programs	Number of students and residents
Dental	56*	17,800*
Dental residents	726*	5257*
Dental hygiene	265†	13,458†
Dental assisting	259†	7304†
Dental laboratory	24†	517†

*Dental Education At-a-Glance, Washington, DC, 2004, American Dental Education Association.
†Allied Dental Education At-a-Glance, Washington, DC, 2004, American Dental Education Association.

estimated $65.6 billion spent on dental care was paid by public dollars in 2001.[16,82] That proportion has been declining since the 1960s. Sources of funding for state oral health programs are varied and include state and federal revenue streams. State oral health programs are supported by federal funding from two main sources[83]:

- Maternal and Child Health Block Grant, Maternal and Child Health Bureau (MCHB) of the HRSA
- Preventive Health Services Block Grant of the CDC

MCHB uses the construct of a pyramid to describe the four levels of core public health services for the population served by Maternal and Child Health (MCH) programs.[84] Figure 5-9 illustrates the MCH pyramid of public health services. Starting at the base, these are (1) infrastructure building services, (2) population-based services, (3) enabling services, and (4) direct health care (gap-filling) services. Infrastructure-building and population-based services provide the broad foundation upon which enabling and direct care services rest. The MCH health services pyramid provides a useful framework for understanding programmatic directions

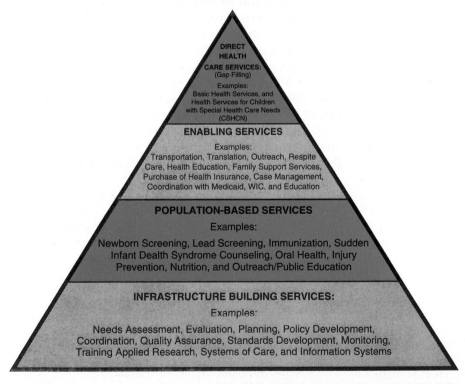

DIRECT HEALTH CARE SERVICES: (Gap Filling)
Examples:
Basic Health Services, and Health Services for Children with Special Health Care Needs (CSHCN)

ENABLING SERVICES
Examples:
Transportation, Translation, Outreach, Respite Care, Health Education, Family Support Services, Purchase of Health Insurance, Case Management, Coordination with Medicaid, WIC, and Education

POPULATION-BASED SERVICES
Examples:
Newborn Screening, Lead Screening, Immunization, Sudden Infant Death Syndrome Counseling, Oral Health, Injury Prevention, Nutrition, and Outreach/Public Education

INFRASTRUCTURE BUILDING SERVICES:
Examples:
Needs Assessment, Evaluation, Planning, Policy Development, Coordination, Quality Assurance, Standards Development, Monitoring, Training Applied Research, Systems of Care, and Information Systems

Source: Maternal and Child Health Bureau. Strategic Plan: Fiscal Year 2003-2007. Rockville, MD: Maternal and Child Health Bureau, 2003.

Figure 5-9 Key public health services delivered by Maternal and Child Health (MCH) Agencies.

Box 5-1   DENTAL PUBLIC HEALTH INFRASTRUCTURE AND CAPACITY IN THE UNITED STATES

- 34 full-time state dental directors and a total of 418 full-time equivalent positions in states
- 473 local health departments with dental programs
- 855 community-based low-income dental clinics
- 290 school-based or school-linked dental programs

Adapted from Association of State and Territorial Dental Directors: Building Infrastructure and Capacity in State and Territorial Oral Health Programs, 2000.

and resource allocation by the Bureau and its partners as they work collaboratively to carry out the mission and accomplish the goals of MCHB.

Federal, state, and local governments support a wide array of oral health programs that may include direct care services.[1,85] Box 5-1 describes the personnel related to the dental public health infrastructure and capacity in the United States for 2000.[84] The downturn in the economy has contributed to major budget constraints for federal, state, and local government agencies in recent years. This comes at a time when the incomes of many families are stressed and an increase has occurred in the oral health needs of many children and adults as well as those in vulnerable population groups. The infrastructure and capacity of many dental public health programs at the national, state, and local levels are limited and stretched compared with the oral health needs in states and communities.[84]

Recently published reports reviewed the challenges faced in ensuring a viable dental public health infrastructure as well as state- and community-based programs to ensure access to dental care for the underserved population in the United States.[86,87] One study examined a number of components, including stresses on state health departments, community and migrant health centers, and U.S. Public Health Services Commissioned Corps.[86] The American Dental Association Report emphasized the need for adequate reimbursement levels, less complex administrative requirements, effective provider and patient outreach, and care coordination. The ADA report outlined model public health interventions and safety net delivery systems to improve access to dental care for vulnerable population groups.[87] The report by Tomar reviewed education by assessing the needs of schools of dentistry, programs in dental hygiene, schools of public health, advanced training in dental public health residencies, and preventive research centers.[85] The report noted inadequacies of the workforce that contributed to problems with dental public health capacity. This included lack of board-certified public health dentists and lack of diversity among the dental workforce and students.[85] Also, regulatory issues related to state boards of dental examiners and state practice acts regarding dental hygiene practice were evaluated in the reports.[85]

FUTURE DIRECTIONS

Healthy People 2000 outlined oral health benchmarks for the United States, and some oral health indicators showed promise of improvements in the 1990s. The National Oral Health Objectives in *Healthy People 2010* provide the road map for the next decade. Political will is critical at the national, state, and local levels for improved oral health outcomes to come to fruition in 2010. Resources are crucial for the development and maintenance of effective dental public health programs to effectively promote oral health and prevent oral diseases. Oral health programs at the national, state, and local levels need the following key elements to be better prepared to achieve the *Healthy People 2010* objectives:

- A workforce appropriately trained and competent in dental public health representing the diversity of the United States
- Adequate workforce and sufficient administrative presence with skilled staff and leadership from full-time oral health program directors
- Collaborative oral health planning that integrates evidence-based public health principles and practices
- Support of informed policy makers to develop and promote oral health policies
- Strong public-private partnerships
- Ability to obtain and leverage adequate financial resources
- Legal authority to use personnel in an effective and cost-efficient manner
- Infrastructure and capacity to plan, implement, and evaluate oral health policies, practices, and programs that are sustainable for the foreseeable future
- Population-based interventions to prevent oral diseases in communities
- Health systems interventions to ensure access to oral health care for children and adults

Oral Health in America: A Report of the Surgeon General described the oral health successes of the twentieth century and also discussed the oral health challenges confronting the nation. *A National Call to Action to Promote Oral Health* proposed opportunities to reduce oral health disparities in the twenty-first century. These reports provide the framework that, when combined with political will, can produce oral health improvements for everyone in the United States.

SUMMARY

This chapter has presented the oral health indicators used for tracking and monitoring national oral health objectives. These benchmarks provide an important framework for the assessment of oral health in the United States in the past and in the coming decade. The chapter has described current status and past trends of oral health and access to oral health care services used as key indicators in the United States. Finally, important oral health disparities among population groups based on race and ethnicity, family income, education level, gender, geographic location, and disability have been highlighted in the chapter.

Applying **Your Knowledge**

1. Select an oral health indicator such as dental caries or periodontal disease. For each oral health indicator discuss current status, past trends, and disparities among population groups. Use information presented in the chapter, websites listed in the appendixes, library resources, and the internet for updated information now available to describe the oral health status of the selected indicator.

2. Describe how you would use the information found on the selected oral health indicator to plan, implement, and evaluate public health programs in your role as:
   a. State Dental Director
   b. County Oral Health Director
   c. Dental Director in a Community Health Center

DENTAL HYGIENE COMPETENCIES

Reading the material in this chapter and participating in the activities of Applying Your Knowledge will contribute to the student's ability to demonstrate the following competencies:

Health promotion and disease prevention

HP.4 Identify individual and population risk factors and develop strategies that promote health-related quality of life.

Community involvement

CM.1 Assess the oral health needs of the community and the quality and availability of resources and services.

Patient/client care

PC.1 Systematically collect, analyze, and record data on the general, oral, and psycho-social health status of a variety of patients or clients using methods consistent with medicolegal principles.

PC.2 Use critical decision making skills to reach conclusions about the patient's or client's dental hygiene needs based on all available assessment data.

PC.5A Determine the outcomes of dental hygiene interventions using indexes, instruments, examination techniques, and the patient's or client's self-report.

Community Case

As the State Dental Director, you are working with a state oral health coalition to plan a statewide oral health survey. You decide to review the current status of key oral health indicators from information you have for the nation and various states. This information is presented in Table A and the graph in Figure B.

1. Based on the information in Table A, which state has the highest rate of untreated tooth decay?
   a. New Mexico
   b. Wisconsin
   c. Delaware
   d. Arkansas
   e. Utah
2. Based on the information in Table A, which state has the lowest rate of untreated tooth decay?
   a. Maine
   b. New Hampshire
   c. Missouri
   d. Washington
   e. Vermont
3. Based on the information in Table A, which state does not meet the national oral health objective of 33% of third-grade children with untreated tooth decay by 2010?
   a. Delaware
   b. Arkansas
   c. Missouri
   d. Washington
   e. New Hampshire
4. Based on the information in the bar graph in Figure B:
   White children 6 to 11 years of age in 1988-1994 had more than two times the rate of dental sealants than their Mexican American counterparts.
   African American children 6 to 11 years of age in 1988-1994 had the highest rate of dental sealants.
   a. The first statement is true and the second statement is false
   b. The first statement is false and the second statement is true
   c. Both statements are true
   d. Both statements are false
5. Based on the information in the bar graph in Figure B, which group of 6- to 11-year-old children had the greatest need for dental sealants in 1999-2000?
   a. White children
   b. Mexican American children
   c. African American children
   d. All of the groups had the greatest need for dental sealants
   e. Mexican American and African American children have the same need

Table A   **Percentage of third-grade students with untreated tooth decay**

State	School Year	Percent (%) with Untreated Tooth Decay
Arkansas	2001–2002	42.1
Delaware	2001–2002	30.9
Maine	1998–1999	20.4
Missouri	1999–2000	23.0
New Hampshire	2000–2001	21.7
New Mexico	1999–2000	37.0
Utah	2000–2001	23.0
Vermont	2002–2003	16.1
Washington	1999–2000	20.5
Wisconsin	2001–2002	30.8

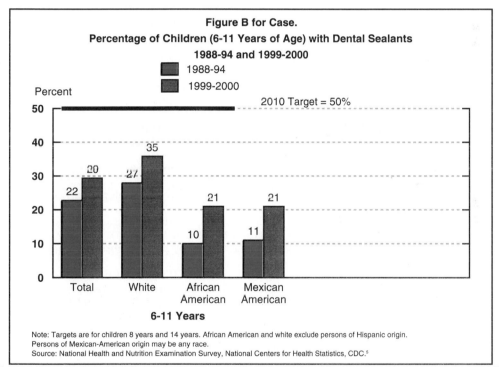

Figure B for Case.
Percentage of Children (6-11 Years of Age) with Dental Sealants
1988-94 and 1999-2000

- 1988-94
- 1999-2000

Percent

2010 Target = 50%

Total: 22, 20
White: 27, 35
African American: 10, 21
Mexican American: 11, 21

6-11 Years

Note: Targets are for children 8 years and 14 years. African American and white exclude persons of Hispanic origin. Persons of Mexican-American origin may be any race.
Source: National Health and Nutrition Examination Survey, National Centers for Health Statistics, CDC.[5]

Figure B Percentage of children 6 to 11 years of age with dental sealants, 1988-1994 and 1999-2000.

References

1. U.S. Department of Health and Human Services: Oral Health in America: A Report of the Surgeon General. Rockville, Md, U.S. Department of Health and Human Services, National Institute of Dental and Craniofacial Research, National Institutes of Health, 2000.
2. U.S. Department of Health and Human Services: Healthy People 2000: National Health Promotion and Disease Prevention Objectives. Washington, DC, U.S. Department of Health and Human Services, 1990.
3. National Centers for Health Statistics, Centers for Disease Control and Prevention: Healthy People 2000 Progress Review: Briefing Book Materials–Objective Charts and Disparity Charts for Focus Area 13—Oral Health, December 15, 1999.
4. U.S. Department of Health and Human Services: Healthy People 2010: Understanding and Improving Health, 2nd ed. Washington, DC, U.S. Department of Health and Human Services, 2000.
5. National Centers for Health Statistics, Centers for Disease Control and Prevention: Healthy People 2010 Progress Review: Briefing Book Materials–Data Summary Table for Focus Area 21—Oral Health, March 17, 2004.
6. U.S. Department of Health and Human Services: A National Call to Action to Promote Oral Health. Rockville, Md, U.S. Department of Health and Human Services, Public Health Service, Centers for Disease Control and Prevention, National Institutes of Health, National Institute of Dental and Craniofacial Research, May 2003.
7. Cohen LK, Gift HC (eds): Disease Prevention and Oral Health Promotion: Socio-dental Sciences in Action. Copenhagen, Munksgaard, 1995.
8. Task Force on Community Preventive Services: Promoting Oral Health: Interventions to Prevent Dental Caries, Oral and Pharyngeal Cancers, and Sports-Related Craniofacial Injuries: A Report on the Recommendations of the Task Force on Community Preventive Services. Morb Mortal Wkly Rep 50(RR-21):1-13, 2001.
9. Task Force on Community Preventive Services: Strategies for Reducing Exposure to Environmental Tobacco Smoke, Increasing Tobacco-Use Cessation, and Reducing Initiation in Communities and Health-Care Systems: A Report on Recommendations of the Task Force on Community Preventive Services. Morb Mortal Wkly Rep 49(RR12):1-11, 2000
10. Centers for Disease Control and Prevention: Recommendation for Using Fluoride to Prevent and Control Dental Caries in the United States. Morb Mortal Wkly Rep 50(RR-14):1-42, 2001.
11. U.S. Preventive Services Task Force: Guide to Clinical Preventive Services, 2nd ed. Baltimore, Md, 1996.
12. Gift HC, Reisine ST, Larch DC: The social impact of dental problems and visits. Am J Public Health 82:1663, 1993.
13. Acs G, Lodolinni G, Kaminski S, et al: Effect of nursing caries on body weight in a pediatric population. J Pediatr Dent 14:302, 1992.
14. Chen M, Andersen RM, Barmes DE, et al: Comparing Oral Health Care Systems: A Second International Collaborative Study. Geneva, World Health Organization, 1997.
15. Centers for Disease Control and Prevention, National Center for Health Statistics: Data 2010: Oral Health Focus Area Summary, August 28, 2004.
16. Dental, Oral and Craniofacial Data Resource Center: Oral Health U.S., 2002: Bethesda, Md, 2002.
17. Truman BI, Gooch BF, Evans CA Jr. (eds): The Guide to Community Preventive Services: Interventions to Prevent Dental Caries, Oral and Pharyngeal Cancers, and Sports-Related Craniofacial Injuries. Am J Prev Med 23(1 Supp), 2002.
18. Task Force on Community Preventive Services: The Guide to Community Preventive Services: Tobacco Use Prevention and Control. Am J Prev Med 20(2 Supp):1, 2001.
19. Bertness J, Holt K: Promoting Awareness, Preventing Pain: Facts on Early Childhood Caries (ECC), 2nd ed. Washington, DC: National Maternal and Child Oral Health Resource Center, 2004.
20. Reisine S, Douglas JM: Psychological and behavioral issues in early childhood caries. Community Dent Oral Epidemiol 26:32, 1998.
21. Vargas CM, Crall JJ, Schneider DA: Sociodemographic distribution of pediatric dental caries: NHANES III, 1988-1994. J Am Dent Assoc 129:1229, 1998.
22. Macek MD, Heller KE, Selwitz RH, Manz MC: Is 75 percent of dental caries really found in 25% of the population. J Public Health Dent 64:20, 2004.

23. Winn DM, Brunelle JA, Selwitz RJ, et al: Coronal and root caries in the dentition of adults in the United States, 1988-1999 (special issue). J Dent Res 75:642, 1996.
24. Centers for Disease Control and Prevention, National Center for Health Statistics: Healthy People 2000 Review, 1998-1999. Hyattsville, Md, Public Health Service, 1999.
25. Gift HC, Corbin SB, Nowjack-Raymer RE: Public knowledge of prevention of dental disease. Public Health Rep 109:397, 1994.
26. Centers for Disease Control and Prevention: Populations Receiving Optimally Fluoridated Public Drinking Water—United States, 2000. Morb Mortal Wkly Rep 51(7):144-147, 2002.
27. American Dental Association. 1998 Consumers' Opinions Regarding Community Water Fluoridation. Chicago, American Dental Association, 1998.
28. Centers for Disease Control and Prevention: Knowledge of the purpose of community water fluoridation: United States, 1990. Morb Mortal Wkly Rep 41:919, 1992.
29. Centers for Disease Control and Prevention, National Center for Health Statistics: Healthy People 2000 Review, 1999-2000. Hyattsville, Md, Public Health Service, 1999.
30. Centers for Disease Control and Prevention: Preventing and controlling oral and pharyngeal cancer: Recommendations from a national strategic planning conference. Morb Mortal Wkly Rep 47(RR14):1, 1998.
31. American Cancer Society: Detailed guide: oral cavity and oropharyngeal cancer—what are the key statistics about oral cavity and oropharyngeal cancer? Atlanta, American Cancer Society, 2004.
32. American Cancer Society: Cancer facts and figures. Atlanta, American Cancer Society, 2004.
33. National Centers for Health Statistics, Centers for Disease Control and Prevention: Healthy People 2010 Progress Review: Briefing Book Materials–Data Summary Table for Focus Area 3—Cancer, October 16, 2002.
34. Silverman S. Oral Cancer, 5th ed. Atlanta, American Cancer Society, 2003.
35. Surveillance, Epidemiology, and End Results (SEER) Program: SEER Stat Databases. Bethesda, Md, National Cancer Institute, DCCPS, Surveillance Research Program, Cancer Statistics Branch, April 2004.
36. U.S. Cancer Statistics Working Group: United States Cancer Statistics: 2000 Incidence. Atlanta, Department of Health and Human Services, Centers for Disease Control and Prevention and National Cancer Institute, 2003.
37. National Centers for Health Statistics, Centers for Disease Control and Prevention: Healthy People 2010 Progress Review: Briefing Book Materials–Data Summary Table for Focus Area 27—Tobacco, May 14, 2003.
38. Horowitz AM, Nourjah PA, Gift HC: U.S. adult knowledge of risk factors and signs of oral cancers: 1990. J Am Dent Assoc 126:39, 1995.
39. Brunelle JA, Bhat M, Lipton JA: Prevalence and distribution of selected occlusal characteristics in the U.S. population, 1988-1991 (special issue). J Dent Res 75:706, 1996.
40. Kaste LM, Gift HC, Bhat M, Swango PA: Prevalence of incisor trauma in persons 6 to 50 years of age: United States, 1988-1991 (special issue). J Dent Res 75:696, 1996.
41. U.S. Department of Health and Human Services, Public Health Service (USDHHS, PHS): Review of Fluoride: Benefits and Risks. Report of the Ad Hoc Subcommittee on Fluoride. Washington, DC, USDHHS, PHS, February 1991.
42. U.S. General Accounting Office: Oral Health: Factors Contributing to Low Use of Dental Services by Low-Income Populations. Washington, DC, U.S. General Accounting Office, September 2000.
43. Children's Dental Services under Medicaid: Access and Utilization (No. OE1-09-93-00240). San Francisco, U.S. Department of Health and Human Services, Office of the Inspector General, 1996.
44. Edelstein BL, Manski RJ: Pediatric dental visits during 1996: An analysis of the federal Medical Expenditure Panel Survey. Pediatr Dent 22:17, 2000.
45. Mueller CD, Shur CL, Paramore LC: Access to dental care in the United States. J Dent Educ 129:429, 1998.
46. Newacheck PW, Hughes DC, Hung Y-Y, et al: The unmet health needs of America's children. Pediatrics 105(Suppl):989, 2000.
47. Kenney GM, Ko G, Ormond BA: Gaps in Prevention and Treatment: Dental Care for Low-income Children. Washington, DC, The Urban Institute, New Federalism, National Survey of America's Families Series B (No. B-15), April 2000.
48. U.S. General Accounting Office: Dental Disease Is a Chronic Problem Among Low-Income Populations. Washington, DC, U.S. General Accounting Office, April 2000.

49. Children's Dental Health Project: Preserving the Financial Safety Net by Protecting Medicaid and SCHIP Dental Benefits. Washington, DC, Children's Dental Health Project, September 2003.

50. Vargas CM, Isman RE, Crall JJ: Comparison of children's medical and dental insurance coverage by sociodemographic characteristics, United States, 1995. J Public Health Dent 262:38, 2002.

51. Center for Policy Alternatives: Dental Coverage under Medicaid. Washington, DC, Center for Policy Alternatives, September 1999.

52. Kenney GM, Haly JM, Tebay A, et al: Children's Insurance Coverage and Service Use Improve. Washington, DC, The Urban Institute, New Federalism, National Survey of America's Families, Snapshots of America's Families III, No. 1, 2003.

53. Newacheck PW, Peraly M, Hughes DC. The roles of Medicaid in ensuring children's access to care. JAMA 280:1789, 1998.

54. Office of the Inspector General, U.S. Department of Health and Human Services: Children's Dental Services under Medicaid: Access and Utilization (No. OE1-09-93-00240). San Francisco, U.S. Department of Health and Human Services, Office of the Inspector General, 1996.

55. Health Care Financing Administration, U.S. Department of Health and Human Services: Innovative Management of Dental Decay for Young Children Enrolled in Medicaid and Children's Health Insurance Program (CHIP), Grant Demonstration Program Announcement. Baltimore, Md, Health Care Financing Administration, U.S. Department of Health and Human Services, May 2000.

56. Kanellis MJ, Damiano PC, Momany ET: Medicaid costs associated with hospitalization of young children for restorative dental treatment under general anesthesia. J Public Health Dent 60:28, 2000.

57. Griffin SO, Gooch BF, Beltran E, et al: Dental services, costs, and factors associated with hospitalization for Medicaid-eligible children. J Public Health Dent 60:21, 2000.

58. American Dental Association: Proceedings: Report of Achieving Improvement in Medicaid (AIM) for Change Medicaid Conference, Chicago, American Dental Association, August 2-3, 1999.

59. Spisak S, Holt K (eds): Building Partnerships to Improve Children's Access to Medicaid Oral Health Services: National Conference Proceedings. Arlington, Va, National Maternal and Child Oral Health Resource Center, 1999.

60. American Dental Association: State Innovations to Improve Dental Access for Low-Income Children: A Compendium. Chicago, American Dental Association, 2003.

61. American Dental Association: Policy Brief Series: Increasing Access to Medicaid Dental Services for Children Through Collaborative Partnerships. Chicago, American Dental Association, 2004.

62. Association of State and Territorial Dental Directors: Best Practices Approaches for State and Community Oral Health Programs: Access to Oral Health Care—Workforce Development. Jefferson City, Mo, Association of State and Territorial Dental Directors, 2003.

63. Crall JJ: Children's oral health services: Organization and financing considerations. Ambul Pediatr 2:148, 2002.

64. Valachovic RW: Dental workforce trends and children. Ambul Pediatr 2:154, 2002.

65. American Dental Association: Distribution of Dentists in the United States by Region and State, 1995. Chicago, American Dental Association, 1997.

66. Brown LJ, Lazar V: Workforce trends that influence the dental service capacity. J Am Dent Assoc 129:619, 1998.

67. U.S. Census Bureau. Current population reports, 1999.

68. American Dental Association: Distribution of Dentists in the United States by Region and State, 1998. Chicago, American Dental Association, January 2000.

69. American Association of Dental Schools: Trends in Dental Education 2000: The Past, Present and Future of the Profession or the People It Serves. Washington, DC, American Association of Dental Schools, January 1999.

70. Health Resources and Services Administration: United States Health Workforce Personnel Fact Book. Rockville, Md, U.S. Department of Health and Human Services, 2000.

71. Joshua OJ, Mertz E, Grumbach K. Dental Professional Shortage Area Methodology: A critical review. San Francisco, University of California at California Center to Address Disparities in Children's Oral Health and UCSF Center for California Workforce Studies, 2002.

72. Health insurance report: Second-class medicine. Consumer Reports, September 2000, 42-50.

73. Barnett WS, Brown KC: Dental Health Policy Series: Issues in Children's Access to Dental Care under

Medicaid. Chicago, American Dental Association, April 2000.

74. American Dental Education Association: President's Commission: Improving the Oral Health Status of All Americans: Roles and Responsibilities of Academic Dental Institutions: The Report of the ADEA President's Commission. Washington, DC: American Dental Education Association, 2003.

75. Brown LJ, Lazar V: Minority Dentists: Why Do We Need Them? Washington, DC, Closing the Gap, Office of Minority Health, July 1999.

76. American Dental Association: Future of Dentistry: Today's Vision, Tomorrow's Reality. Chicago, American Dental Association, Health Policy Resources Center, 2001.

77. American Dental Hygienists' Association: Future of Dental Hygiene Report. Chicago, American Dental Hygienists' Association, (in press).

78. National Centers for Health Statistics, Centers for Disease Control and Prevention: Healthy People 2010 Progress Review: Briefing Book Materials–Data Summary Table for Focus Area 1—Access to Quality Health Services, June 4, 2002.

79. American Dental Education Association: Dental Education At-A-Glance. Washington, DC, American Dental Education Association, 2004.

80. Haden NK, Morr KE, Valachovic RW: Trends in allied dental education: an analysis of the past and a look to the future. J Dent Educ 65:480, 2001.

81. American Dental Association: Medicaid and Dental Care for Children: A Review of the Literature. Chicago, American Dental Association, Health Policy Resources Center, 2003.

82. U.S. Census. Statistical Abstract of the United States. Washington, DC, U.S. Census, 2003.

83. Association of State and Territorial Dental Directors: Synopsis of State and Territorial Dental Public Health Programs. Jefferson City, Mo, Association of State and Territorial Dental Directors, 2004.

84. Maternal and Child Health Bureau, Health Resources Services Administration: Strategic Plan: Fiscal Year 2003-2007. Rockville, Md: Maternal and Child Health Bureau, HRSA, 2003.

85. Association of State and Territorial Dental Directors: Building Infrastructure and Capacity in State and Territorial Oral Health Programs. Jefferson City, Mo, Association of State and Territorial Dental Directors, 2000.

86. Tomar SL: Assessment of the dental public health infrastructure in the United States. Gainesville, Fla: University of Florida College of Dentistry, July 2004 (Contract number 263-MD-012931, National Institute of Dental and Craniofacial Research, National Institutes of Health).

87. American Dental Association: State and community models for improving access to dental care for the underserved—a white paper. Chicago, Ill: American Dental Association, October 2004.

6

Oral Health Programs in the Community

Sherry R. Jenkins, RDH, BS
Kathy Voigt Geurink, RDH, MA
Linda Altenhoff, DDS

Objectives

Upon completion of this chapter, the student will be able to:

- Identify oral health programs at the national, state, and local level
- Discuss the essential public health services for oral health
- Describe the four phases of organizing an effective community oral health program
- Define goals and objectives
- Explain how program goals and objectives are used in program planning, implementation, and evaluation
- Discuss the benefits of primary prevention programs, including fluoridation, sealants, and oral health education
- Describe the importance of community water fluoridation as a public health measure
- Identify the different funding streams and structures for obtaining dental services through public health systems

Key Terms

Essential Public Health Services
  for Oral Health
Oral Health Coalition
Assessment

Planning
Implementation
Evaluation
Goals

Objectives
Community Water Fluoridation
Sealants
Oral Health Education

OPENING STATEMENT

Community Oral Health Programs

- Community Dental Sealant Programs

- Tobacco Cessation and Spit Tobacco Programs

- Water Fluoridation Programs

- Oral Health Coalitions

- Early Childhood Caries Programs

- Geriatric Dental Programs

- School Fluoride Mouth Rinse Programs

- School-Based Oral Health Programs

- Needs Assessment and Oral Health Surveys

GENERAL HEALTH AND ORAL HEALTH

The mission of public health is to "fulfill society's interest in assuring conditions in which people can be healthy."[1] Without public health, including community oral health, society as a whole suffers because of lost productivity, decreased learning among our school-age children as a result of health-related absences, and increased health care costs. Surgeon General David Thatcher, in the May 2000 Surgeon General's Report,[2] refers to dental disease as a "silent epidemic that restricts activities in school, work, and home, and often significantly diminishes the quality of life." He further states:

> To improve the quality of life and eliminate health disparities demands the understanding, compassion, and will of the American people. There are opportunities for all health professionals and communities to work together to improve health.[2]

This chapter discusses community oral health programs as opportunities for achieving improved oral health and, consequently, overall health.

NATIONAL, STATE, AND LOCAL PROGRAMS: ROLE OF THE HEALTH DEPARTMENT

National Level

National, state, and local dental public health programs have similar roles but widely varying organizational schemes. Nationally, several governmental programs are involved in oral health promotion.

Among these programs are the U.S. Department of Health and Human Services (DHHS), the federal government's principal agency for protecting the health of all Americans and providing essential services, especially for people who are least able to help themselves. DHHS is the largest grant-making agency in the federal government (~60,000 grants per year). DHHS works with state and local governments and funds services at the local level through state or county agencies or through private sector grantees. DHHS also provides regulatory oversight and monitoring of the expenditures made by grantees. DHHS has multiple public health service operating divisions, including:

- National Institutes of Health (NIH)
- Food and Drug Administration (FDA)
- Centers for Disease Control and Prevention (CDC)
- Indian Health Service (IHS)
- Health Resources and Services Administration (HRSA)

State Level

Approximately two thirds of the states have full-time state dental directors who provide leadership and guidance in the planning, funding, and implementation of oral health promotion programs for the residents of the states that they serve. These programs vary in their scope of services and organization across the United States.

A state's program may include, in addition to the state dental director, regional dental directors, public health educators, clinical dentists, dental hygienists, and dental assistants who provide oral health services to underserved populations. These public professionals also promote oral health through educational programs in public and private schools and through collaborative efforts with dental and dental hygiene schools; Head Start centers; Women, Infant, and Children (WIC) programs; county and city health departments; community-based organizations; faith-based organizations; civic groups; and local dental providers and dental hygienists.

Private practice dental hygienists, through collaboration with state-sponsored oral health promotions, can serve in the roles of Educator/Health Promoter and Consumer Advocate in addition to their role as Clinician, therefore positively affecting the oral health of a greater population base.

Local Level

Individual county and city health departments across the nation have recognized the need within their communities for the provision of oral health services to various members of their populations. Many of these clinics are federally funded, offering services on a sliding scale fee schedule and accepting clients who receive public assistance through Medicaid. These clinics employ both public health dentists and dental hygienists and sometimes have supplemental clinical coverage provided by local dental professionals.

Hours of operation are also tailored to best meet the needs of the population that they serve. The clinics provide diagnostic, preventive, and restorative oral health services to older adults and to the indigent population and the working poor.

Essential Public Health Services for Oral Health

The core public health functions of assessment, policy development, and assurance shape the basic practice of public health at state and local levels. These core public health functions and the essential public health services (see Chapter 1) provided input into the **Essential Public Health Services for Oral Health** developed by the Association of State and Territorial Dental Directors (ASTDD) (Box 6-1).[3] These guidelines describe the roles of state oral health programs and have been used in the development and evaluation of public health activities at the state level.

Many states have developed programs that include the essential services for oral health. For example, in the State of Washington the *Smile Survey* was initiated to provide statewide screenings for children to assess the status of their oral health and to identify problems. Preventive programs such as sealants and oral health education have followed as an answer to the problem of tooth decay. In addition, the Washington State Oral Health Coalition was formed in 1993. A *coalition* is a diverse group of individuals, organizations, and agencies that unite to reach a common goal. An **oral health coalition** is therefore a cooperative effort on the part of many individuals and organizations to build systems and develop programs that improve community oral health.

The Washington State Oral Health Coalition has proved to be an excellent means of bringing dedicated professionals together to resolve oral health issues through policy development. This coalition is also involved in continual assessment of oral health and in the assurance of oral health solutions. More than 20 different locations in Washington have established oral health coalitions, with representation from consumers, schools, community clinics, health care and dental providers, health departments, and agencies that come in contact with low-income and minority populations. Anyone interested in achieving the goal of optimal oral health for Washington residents is invited to join. The strength and unity of a coalition make this goal attainable. The Washington Department of Health and the U.S. DHHS have developed a document, *Community Roots for Oral Health: Guidelines for Successful Coalitions,* available to people interested in forming an oral health coalition to improve the oral health of residents in their community (Box 6-2).[4]

ASSESSMENT, PLANNING, IMPLEMENTATION, AND EVALUATION

Four components are necessary in initiating an oral health program: **assessment, planning, implementation,** and **evaluation.** Dental hygienists in private practice and in the community use these components to deliver oral health care. Community health extends the role of the dental hygienist from the traditional private practice to the community as a whole.

BOX 6-1   ESSENTIAL PUBLIC HEALTH SERVICES FOR ORAL HEALTH

Assessment

- Assess oral health status and needs so that problems can be identified and addressed
- Analyze determinants of identified oral health needs, including resources
- Assess the fluoridation status of water systems and other sources of fluoride
- Implement an oral health surveillance system to identify, investigate, and monitor oral health problems and health hazards

Policy Development

- Develop plans and policies through a collaborative process that supports individual and community oral health efforts to address oral health needs
- Provide leadership to address oral health problems by maintaining a strong oral health unit within the health agency
- Mobilize community partnerships between and among policy makers, professionals, organizations, groups, the public, and others to identify and implement solutions to oral health problems

Assurance

- Inform, educate, and empower the public regarding oral health problems and solutions
- Promote and enforce laws and regulations that protect and improve oral health, ensure safety, and ensure accountability for the public's well-being
- Link people to needed population-based oral health services, personal oral health services, and support services, and assure the availability, access, and acceptability of these services by enhancing system capacity, including directly supporting or providing services when necessary
- Support services and implementation of programs that focus on primary and secondary prevention
- Assure that the public health and personal health workforce has the capacity and expertise to effectively address oral health needs
- Evaluate effectiveness, accessibility, and quality of population-based and personal oral health services
- Conduct research and support demonstration projects to gain new insights and applications of innovative solutions to oral health problems

Adapted from Association of State and Territorial Dental Directors: Guidelines for State and Territorial Oral Health Programs, 1997.[2]

In this setting the community is viewed as the patient. The community survey is comparable to the patient's examination for assessment. The program plan and implementation are similar to the treatment plan and treatment of the patient. Evaluation and review of the program can be compared to the evaluation of the patient's treatment (Box 6-3).

BOX 6-2   ORAL HEALTH COALITIONS

- Provide public recognition and visibility
- Leverage resources; expand the scope and range of services
- Provide a comprehensive approach to programming
- Enhance clout in advocacy and resource development
- Enhance competence
- Avoid duplication of services, and fill gaps in service delivery
- Accomplish what single members cannot

Adapted from Children's Alliance: Washington State Oral Health Coalition. Available from http://www.doh.wa.gov/ [4]

BOX 6-3   COMPONENTS NECESSARY FOR INITIATING AN ORAL HEALTH PROGRAM

Community			Private Practice
Community survey	$\longrightarrow$	ASSESSMENT	$\longleftarrow$ Patient exam
Plan the program	$\longrightarrow$	PLANNING	$\longleftarrow$ Plan patient treatment
Conduct the program	$\longrightarrow$	IMPLEMENTATION	$\longleftarrow$ Treat the patient
Review program/evaluate	$\longrightarrow$	EVALUATION	$\longleftarrow$ Evaluate patient treatment

With increased emphasis on improving public access to oral health care, the responsibilities of the dental hygienist to promote oral health in the community take on renewed importance. Therefore it is important that the dental hygienist understand the basic concepts of assessment, planning, implementation, and evaluation as they apply to oral health programs.

Definitions of the components of initiating an oral health program follow[5]:

1. *Assessment* is an organized and systematic approach to identify a target group and to define the extent and severity of oral health needs present.
2. *Planning* is an organized response to reduce or eliminate one or more problems.
3. *Implementation* includes the process of putting the plan into action and monitoring the plan's activities, personnel, equipment, resources, and supplies. This step should include feedback from personnel and participants as well as ongoing evaluation mechanisms.
4. *Evaluation* is the method of measuring results of the program against objectives developed during the early planning stages. This process is ongoing and should identify problems and solutions to assist in revising the program as needed.
   a. *Formative evaluation,* or the internal evaluation of a program, is an examination of the processes or activities of a program as they are taking place.
   b. *Summative evaluation* involves judging the merit or worth of a program after it has been in operation. This step is an attempt to determine whether a fully operational program is meeting the goals for which it was developed.

The above components are portrayed in the planning cycle model in Figure 3-4. The model provides a continuous cycle of steps to assess, plan, implement, and evaluate.[6]

Assessment

Assessing the relative importance of needs can be a complex process. It depends on human values, some of which are universally agreed upon and others that are more controversial. For example, a need that involves life or death generally receives higher priority; however, a choice between a health need that might affect the lives of a few people and one that affects the lives of large numbers of people is less clear-cut. Although many would argue that the needs of larger numbers must take priority, others want to consider factors such as age and the future impact on society. For example, a community may need to decide about initiating a free influenza vaccine program for its older population, enhancing the immunization program for children, or adding a clinic offering reduced dental care for indigent families (see Guiding Principles).

GUIDING PRINCIPLES

Establishing Health Priorities
- What is the magnitude of the problem? (Does it cause death or disability?)
- How many people are affected (one person, small community, whole country)?
- What types of resources are available (personnel, money, facilities, technology)?
- What has already been done in the community?
- What are the prevailing attitudes toward the problem?
- Which groups are expressing the most interest in the problem?
- What are the legal constraints?

Compounding the problem of establishing the priorities of health needs is the fact that each community is unique, with its own values and ideas. If a community's basic need for food and security are not being met, dental needs assume a low priority. An issue that often arises is the idea that if a community's perception of needs is adhered to exclusively, actual clinical health problems may go untreated because the people are not knowledgeable about many areas of health care. The solution to this dilemma involves striking a delicate balance between negligence and overzealousness. Although it is unethical to impose one's own perceptions on a community, it is the professional's responsibility to inform people of existing problems and their consequences.[7]

A needs assessment can identify the problem. The assessment provides information not only about the problem but also about the community itself. The data collected can be used to develop a community profile that will assist in finding the appropriate solution. Conducting a needs assessment for a community can be expensive with regard to labor and time. If funds are not available, coordination with other agencies interested in obtaining similar health information on the given population may be the solution.

Another possibility is to investigate dental surveys that have been done by other organizations. Dental surveys are conducted by professionals at dental schools, local and state health departments, and community health centers. Coordination with other agencies and organizations to know what has been done and what needs to be accomplished can prevent duplication of services.[8] Data can be obtained and analyzed by various methods (see Chapter 3). After the needs assessment is performed, developing the appropriate goals and objectives is the next step.

Planning

Developing goals, objectives, and program activities is part of the planning process. During this stage it is essential to have community involvement and participation. The formulation of program goals and objectives is an active process, offering specific proposals for changes to be made in the community. These changes address the specific problems identified in the needs assessment.

Goals

Goals provide a broadly based statement of what changes will take place, from which specific objectives are developed, for example: The school-based fluoride mouth rinse program will improve the oral health of school-aged children.

Objectives

Objectives are more specific than goals; they describe, in a measurable way, the desired end result of program activities. They should tell the learner what he or she needs to do to be successful.

The *performance verb* is the key to a measurable objective (Box 6-4); it is an action word, such as "write," "demonstrate," or "recite." Other elements of the objective are the *condition*, which tells under what circumstance the activity occurs, and the *criterion*, which tells how well the activity must be performed. The performance verb is essential in writing a measurable objective. The inclusion of a condition and a criterion makes the objective more specific and useful to the learner. In summary:

1. A *performance verb* tells the activity and outcome.
2. A *condition* tells under what circumstance the outcome will occur.
3. A *criterion* tells how well the action and outcome must be accomplished to be effective.

An example of an objective for the aforementioned goal would be as follows: Upon completion of today's six-step demonstration of how to rinse, the children will demonstrate the six steps without error.

Box 6-4   PERFORMANCE VERBS FOR WRITING BEHAVIORAL OBJECTIVES

Analyze	Examine	Map	State
Apply	Estimate	Measure	Sort
Attempt	Explain	Observe	Spell
Adjust	Express	Organize	Try
Brush	Find	Perform	Test
Calculate	Form	Practice	Unite
Categorize	Gather	Predict	Weigh
Choose	Group	Plan	Write
Classify	Hypothesize	Produce	
Complete	Identify	Prove	
Create	Invent	Record	
Copy	Join	Recognize	
Describe	Keep	Repeat	
Define	Label	Select	
Design	List	Show	
Demonstrate			

Performance verb: demonstrate
Condition: upon completion of today's six-step demonstration
Criterion: without error

Another example of a measurable objective: Upon completion of the calibration exercise, the three examiners will record their findings with an 85% accuracy.

Performance verb: record
Condition: upon completion of the calibration exercise
Criterion: 85% accuracy

Once the problem has been identified and program goals and objectives have been established with a description of a solution, the next step is to state how to bring about the desired results. This area of program planning, referred to as *program activities,* describes how the objectives will be accomplished.

In planning these program activities, one must carefully consider the type of *resources* available as well as program *constraints*. For example, in planning a school fluoride mouth rinse program in which the chosen activity would be weekly rinsing, resources might include selecting (1) the site at which the rinsing is conducted, (2) personnel, (3) supplies, and (4) the financial means to pay for the supplies. Constraints might include (1) availability of dental personnel to conduct screenings, (2) negative attitudes from some parents, (3) the amount of time it takes to rinse, or (4) lack of funding.

Planning is a crucial element to a successful program. A community oral health program that is well planned, with specific activities and consideration to resources and constraints, is usually successful in terms of implementation.

Implementation

The process of putting the plan into action, the implementation phase, is ongoing and should be supervised and evaluated to ensure program effectiveness. Implementation, like planning, involves individuals, agencies, and the community working together. The strategy should answer the following questions[8]:

1. Why: the effect of the objective to be achieved
2. What: the activities required to achieve the objective
3. Who: the individuals responsible for each activity
4. When: the chronologic sequence of activities
5. How: the materials, media, methods, and techniques to be used
6. How much: a cost estimate of materials and time

For ease in addressing these questions, many community oral health programs begin on a small scale. Using a smaller population with the intent to expand later is called *pilot testing.* In a pilot test for a fluoride mouth rinse program, for instance, only one school would be involved the first year and the program would be expanded to include two or more schools the following year. This implementation strategy allows for an opportunity to test the program's effectiveness and provides ease in control and monitoring of the program activities. A pilot program provides useful information and enables decisions to be made about the future of the program. Piloting is a form of evaluating the implementation.

Evaluation

Evaluation is a judgment of merit or worth about the program. The first step is to review the program goals and then to examine the specific measurable objectives. To evaluate the effectiveness of health programs, specific measurement instruments must be set up for collection of data on the attainment of each program objective. The data that are obtained through measuring the objectives are called measurable outcomes. Each objective should be reviewed to determine how well it is meeting the program goals. The bottom line in evaluation is accountability—to consumers, providers, and all involved agencies. Evaluation determines whether the program accomplishes what it was designed to accomplish (e.g., were the objectives of this study or program successfully met? If not, why not?). Summarizing what went well and what did not, or drawing conclusions based on intuition, is not adequate; the objectives themselves must be specifically addressed.

Inherent in this approach is the possibility of attaining a negative outcome, that is, the conclusion that the objectives have not been met. At the same time, however, this does not mean that the program has been a failure. If a program is evaluated properly so that negative outcomes become learning experiences and indicators of future programming and research, in some sense it has been a success.[7] Formative evaluation during the implementation process can point out problems and identify opportunities to correct program deficiencies early on. With ongoing evaluation and change, the summative evaluation (end result) may in fact measure a program with initial problems as successful.

Program evaluation is an example of *applied research*. *Basic (clinical) research* (see Chapter 7) involves inquiry into the truth about facts, behaviors, relationships, and principles. Applied research is concerned with these same concepts but emphasizes the application of the knowledge and developing solutions to problems. For example, a basic researcher would be concerned with the effectiveness of the fluoride mouth rinse on the teeth and which concentration to use. A program evaluator would be concerned with the effect of the program operation and its ability to meet the program objectives. The fundamental purpose of program evaluation is to assist in decision making on the effectiveness of the program in its entirety and to reassess the program and make necessary changes to make the program more effective.

Dental hygienists play a role in assessing, planning, implementing, and evaluating community oral health programs. The dental hygienists who have chosen careers as state dental directors, public health educators, or promoters have played an important role in the advancement of dental public health, but there is much more that can be accomplished by all of the dental hygiene profession. By knowing how to organize an effective community oral health program and becoming involved in its implementation, dental hygienists can have an impact in reaching the goal of optimal oral health care for all people.

PRIMARY PREVENTION PROGRAMS: FLUORIDATION, SEALANTS, ORAL HEALTH EDUCATION

Community Water Fluoridation

Community water fluoridation is the addition of a controlled amount of fluoride to the public water supply with the intent to prevent dental caries in the population. Fluoridation has been recognized as one of the major public health measures of the twentieth century:

> At the turn of the century most Americans could expect to lose their teeth by middle age. That situation began to change with the discovery of the properties of fluoride and the observation that people who lived in communities with naturally fluoridated drinking water had far less dental caries than people in comparable communities without fluoride in their water supply.[2]

In the 1920s, Dr. Frederick McKay first noticed that people living in regions of Colorado had brown stain on their teeth (*fluorosis,* or mottled enamel) but few, if any, caries. In the 1930s, Dr. Trendley Dean conducted epidemiologic studies to prove the relationship of dental fluorosis, concentration of fluoride in the water, and reduction of dental caries.

Fluoride is the thirteenth most abundant natural element; it is found in rocks, soil, fresh water, and ocean water. Therefore trace amounts of fluoride are found in all natural water sources. As a result of the general availability of public water sources to most people, the adjustment of the natural fluoride content found in the water to levels optimal for combating oral disease has proved to be a successful public health measure. This approach provides fluoride to the population, with minimal regard to socioeconomic factors, in a passive vehicle for the consumer. Water fluoridation, accomplished in this manner, results in improved oral health, reduced expenditures for dental restorative procedures, and decreased absences from school and work resulting from oral pain, with a resultant increase in learning and productivity.

The first city in the United States to adjust the fluoride content in the community water supply was Grand Rapids, Michigan, in the 1940s. Subsequent studies of adjusted fluoridation demonstrated that 50% to 70% of caries were prevented in the permanent teeth of children. Today, decay reduction rates in fluoridated communities are approximately 8% to 37% for children, and 20% to 40% for adults.[9]

Figure 6-1 correlates the percentage of the population residing in areas with fluoridated community water systems and the mean number of decayed, missing (because of caries), or filled permanent teeth (DMFT) among children aged 12 years in the United States from 1967 to 1992. The average number of DMFT steadily declined from 1967 to 1992 because of populations residing in fluoridated communities.[10]

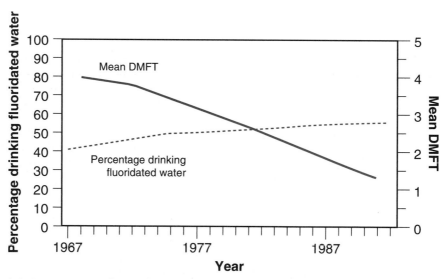

Figure 6-1 Percentage of population residing in areas with fluoridated water systems and with decayed, missing, or filled permanent teeth (DMFT) among children aged 12 years, 1967 to 1992. *(Data from Centers for Disease Control and Prevention [CDC]: Fluoridation Census, 1993; CDC, Third National Health and Nutrition Examination Survey, 1988 to 1994; National Center for Health Statistics, 1974 and 1981; and National Institute of Dental Research, 1989.)*

Fluoridated Communities

In the 1950s and 1960s many states and cities were quick to implement fluoridation programs. In following years this trend began to level off. Fluoridation decisions are currently left to states and frequently to local governments and city councils. The expansion of fluoridation therefore is not easily accomplished and requires decisions at various levels. Recent increases in community water fluoridation can be attributed to the emphasis on its importance in caries prevention as discussed in the 2000 Surgeon General's Report, *Oral Health in America,* and its recognition in the *Healthy People 2010 Objectives.*[11]

Almost 162 million U.S. residents currently benefit from water fluoridation. As of 2000 the total population receiving water fluoridation rose from 55.9% to 57.6%. The *Healthy People 2010* objective for community water fluoridation is an increase in the proportion of community water systems optimally fluoridated; the target is 75% of the population. Figure 6-2 shows the percent of the U.S. population on public water systems served by fluoridation in 2000. Currently 65.8% of the U.S. population on public water supplies receive fluoridated water. Box 6-5 shows the population served by water fluoridation in the United States.[11]

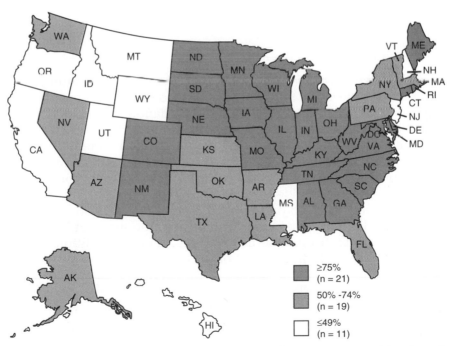

Figure 6-2 Proportion of people who have public water systems served by fluoridation in 2000. *(From Centers for Disease Control Fluoridation Census. Atlanta, 2000.)*

Box 6-5   Population served by water fluoridation in the United States as of April 1, 2000

Total U.S. population	281,421,906
Total U.S. population on fluoride drinking water systems	162 million
% of U.S. population receiving fluoridated water	57.6%
% of U.S. population on public water supply system receiving fluoridated water	65.8%

Adapted from http://www.cdc.gov/nohss.

Cost of Water Fluoridation

It has been calculated that the mean annual per capita cost of community water fluoridation ranges from $0.68 for systems with a population over 50,000 and $0.98 for systems with a population base between 10,000 and 50,000 to $3.00 for systems with fewer than 10,000 people[11] (Table 6-1). The lifetime cost of fluoridation per person is less than the cost of one dental filling. With the escalating cost of health care, fluoridation remains a preventive measure of minimal cost. In determining the economic importance of fluoridation, we should remember that the cost of treating dental disease is paid not only by the affected individual but also by the public through health departments, health insurance premiums, and federally supported programs such as Medicaid.

Optimal Amounts of Fluoride

Several states have fluoridation projects that assist communities in their efforts to assess the need for fluoridation and to design and implement fluoridation of their public water systems. The state fluoridation staff also provides training and technical assistance for local water facility operators.

When the water supply is being fluoridated in a community, climatic temperature and consumption of water are taken into consideration. The recommended levels for water fluoridation in the United States range from 0.7 to 1.2 parts per million (ppm) of fluoride, depending on the average daily temperature for that area. This range is based on the hypothesis that water consumption increases with increasing climatic temperature. This assumption may not be as accurate as earlier research indicates because of the increased use of air conditioning and the increased consumption of soft drinks and bottled water.[12]

Table **6-1**   **Estimated annual per capita cost for community water fluoridation**

Community size:	Cost/person
<10,000 (small systems)	$3.00
10,000-50,000 (medium systems)	$0.98
>50,000 (large systems)	$0.68

Examples of Community Water Fluoridation Programs

Indiana

An example of a state that has successfully adopted fluoride into its community water systems is Indiana. The Indiana State Department of Health has given community water fluoridation a high priority and had reached the *Healthy People 2010* objective of 75% fluoridation in the 1970s.[13] Grant monies were applied for and secured from departments within the U.S. Public Health Services. As a result of the efforts of dedicated professionals, including dental hygienists fulfilling the roles of Educators, Consumer Advocates, and Change Agents, the state is 98% fluoridated.

The successful implementation of this program can be attributed to effective planning, implementation, and evaluation procedures. In the planning stage, assessment of the community needs and feasibility studies were conducted. The cooperative efforts of professionals, city officials, and citizens resulted in positive voluntary voting for the implementation of fluoride. Important evaluation measures of the program are the surveillance visits to monitor the amount of fluoride levels in the community drinking water.

More than 1500 surveillance visits are conducted per year to ensure that optimal fluoride levels are maintained. Because of this monitoring, 98% of the 262 fluoridating Indiana communities and 92% of the 56 fluoridating Indiana schools routinely have optimal fluoride levels. Ongoing DMFS surveys convey the successful results of reduced dental decay.[13]

California

Another state that illustrates a successful effect of a unified effort to implement fluoridation is California. The California Task Force was developed in 1993 and consisted of members from organizations such as the California Dental Association, the California Department of Health, the California Dental Hygiene Association, the California Public Health Association, and the California Dental Health Foundation. The task force created a plan to implement fluoridation in the entire state. Whereas only 17% of California was fluoridated in 1993, today more than 35% of the communities are fluoridated.[14]

For further information on these programs and other state coalitions and task force plans, see Resources at the end of this chapter.

Other Fluoride Programs

Mouth rinse programs

In communities where a public water source is not available or where water fluoridation is undesired for various reasons, school-based fluoride mouth rinse programs have been implemented and offer the benefits of fluoride in a structured environment. Such programs are a popular and cost-effective means of providing fluoride benefits for children. Participation by children in a school-based program requires parental permission and oversight by a licensed dentist.

The mouth rinse program is administered by school personnel or volunteers on a weekly basis to participating children. The children rinse for 60 seconds with 10 ml of 2% sodium fluoride. The fluoride rinse is then expectorated into a paper cup, a napkin is placed inside the cup to absorb the solution, and the cup is discarded. The procedure takes less than 5 minutes.

School water supply

Another means of providing fluoridation for school children in nonfluoridated communities is adding fluoride to the school water system. The amount of fluoride added to the school water is 4.5 times the optimal amount that would be added to the community water. This method is not as readily selected because the amount of water consumed cannot be monitored easily. Limited evidence of effectiveness and difficulties with implementation and operation have led schools to seek alternative preventive methods.

Dietary fluoride supplements

The use of dietary fluoride supplements is another popular way of providing fluoride to children. These supplements are available only by prescription and are intended for use by children living in nonfluoridated areas to increase their fluoride exposure to a level equivalent to children who live in optimally fluoridated areas.

Supplements are available in two forms: (1) drops for infants aged 6 months and older and (2) chewable tablets for children and adolescents. To decrease the risk of dental fluorosis in permanent teeth, fluoride supplements should be prescribed only for children living in nonfluoridated areas. The need for continuation of fluoride supplements should be reevaluated in the event of a child's change of residence.

The correct dosage is based on the child's age and the existing fluoride level in available drinking water sources (Table 6-2).[15] The water sources to be considered should include:

- Water in the home
- Bottled water

Table **6-2**   **Dietary fluoride supplement schedule***

| Age | Fluoride Ion Level in Drinking Water (ppm[†]) | | |
	<0.3 ppm	0.3-0.6 ppm	>0.6 ppm
Birth-6 mo	None	None	None
6 mo-3 yr	0.25 mg/day[‡]	None	None
3-6 yr	0.50 mg/day	0.25 mg/day	None
6-16 yr	1.0 mg/day	0.50 mg/day	None

Copyright © 2001 American Dental Association. Available from http://www.ADA.org.
*Approved by the American Dental Association, American Academy of Pediatrics, and American Academy of Pediatric Dentistry.
[†]1.0 part per million (ppm) = 1 milligram/liter (mg/L).
[‡]2.2 mg of sodium fluoride contains 1 mg of fluoride ion.

- Water at a school or a day care center
- After-school care sources

The need for compliance over an extended period of time is a major procedural and economic disadvantage of community-based fluoride supplement programs. This liability makes them impractical as an alternative to water fluoridation as a public health measure. Although total costs of the purchase of supplements and administration of a program are small, compared with the installation and startup costs associated with fluoridation equipment, the overall cost of supplements per child is much greater than the per capita cost of community water fluoridation. Additionally, community water fluoridation provides decay prevention and oral health benefits for the entire population regardless of age, socioeconomic status, educational attainment, or other social variables. This is particularly important for families and individuals who do not or cannot access regular oral health services.

Fluoride varnishes

Developed in Europe during the 1960s, fluoride varnishes were introduced into the United States in 1994 and remain in wide use within Europe and Canada. The varnish is applied by an operator, with a recommended twice-yearly reapplication for optimal benefit. The varnish is not intended to be permanent, like a sealant, but to hold the fluoride in contact with the tooth for a period of time. Duraflor, approved by the Food and Drug Administration (FDA), has gained popularity in the United States.

Varnishes may be used to prevent root surface caries on adults with gingival recession. They offer easy applicability of fluoride for disabled children or hospitalized patients.[16] Studies in Europe have demonstrated their efficacy.[17] Whether varnishes should be the choice of clinical programs in communities with high caries rates or whether they are better for patients on an individual basis is currently being studied.

An example of using fluoride varnish to prevent early childhood caries is a program implemented by The Division of Dental Health, Virginia Department of Health. This program is funded by a Health Resources and Services Administration (HRSA) Collaborative Systems Grant. The primary focus of the program is to train dental and nondental (medical) providers to use an oral health risk assessment tool and place fluoride varnish on the teeth of children under the age of 3. Grant funds are also supporting development of educational materials targeting the Medicaid eligible population. Other partners collaborating on the grant include the Division of WIC and Community Nutrition Services, Early Head Start, Virginia's Department of Education, University of Virginia School of Medicine, Department of Medical Assistance Services, and Virginia Commonwealth University School of Dentistry. The Division of Health, Virginia Department of Health also provides other dental services for the residents of Virginia including a school fluoride mouth rinse program and a statewide oral health education program. For more information on oral health programs in Virginia, visit the website listed at the end of the chapter.[18]

Additional Fluoride Sources

The introduction of *systemic* fluoride through water, vitamins, and tablets during the enamel formation phase of both primary and permanent teeth of children, in utero and post partum, provides for optimal dental decay preventive benefits through fluoride ion exchange and resultant denser enamel matrix. Fluoride is provided *topically* through toothpaste, mouth rinses, and professionally prescribed fluoride gels, pastes, rinses, and varnishes. The benefits associated with topical fluoride include the remineralization of early incipient lesions. The effectiveness of various fluoride sources in the reduction of dental caries is shown in Box 6-6.[19]

With all the additional sources of fluoride available today, the prevalence of caries has decreased but the prevalence of dental fluorosis has increased in both fluoridated and nonfluoridated communities. Factors associated with increased fluorosis today are[19]:

- Early use of fluoride toothpaste
- Use and misuse of dietary supplements
- Consumption of infant formula containing fluoride

Health care professionals such as dentists, dental hygienists, and physicians are important sources of information for patients regarding the use of fluoride-containing products such as toothpaste and may be able to help reduce the prevalence of enamel fluorosis by educating the public on the appropriate use of these products.

Even though other sources of fluoride are available and despite the increased risk of fluorosis, community water fluoridation remains the most cost-effective, the most practical, and the safest means of preventing tooth decay.

Antifluoridationists

Antifluoridationists are opponents of community water fluoridation. Their reasons include individual rights, safety, government mistrust, and religious freedom. The

---

Box 6-6   COMMUNITY WATER FLUORIDATION, EARLY STUDIES

- **Community water fluoridation:** Early studies: 50% to 70% reduction in caries, currently 20% to 40% reduction in caries due to additional availability of other fluoride sources
- **Mouth rinses:** Studies in the 1970s and 1980s demonstrated a reduction in caries ranging from 20% to 50%
- **Fluoride tablet supplements:** Controlled trials in the United States in the 1970s indicated approximately a 20% to 28% reduction
- **Toothpaste:** In clinical trials done between 1945 and 1985, 23% to 32% reduction in caries

Community water fluoridation, early studies: 50% to 70% reduction in caries, currently 8% to 37% in children and 20% to 40% in adults.

Data from Milgram P, Reisine S: Oral health in the United States: The post-fluoride generation. Annu Rev Public Health 21:403-406, 2000.

arguments against fluoridation do not have any merit based on scientific knowledge. The economic and health benefits of fluoridation for millions of Americans have been confirmed in numerous studies by renowned scientists.[16,20]

Antifluoridationists attempt to appeal to people's emotions. They provide inaccurate, false information to the public and to the elected officials and attempt to link adverse health effects with fluoridation. Dental hygienists, in the roles of educators and resource persons, can influence the public knowledge about the benefits of fluoridation in their community and can provide scientific, accurate information to the community officials.

For antifluoridationists to be defeated, community education must be executed in a well-planned, unified manner. As active members of the American Dental Hygienists Association and the local components, dental hygienists become an effective force that can have an impact on the community. An organized plan of action can make a difference. Being aware of the issues and being well versed on fluoridation studies and cognizant of the political process are necessary steps in winning a fluoridation campaign. Dental hygienists also work as *Change Agents* in promoting the legislative approval of fluoridation.

Some states and cities have taken administrative action to implement fluoridation; this means that state legislatures and the city council or commission, because of the public health benefits, have voted for fluoridation. People usually prefer to have a voice in the decision making process; however, if fluoride is on the ballot, people need to be educated on the issue to make a wise decision. Education is the key to the success in reaching the *Healthy People 2010* goal of fluoridation for 75% of the population in the United States.

Dental Sealants

An effective primary preventive strategy, commonly used to protect permanent molars from decay, is the application of dental **sealants.** Although the percentage of school-aged children with sealants has risen in recent years as the public and private sectors have been using the procedure, as dental insurance has paid for the sealants, and as parents have requested sealants for their children, no increase in use has occurred among children in low-income populations. One goal of *Healthy People 2010* is to have 50% of children receiving dental sealants on their permanent molars. According to the 1988-1994 baseline data, only 23% of 8-year-old children and 15% of 14-year-old adolescents had dental sealants on their permanent molars.[21]

To help reach the goal of 50% of children having dental sealants, many states have instituted school-based dental sealant programs. In some programs mobile dental vans are sent to schools and the sealants are applied in the van. In other programs portable equipment is transported from school to school and is set up in available spaces. Students are then brought to the designated room for the procedure.

Sealant programs generally focus on 6- to 8-year-olds and 12- to 14-year-olds because the first and second molars usually erupt during these years. Placing sealants on these teeth shortly after their eruption protects them from development of caries in areas where food and bacteria are retained. If sealants were applied routinely to susceptible tooth surfaces in conjunction with the appropriate use of fluoride, most tooth decay in children could be prevented.

The "Seal a Smile" program in Wisconsin is an example of a primary prevention program to promote dental sealants to all children who need them. Funded by a grant from the CDC, the program is part of an initiative called "Healthy Smiles for Wisconsin." The goal of the Healthy Smiles for Wisconsin Coalition is that no child in that state should go without adequate oral health care, preventive services, or education. The organization has developed a planning guide for communities wanting to set up a Seal a Smile Program. The guide is free of charge and provides a step-by-step plan for starting a sealant program.[22]

Oral Health Education

Health education is the process of teaching people about health. The scope of health education may include educational activities for children, parents, policy makers, or health care providers. Educational programs are developed and presented in many different formats and settings.

Oral health education is a learning experience directed at helping people prevent oral disease. Oral health education can be presented directly to the clients through individual or group activities, such as health fairs, or in school curricula (Figure 6-3). The intent of oral health education is to assist people in making

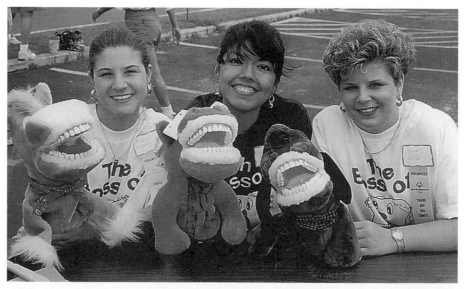

Figure 6-3 Dental hygiene students use puppets to present oral health education at a health fair.

decisions about their oral health and to choose behaviors conducive to maintaining this health.

For health education to be effective, the participant must be actively involved in the learning process. The cognitive model alone (attitude + knowledge = behavior change) has been ineffective in producing change. The educator must consider many factors that influence learners and their behavior. Both internal and external factors should be considered in developing an oral health educational program (Box 6-7). Patient attitudes and environment affect behaviors and the possibility of change. The outcome of the oral health education process will be successful only if all factors are considered.

With regard to the sociodemographic factor of age, most dental education programs have been implemented for children. Oral health education for children is a priority because of the high prevalence of dental caries in this group. If a society free of dental disease is the goal, educational programs must be targeted for the future of society—the children. The school system therefore continues to be the setting used to implement large-scale oral health education programs. The school-based oral health education program remains an important component of the goal of optimal oral health for all citizens. Oral health education should be an integral component of all school health education curricula.

Other opportunities for oral health education can be accessed through faith-based, community-based, and social service organizations such as the WIC Program, Head Start, Lions' Clubs, and Rotary Clubs. These organizations present opportunities for oral health education on a diversity of topics such as:

- Prenatal and postnatal oral health education for parents, infants, and toddlers
- Oral health concerns of special care patients
- Oral health education for older adults
- Oral health effects of tobacco and oral cancer information

Oral health educational programs can be given through health care facilities, such as hospitals and clinics, and long-term care facilities, such as nursing homes and alternative care centers. Specialty groups such as the 4-H Clubs, Future Farmers

BOX 6-7   FACTORS THAT INFLUENCE THE DENTAL EDUCATION PROCESS

Individual Factors (internal)

- Education level
- Beliefs, values, perceptions
- Age, income, race, and other sociodemographic factors

Environmental Factors (external)

- Intrapersonal interactions with family and peers
- Community influences, including cultural norms and public policy
- Technology to deliver the information

Data from various websites for state oral health programs. See list at end of chapter.

BOX 6-8 GAGLIARDI'S FIVE-STEP LESSON PLAN

Components of a Lesson Plan
1. Anticipatory planning (introduction of the lesson and materials needed)
2. Objectives (what the student will gain from this lesson)
3. Instruction/information (the bulk of the lesson that is new and exciting for the student)
4. Guided practice activities (to reinforce the information taught)
5. Closure (restatement of the objectives to test knowledge)

Adapted from Gagliord L: Dental Health Education: Lesson Planning and Implementation. Connecticut, Appleton and Lange, 1999.

of America, sports clubs, and youth organizations welcome educational programs. See Chapter 8 for additional information on health promotion.

When planning to provide a presentation to a selected population, the first step would be to develop a lesson plan. A Five-Step Lesson Plan described by Gagliardi includes: Preparation, Anticipatory planning, Objectives, Instruction/information, Guided practice activities, and Closure as seen in Box 6-8.[23] An example of a lesson plan using the five steps can be seen in Figure 6-4.

State Oral Health Programs

Box 6-9 presents a synopsis of the most common oral health programs offered in various states. The most common programs are in the areas of fluoridation, sealants, early childhood caries, health education and promotion, and tobacco cessation.[24] Examples of successful programs in the fluoride arena and in the placement of sealants have been provided.

In the area of early childhood caries, the Texas Department of Health has implemented an oral health education program called "Take Time for Teeth." In this program outreach workers, educators, and health care providers are taught a standardized oral health message that emphasizes preventive oral health practices at an early age. The people trained are chosen because they interact with the population targeted, that of children and families. Topics include:
1. Dental checkups for pregnant women.
2. Recognition of "white spots" and how to prevent baby bottle tooth decay.
3. The benefits of taking a child to the dentist every 6 months beginning at age 1 year.
4. The importance of dental sealants in preventing tooth decay.

The long-term goal of this statewide program is to have a positive impact on oral health status and to facilitate a positive behavioral change relating to oral health and prevention.[25]

A national tobacco cessation program is the National Spit Tobacco Education Program (NSTEP), funded by the Robert Wood Foundation and administered by the

---

Brushing Lesson Plan for Kindergarten

Preparation: Have available in a paper bag various types of brushes. Puppets with teeth or large mouth model and large toothbrush. Toothbrush for each student.

1. **Anticipatory planning**
   Describe the importance of a healthy mouth and teeth:
   > What do we do with our mouths (talk, eat, smile, etc.)?
   > How can we take care of our mouths and teeth (brushing, flossing, eating healthy, and going to the dentist)?

2. **Objectives**
   Students will be able to:
   > Demonstrate how to hold a toothbrush.
   > Explain that at least twice daily brushing of teeth is necessary for good oral health.

3. **Instruction/information**
   Review types of brushes (pull from paper bag).
   Describe a brushing technique and sequence.
   Go over use of toothbrush and general rules:
   > Do not share toothbrushes
   > Keep toothbrush clean; storage
   > Replace when worn or if you have been sick
   > Never walk around with toothbrush in your mouth

4. **Guided practice activities**
   Demonstrate brushing on puppet.
   Divide students into groups and have them each brush the puppet's teeth.

5. **Closure**
   Reinforce importance of brushing at least twice daily.
   Emphasize importance of having a good, clean toothbrush.

Figure 6-4 Sample lesson plan.

Oral Health America and supported by Major League Baseball. The goal is to educate young people on the dangers of using spit tobacco. Tobacco is presented as a potentially dangerous drug that can cause oral cancer. NSTEP and its partnerships with public, private, and voluntary groups, including the dental and medical professions, are helping Americans to stop using tobacco. The program uses television, radio, print, and public service announcements featuring baseball celebrities to send its

Box 6-9   Synopsis of state oral health programs

Access to Dental Care Programs
Prevent Abuse and Neglect through Dental Awareness (PANDA) Program
Children Forensic Identification team
Community Dental Sealant Programs*
Community Oral Health Systems Development
Community Water Fluoridation*
Dental Screening Programs*
Early Childhood Caries and Baby Bottle Tooth Decay Programs*
Fee-For-Service Programs for Indigent Children
Fluoride Supplement Programs
Head Start Grantees Reviews
Mouth Guard and Injury Prevention Programs
Needs Assessment and Oral Health Surveys*
Old Age Pensioners Dental Program
Oral Health Assurance
Oral Health Education and Promotion Programs*
Oral Health for School Nurses Program
Private Well Water Testing Program
School Fluoride Mouth Rinse Programs*
Tobacco Cessation and Spit Tobacco Programs*
Treatment Clinics and Mobile Dental Units

*The most common programs.

message into the community.[26] For additional information on oral health programs, refer to the Resources at the end of the chapter.

As oral health professionals, dental hygienists are educated to incorporate prevention and oral health education into every patient encounter. The dental hygienist in the role of Educator/Health Promoter uses the knowledge of primary preventive measures (e.g., fluorides, sealants, and oral hygiene care) to inform people on how to improve their oral health. Keeping updated on available resources and health education programs for special populations in the community assists the dental hygienist in the roles of Resource Person and Consumer Advocate.

School-Based Oral Health Program

A comprehensive school-based program such as "A Rural School-Based Oral Health Program for South Texas" provides services in the prevention, treatment, and education components. This program was formed as a collaboration with Methodist Healthcare Ministries, University of Texas Health Science Center at San Antonio (UTHSCSA), Texas Department of Health, and two independent school districts and

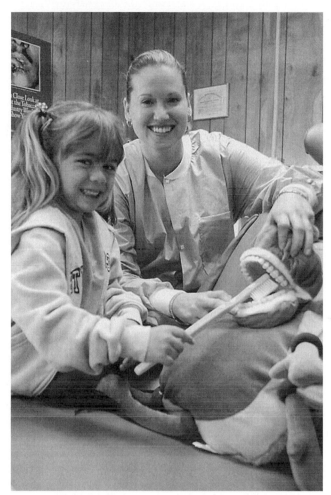

Figure 6-5 Dental hygiene student and first-grader practice oral hygiene skills.

was funded in part through a grant from the Robert Wood Johnson Foundation. The comprehensive model focuses on the prevention, treatment, and education needs of children as they relate to oral health. The prevention component includes annual assessments, sealants, fluoride treatments, mouth guard fabrication for sports, oral hygiene instruction, nutrition, tobacco use, and early intervention programs. The treatment component includes essential services such as emergency, diagnostic, preventive, and restorative care. Referrals are established for children requiring specialty care. Oral health education is being incorporated into the curriculum at the schools. UTHSCSA Dental Hygiene faculty and students are helping to provide the treatment and educational services to children at the school-based health center (Figure 6-5).

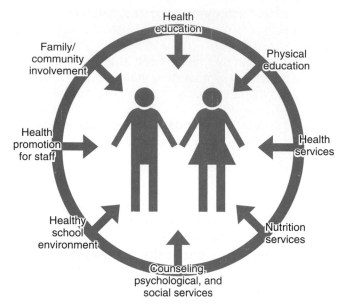

Figure 6-6 Oral health integrated into coordinated school health programs.

The success of a school-based oral health program such as "A Rural School-Based Oral Health Program for South Texas" depends on the integration of the program with other school health programs. The Division of Adolescent and School Health (DASH) has endorsed eight interactive components as essential elements of a coordinated school health program[27] (Figure 6-6). The school can therefore be the facility where families, health care workers, youth organizations, and teachers can interact to maintain the well-being of young people.

SECONDARY AND TERTIARY PREVENTION PROGRAMS

Treatment Component

For better understanding of the impact of public health on dental disease, one must remember that dental diseases are not reversible and are not self-curing. Although primary preventive procedures are very successful in reducing the prevalence and incidence of the major dental diseases, prevention has not been able to eliminate them. Approximately 60% of Americans visit a dental office yearly.[28] Cost is a major reason why people do not see a dentist. People often wait to visit a dentist only in emergencies. Financial barriers and geographic access become reasons why people do not receive primary prevention and are thus in need of secondary or tertiary treatment of dental disease. Therefore, in addition to a preventive component, a treatment component is an essential element of a public oral health program.

Delivery of dental care in public health dental clinics can include fixed dental clinics, which may be run by federal, state, county, city, or private not-for-profit organizations. The practice of clinical dentistry in the public health setting is also accomplished through mobile clinics (vans) or with the use of portable dental equipment (see Chapter 2). Secondary and tertiary levels of prevention include the treatment of dental disease for people of all ages and with diverse backgrounds.

Services for Older Adults

An expanding population in need of both primary prevention and secondary and tertiary care is the elderly in our communities. Between 1990 and 1994, the number of older adults increased 11-fold (from 3 million to 33 million). These people are now the fastest growing segment of the population in the United States. The U.S. Census Bureau projects that the number of persons aged 65 and older will more than double, by the middle of the twenty-first century, to approximately 80 million. In 1994, one in eight Americans were over 65 years of age; by the year 2030, one in five are expected to be in this category.[29]

The elderly not only are living longer but also are keeping their natural teeth; they are therefore in need of dental services and a means to pay for the services. As the income of older people declines with retirement, insurance programs eliminate the dental component for persons older than 70 years, and Medicare does not cover dental services. In the role of Change Agent and Consumer Advocate, dental hygienists can actively participate in supporting legislation to include dental as a component of health care for the elderly.

An example of a program for elderly dental care at reduced cost is the "Apple Tree Geriatric Dental Program." Apple Tree provides both primary educational services along with secondary restorative treatment and tertiary services that include making and fitting partials and dentures. This program began in Minnesota in 1986, when a few dental professionals recognized the problems of access to care in the aging population. The program was initiated in an effort to bring oral health to older adults. The program works with state and local authorities to establish mobile sites and to seek funding sources for dental care. The program has expanded to include patients with special needs, children with disabilities, and indigent families. Apple Tree Programs are located in Minnesota and in North Carolina. More than 95 locations are available where numerous dental professionals provide oral health care to persons with special needs.[30]

With the growing elderly population, it is apparent that there is a need for more community oral health programs similar to Apple Tree and a need for dental professionals to study the social, demographic, health, and economic characteristics of today's elderly citizens.

FINANCING PROGRAMS

The financing of public oral health has gone through transitions during the 1990s and will continue to change in the future. The change, it is hoped, will include expanding services to various population groups.

At present, funding for programs addresses the health issues of women and children and is accomplished through numerous federal initiatives. These public programs are concerned with the health and well-being of pregnant women and children; they not only cut across multiple agencies but also have multiple federal and state funding streams. The private sector and the business community work with state governors on initiatives that strive to improve health status and strengthen families. Public financing programs for oral health care are defined in Table 6-3.[31]

Federal Initiatives

Federal initiatives that provide funding to states for programs addressing women and children's oral health issues include:
- Maternal and Child Health Services Block Grants (Title V)
- Special Supplemental Nutrition Program for Women, Infants, and Children (WIC)
- State Children's Health Insurance Program (S-CHIP) through Title XXI
- Medicaid (Title XIX)
- Administration for Children and Families (ACF)

Table 6-3   Public financing of oral health care

Program	Explanation
• **Medicaid** (funded jointly by federal and state governments)	Comprehensive dental services for children under the Early and Periodic Screening, Diagnosis, and Treatment (EPSDT) program.
• **State Children's Health Insurance Plan** (funded jointly by federal and state governments)	Provides no direct legislative mandate for dental services but supports the inclusion of oral health care in each state's program
• **Medicare** (funded by federal government)	Medical insurance program for the elderly that does not cover dental care except when dental services are directly related to the treatment of the medical condition.
• **Head Start** (funded by federal government)	The dental component of Head Start includes mandated screening and referrals for necessary care. Some programs also provide fluoride treatments and pay for dental care for children who are not covered by Medicaid. All programs require that the children brush their teeth after eating meals provided by Head Start.

Block Grants

Maternal and Child Health Services Block Grants (Title V grants) provide funding to states for the provision of prenatal care for women, primary and preventive care for children, and health and supportive services for children with special health care needs.

Women, Infants, and Children's Program

The Women, Infants, and Children's (WIC) program provides grants for supplement foods, health care referrals, and nutritional education for low-income pregnant, breast-feeding, and non-breast-feeding women in addition to infants and children found to be at nutritional risk.

State Children's Health Insurance Plan

CHIP provides funding through Title XXI grants to develop comprehensive health insurance coverage for children not covered by Medicaid or other third-party health insurance. CHIP can provide for oral health services and traditional medical services.

Medicaid

Medicaid, or Title XIX, is a joint state-federal financed program that is administered by the states to provide medical assistance for the poor. In many states the Medicaid program has ventured into the Managed Care health arena in an effort to reduce health care expenditures while maximizing preventive health measures.

Administration for Children and Families

Administration for Children and Families (ACF), an agency of DHHS, is responsible for 60 programs that provide assistance to needy children and families, including the administration of the Medicaid program. Head Start, another program under ACF administration, serves approximately 900,000 preschool children annually. Head Start provides for medical and oral health screening and treatment of conditions identified for enrolled children. It also includes daily oral hygiene activities and weekly oral health curricula.

The provision of oral health services to individuals who fall outside the eligibility guidelines for entitlement programs such as Medicaid are often addressed through voucher or fee-for-service programs. These may be administered by state health departments, by state dental associations, or through private entities. Many of the fee-for-service programs provide for emergency oral health services for school-aged children. These programs use *nominators*, who are generally school nurses or social workers and are familiar with the economic status of the families seeking services. Although the initiation of the fee-for-service program is generally due to an emergent cause, providers are encouraged to try to meet all of the oral health needs of the patient within the guidelines of the program.

Donated Dental Services Program

The Donated Dental Services (DDS) Program also addresses the oral health needs of medically compromised, permanently disabled, or elderly people. This program is a joint effort of participating dentists, dental laboratories, and coordinating personnel. It provides one-time, comprehensive oral rehabilitation for qualifying individuals. Begun in Colorado, the DDS Program is branching out into other states as participating providers are identified.

SUMMARY

The various community oral health programs introduced in this chapter offer practicing dental hygiene health care professionals an extension of their private practice experience. Becoming acquainted with the oral health care needs of the community at large—in conjunction with an understanding of the available program and funding resources from the local, state, and national levels—provides an opportunity for dental hygienists to have a positive impact on the overall health of their communities. In this manner dental hygienists serve their profession, colleagues, and patients as Educators, Change Agents, and Consumer Advocates, providing leadership and increased understanding of the relationship between oral health and the health of the community as a whole. Additional resources are available at the end of the chapter.

Applying **Your Knowledge**

1. Research and prepare a report on fluoride concentration levels in existing water supply sources in your community.
2. Have a classroom debate on fluoridation. Appoint people to take pro and con positions, and research your position before the debate. Have a mock city council decide the outcome.
3. Develop a community oral health educational program. Write your goal and measurable objectives. Show all stages of development, including assessment, planning, implementing, and evaluating of the program.
4. Discuss how you, as a private practice dental hygienist, might help implement the core essential public health functions and oral health services in your community.
5. Research the possibility of forming an oral health coalition in your community. Whom would you invite to join the organization? Decide on the goals and objectives of the organization.

DENTAL HYGIENE COMPETENCIES

Reading the material in this chapter and participating in the activities of Applying Your Knowledge will contribute to the student's ability to demonstrate the following competencies:

Community involvement

CM.2 Provide screening, referral, and educational services that allow clients to access the resources of the health care system.
CM.3 Provide community oral health services in a variety of settings.
CM.5 Evaluate reimbursement mechanisms and their impact on the patient's or client's access to oral health care.
CM.6 Graduates will be able to evaluate the outcomes of community-based programs and to plan for future activities.

Health promotion

HP.1 Promote the values of oral and general health and wellness to the public and organizations within and outside the profession.
HP.2 Evaluate factors that can be used to promote patient or client adherence to disease prevention and/or health maintenance strategies.

Community Case

The dental hygiene school in your community has received a 3-year grant to establish a school-based dental program that includes prevention, treatment, and education components. You are the newly employed dental hygienist at the school and will supervise dental hygiene students on-site at the elementary school and in the clinic.

1. You will include all of the components necessary in initiating an oral health program.
   The components include all of the following except which one?
   a. Planning
   b. Assurance
   c. Assessment
   d. Evaluation
   e. Implementation
2. The program goal is to improve the oral health of the school-age children. Which objective that you have written for the second-grade class's educational component would be measurable?
   a. The students will understand the meaning of plaque and how to remove it
   b. The students will label the parts of the tooth accurately on a diagram

     c. The students will know how to brush and floss

     d. The students will remember the cause of tooth decay

     e. The students will completely understand the connection of oral health to general health

3. Which preventive program would you support that would have the most benefit for the school-age children?

     a. School fluoride mouth rinse program

     b. School water fluoridation

     c. Fluoride varnish program

     d. Sealant program

     e. Community water fluoridation

4. Which program would be able to provide funding for dental treatment in the school clinic?

     a. Medicaid

     b. Medicare

     c. Head Start

     d. AppleTree Dental

     e. WIC

5. What is the *Healthy People 2010* goal for the percentage of children receiving dental sealants?

     a. 23%

     b. 15%

     c. 50%

     d. 75%

     e. 100%

Resources: *State Oral Health Programs*

Alabama Department of Health
http://www.adph.org/administration/

Alaska Department of Health and Social Services
http://health.hss.state.ak.us/dfys/

Arizona Department of Health Services
http://www.hs.state.az.us/cfhs/ooh/

Arkansas Department of Health
http://www.healthyarkansas.com/Oral_Health/

California Department of Health Services
http://www.dhs.cahwnet.gov/mcs/psd/omds

Colorado Department of Public Health and Environment
http://www.cdphe.state.co.us/pp/oralhealth/OralHealth.htm

Connecticut Department of Public Health
http://www.oralhealth.state.ct.us/

Delaware Health and Social Services
http://www.state.de.us/dhss/dssc/dentaltrns.html

Florida Department of Health
   http://www.doh.state.fl.us/family/dental/
Georgia Division of Public Health and Environment
   http://www.ph.dhr.state.ga.us/programs/oral/index.shtml
Hawaii Department of Health
   http://www.hawaii.gov/health/family-child-health/dental/index.html
Idaho Department of Health and Welfare
   http://www2.state.id.us/dhw/health/des_programs_health.htm#Health%20Promotion
Illinois Department of Public Health
   http://www.idph.state.il.us/about/ohw.htm
Indiana State Department of Health
   http://www.in.gov/isdh/programs/oral/oral.html
Iowa Department of Public Health
   http://www.idph.state.ia.us/ch/oral_health_content/dh.asp
Kansas Department of Health
   http://www.kdhe.state.ks.us/ohi/
Kentucky Department for Public Health
   http://chs.ky.gov/publichealth/dental.htm
Louisiana Department of Health and Hospitals
   http://www.tulane.edu/~oralhlth/oral.htm
Maine Department of Human Services
   http://www.state.me.us/dhs/ddh/index.htm
Maryland Department of Health
   http://www.fha.state.md.us/oralhealth/
Massachusetts Department of Public Health
   http://www.mass.gov/dph/fch/ooh.htm
Michigan Department of Community Health
   http://www.michigan.gov/mdch/
Minnesota Department of Health
   http://www.dhs.state.mn.us
Mississippi Sate Department of Health
   http://www.msdh.state.ms.us/msdhsite/index.cfm/13,1063,151,html
Missouri Department of Health
   http://www.dhss.state.mo.us/CommunityHealthInitiatives/OHPUindex.html
Montana Department of Public Health and Human Services
   http://www.dphhs.state.mt.us/hpsd/pubheal/healsafe/famheal/dental/index.htm
Nebraska Health and Human Services System
   http://www.hhs.state.ne.us/dental/index.htm
Nevada State Health Division
   http://health2k.state.nv.us/oral/
New Hampshire Department of Health and Human Services
   http://www.dhhs.nh.gov/DHHS/ORALHEALTH/
New Jersey Department of Health and Senior Services
   http://www.state.nj.us/health/fhs/oralhlth.htm

New Mexico Department of Health
http://health.state.nm.us

New York State Department of Health
http://www.health.state.ny.us/

North Carolina Department of Health and Human Services
http://www.communityhealth.dhhs.state.nc.us/dental/

North Dakota Department of Health
http://www.ndmch.com/oral-health/

Ohio Department of Health
http://www.odh.state.oh.us/ODHPrograms/ORAL/Oral1.htm

Oklahoma State Department of Health
http://www.health.state.ok.us/program/dental/index.html

Oregon Department of Human Resources
http://www.ohd.hr.state.or.us/dental/index.cfm

Pennsylvania Department of Health
http://www.ohd.hr.state.or.us/dental/index.cfm

Rhode Island Department of Health
http://www.health.state.ri.us/disease/primarycare/oralhealth/home.htm

South Carolina Department of Health and Human Services
http://www.dhhs.state.sc.us

South Dakota Department of Health
http://www.state.sd.us/doh/OralHealth/index.htm

Tennessee Department of Health
http://www2.state.tn.us/health/oralhealth/index.html

Texas Department of Health
http://www.tdh.state.tx.us/dental/

Utah Department of Health
http://health.utah.gov/oralhealth/

Vermont Department of Health
http://www.healthyvermonters.info/hi/dentalhealth/dentalservices.shtml

Virginia Department of Health
http://www.vahealth.org/teeth/index.htm

Washington State Department of Health
http://www.doh.wa.gov/cfh/mch/cahcp/oral_health.htm

West Virginia Department of Health and Human Resources
http://www.wvdhhr.org/mcfh/ICAH/children_dentistry_program.htm

Wisconsin Department of Health and Human Services
http://dhfs.wisconsin.gov/health/Oral_Health/index.htm

Wyoming Department of Health
http://wdh.state.wy.us/main/programs.asp

References

1. Institute of Medicine Committee for the Study of the Future of Public Health, Division of Health Care Services: A Vision of Public Health in America: An Attainable Ideal. In The Future of Public Health. Washington, DC, 1988, National Academy Press.
2. Oral Health in America: A Report of the Surgeon General, Rockville, Md: U.S. Department of Health and Human Services, National Institute of Dental and Craniofacial Research, National Institutes of Health, 2000.
3. Association of State and Territorial Dental Directors: Guidelines for State and Territorial Oral Health Programs, 1997.
4. Washington State Department of Health: Child and Adolescent Health. Available from *http://www.doh.wa.gov/ chf/mch/cahcp/oral_health.htm* (accessed June 2004).
5. Zarkowski P: Community Oral Health Planning and Practice. In Darby M (ed): Comprehensive Review of Dental Hygiene, 5th ed. St. Louis, Mosby, 2002.
6. Turnock BJ: Public Health: What It Is and How It Works. Gaithersburg, Md, Aspen, 1997.
7. Cormier PP, Levy JI: Community Oral Health. New York, Appleton-Century-Crofts, 1981.
8. Mann ML: Planning for community dental programs. In Gluck GM, Morganstein WM (eds): Jong's Community Dental Health, 5th ed. St. Louis, Mosby, 2003.
9. Newbrun E: Effectiveness of water fluoridation. J Public Health Dent 49:279-89, 1989.
10. Centers for Disease Control and Prevention: Achievements in Public Health, 1900-1999: Fluoridation of drinking water to prevent dental caries. MMWR Morb Mortal Wkly Rep 48(41): 933-940, 1999. Available from *http://www.cdc.gov/mmwr/preview/mmwrhtml/mm4841a1. htm* (accessed June 2004).
11. Community and other approaches to promote oral health and prevent diseases. In Oral Health in America: A Report of the Surgeon General. Rockville, Md, U.S. Department of Health and Human Services, National Institute of Dental and Craniofacial Research, National Institutes of Health, 2000.
12. Heller KW, Sohn W, Burt BA, Ecklund SA: Water consumption in the United States in 1994-96 and indications for water fluoridation policy. J Public Health Dent 59:3-11, 1999.
13. Indiana State Department of Health: Oral Health Programs. Available from *http://www.in.gov/isdh/programs/ ora//oral.html* (accessed June 2004).
14. California Department of Health Services: Oral health programs. Available from *http://www.dhs.cahwnet.gov/ mch/psd/omds* (accessed June 2004).
15. Fluoridation Facts: Dietary Fluoride Supplement Schedule, 1994. Available from *http://www.ada.org/consumer/ fluoride/facts/tables.html*
16. Allukian M Jr, Horowitz AM: Effective community prevention programs for oral diseases. In Gluck GM, Morganstein WM (eds): Jong's Community Dental Health, 5th ed. St. Louis, Mosby, 2003.
17. Helfenstein U, Steiner M: Fluoride varnishes (Duraphat): A meta-analysis. Community Dent Oral Epidemiol 22:1-5, 1994.
18. Virginia Department of Health, Division of Dental Health Services. Available from *http://wwwvahealth.org/ teeth/servden.htm* (accessed June 2004).
19. Milgram P, Reisine S: Oral health in the United States: The post-fluoride generation. Annu Rev Public Health 21:403-36, 2000.
20. Horowitz HS: Why I continue to support community water fluoridation. J Public Health Dent 60:67-71, 2000.
21. Healthy People 2010: National Health Promotion and Disease Prevention Objectives. Atlanta, Centers for Disease Control and Prevention, Health Resources and Services Administration, National Institutes of Health, 1999.
22. Healthy Smiles for Wisconsin: Available at *http://www.healthysmilesforwi.org/sealasmile.htm* (accessed August 26, 2000).
23. Gagliardi L: Dental Health Education: Lesson Planning & Implementation. Connecticut, Appleton and Lange, 1999.
24. Centers for Disease Control and Prevention (CDC): Synopsis of State Oral Health Departments. Atlanta, CDC, Association of State and Territorial Dental Directors, 2000.
25. Texas Department of Health: Take Time for Teeth, Division of Oral Health. Available from *http://www.tdh. state.tx/dental/*.

26. Oral Health America: National Spit Tobacco Education Program (NSTEP). Available from *http://www.nstep.org/ .nstep.shtml* (accessed June 2004).

27. Centers for Disease Control and Prevention, Division of Adolescent and School Health (DASH) Coordinated School Health Program. Atlanta: Centers for Disease Control and Prevention, Division of Adolescent and School Health, 2002. Text: *http://www.cdc.gov/HealthyYouth/CHSP/index.htm* Graphic: *http://www.cdc.gov/ HealthyYouth/images/school_health_model.gif.*

28. Center for Disease Control and Prevention: National Center for Health Statistics. Fastats A to Z, updated January 19, 2000. Available from *http://www.cdc.gov/nchs/fastats/dental.html* (accessed June 2004).

29. Hobbs FB: The Elderly Population. U.S. Census Bureau. Available at *http://www.census.gov/population/www/pop-profile/elderpop.html* (accessed June 2004).

30. Apple Tree Dental Program: Available from *http://www.appletreedental.com* (accessed June 2004).

31. Bailit H, Edelstein B, Tinanoff N: Public financing of dental care: Impact and policy implications. J Dent Educ 63:882-886, 1996.

7

Research

Stacy A. Weil, RDH, MS

Objectives

Upon completion of this chapter, the student will be able to:

- Differentiate between the hypothesis and the null hypothesis of a research study
- Explain the importance of the scientific method in research
- Define a population and a sample as related to research
- Discuss sampling techniques and their uses
- Discuss the difference between the independent and dependent variables
- Use the terms *mean, median,* and *mode* to express the results of data collection
- Define the terms *continuous* and *discrete data* and their respective scales of measurement
- Discuss the uses of various statistical techniques
- Use different types of displays to exhibit data
- Explain the difference between type I and type II errors
- Define probability and statistical significance
- Express the importance of evaluating dental literature
- Explain the criteria for reviewing scientific literature
- Review a scientific journal article relating to dentistry

Key Terms

Hypothesis	Calibrated	Reliability
Null Hypothesis	Validity	Interrater Reliability

Intrarater Reliability

Population

Parameter

Target Population

Sample

Statistic

Pilot Study

Random Sampling

Stratified Sampling

Systematic Sampling

Purposive (Judgmental) Sampling

Convenience Sampling

Experimental Group

Control Group

Independent Variable

Variable

Dependent Variable

Data

Discrete Data

Continuous Data

Nominal

Ordinal

Interval

Ratio

Descriptive Statistics

Inferential Statistics

Mean

Median

Mode

Range

Variance

Standard Deviation (SD)

Correlation

Parametric

Normal Distribution

t-Test

Analysis of Variance (ANOVA)

Nonparametric

Chi-Squared Test

Power Analysis

P Value

Type I alpha (α) Error

Type II beta (β) Error

Refereed

Abstract

OPENING STATEMENT

Questions in Research

- How does a public health team decide that fluoridation in a community's water supply will reduce the incidence of new carious lesions?

- Exactly how much fluoride is required to add to the water to achieve a therapeutic effect without a toxic reaction?

- How would officials determine that dental hygienists might improve the quality of life in older people if they were able to work independently in extended-care facilities?

- How do communities decide to spend money on a program providing dental care to individuals with human immunodeficiency virus (HIV) infection instead of to children with special disabilities?

- Where can dental hygienists readily find employment, and what salary can they expect to earn?

QUESTIONS AND ANSWERS IN RESEARCH

Although dental hygienists may seek the answers to the questions in the Opening Statement, patients may have other concerns, for example:

- Does a particular mouth rinse really reduce plaque buildup?
- Which brand of toothpaste is best?
- Can nonsurgical periodontal therapy provide results comparable to those of a surgical procedure?

Even though students may commonly learn the answers to these questions from instructors or colleagues, it is important to understand where to find reliable answers to these questions independently and to understand the process that provides these answers.

Research via the scientific method is the basis from which these answers are produced. Manuscripts published in reputable scientific journals disseminate the results of independent research. To determine whether the information contained therein is indeed reliable and valid, certain knowledge and skills must be a part of the repertoire of every competent dental hygienist practicing in the dental community. This chapter provides a basic outline of what research entails and a method of evaluating the results of that research.

THE SCIENTIFIC METHOD AND DEVELOPMENT OF A RESEARCH PROBLEM

Understanding the basics of research entails gaining an appreciation for the components of a good research study, that is, understanding how a research idea is formulated, how a study is designed and executed, and how the resulting data are critically evaluated so that one can infer appropriate conclusions. Research can be thought of as a search for truth and the knowledge gained from this search. A true definition of research is a systematic inquiry that uses orderly scientific methods to answer questions or solve problems.[1]

The discoveries provided by research may lead to new knowledge or to the revision of existing knowledge. Dental research involves a systematic search for knowledge about issues relevant to the profession. To increase the chance that research will be valid, reliable, and relevant, the *scientific method*—a series of logical steps starting with the formulation of a problem—is employed (Box 7-1).

Formulation of a Problem (Asking the Question)

The first step in beginning a research study is the formulation of an idea. The idea is usually formed from a question that has been raised by a researcher. The question may arise from a very simple observation or thought. For example, during the clinical phase of dental hygiene education, participants might debate about the following:

1. Which areas of the mouth are most difficult to probe accurately?
2. What are the effects of diet on periodontal disease?

BOX 7-1   THE SCIENTIFIC METHOD

- Formulation of a problem (asking the question)
- Formulation of a hypothesis (a proposed answer to the question)
- Collecting the data (finding existing information related to the question as well as gathering of your own information)
- Analysis and interpretation of the results
- Presentation of the results
- Formulation of conclusion (relationship of results to hypothesis)

3. How can adequate oral health care be maintained by physically and mentally challenged people?

From simple notions such as these, a research question or problem can be formulated.

Examples of a research problem formulated from the previous questions might be as follows:

1. Which quadrant in the human dentition is least accurately probed by the second-year dental hygiene student at University X when using the Periodontal Screening Record (PSR) method of probing?
2. What is the percentage of calories from carbohydrates in the diet of patients exhibiting class II periodontal disease?
3. What effect does modifying the brushing techniques of disabled patients in long-term care facilities have on the gingival bleeding index of these patients?

The research problem should be kept as simple and concise as possible. A successful study often depends on an uncomplicated research design, which results from simple questions.

Formulation of a Hypothesis (a Proposed Answer to the Question)

After a research question is formulated, the next step is the development of a **hypothesis,** a statement that reflects the research question. The hypothesis is stated in positive terms that represent the researcher's prediction or opinion. An example of a hypothesis for the question "Which quadrant in the human dentition is least accurately probed by the second-year dental hygiene student at X University when using the PSR method of probing?" would be as follows: Second-year dental hygiene students at University X using the PSR method are most inaccurate when probing the distal lingual surface of teeth in the upper right quadrant of the mouth.

The research statement is often expressed as a **null hypothesis,** which assumes that there is no statistically significant difference between the groups being studied. An example of a null hypothesis for the preceding question would be as follows:

Second-year dental hygiene students at University X show no difference in the accuracy of probing any tooth in the mouth when using the PSR method.

Once the hypothesis has been formed, data can be collected to prove or disprove the statement.

Collecting Data (Finding Existing Information and Gathering Information Independently)

After a research idea and a hypothesis are initially identified, the relevant available literature is reviewed. By examining an area of general interest, the researcher may be inspired to create a research question to resolve unknown or unexplained portions of the area of interest. Alternatively, when a general topic has been selected, a literature review may help to bring the topic into sharper focus. Emulating the accepted research designs that have been previously validated by others, the researcher can then design a study to evaluate the idea. Analysis of the literature is described later in this chapter.

After review and analysis of the available literature, the researcher can plan how the study will be conducted and how the data will be collected. Many different techniques can be used to collect data (see Chapter 3). During data collection, it is important to use **calibrated** instruments that are both valid and reliable. When examiners are involved in data collection, it is imperative that they be calibrated (i.e., in agreement with a set standard of performance for the data collection). For example, if one examiner notes caries on the occlusal surface of a first molar, a second examiner should also be able to note caries on the occlusal surface of the same first molar.

Validity is concerned with gathering data that have been intended to be collected. For example, if two calibrated dentists are examining children for occlusal caries on first molars, both dentists must examine and record caries only on the occlusal surfaces and only on first molars. They are examining the correct surfaces and collecting data that were intended to be collected.

Reliability refers to the consistency and stability of the data. The data are reliable if the examiners are calibrated and can reproduce the results. Both examiners must find the same three occlusal caries on first molars in child No. 1. If they examine child No. 1 an hour later, they should still find the same three occlusal caries as detected previously.

Interrater reliability refers to two or more examiners being in agreement with their findings. **Intrarater reliability** refers to one examiner being consistent with the findings previously recorded by the same examiner.

In developing the plan for conducting the study, it is important to identify the characteristics of the group involved in the study. Group characteristics are defined by such terms as population, sample, experimental, and control. The term *data*, or information, collected from the study group is defined and used in different ways. These terms and their relationship to the collection of research data are explained next.

Population and Sampling

Population

Population can be defined as the entire group or whole unit of individuals having similar characteristics from which the results of an investigation can be inferred.[2] In regard to numeric characteristics of the population, the term **parameter** is used.

Populations can be very large or very small, depending on the topic to be studied. For example, in the first research question (which quadrant in the human dentition is least accurately probed by second-year dental hygiene students at University X using the PSR method of probing?), one can infer that the total population consists of second-year dental hygiene students. It would be optimal to examine each of these students to arrive at the answer. The second-year dental hygiene students are also known as the **target population,** or the population from whom the information is being collected. Because of time constraints, lack of resources, or financial issues, however, it may be decided that a smaller group within this group can provide the researchers with a significant result.

Sampling

Taking a portion of the population is known as *sampling*. A **sample** is a portion or subset of the entire population that, if properly selected, can provide meaningful information about the entire population. When one is discussing numeric characteristics of samples, the term **statistic** is used.

Samples can be large or small and are chosen to most appropriately reflect the research being done. A large sample usually provides the most accurate representation of the population and increases the exactness and accuracy of the data collected. Occasionally a small sample may be used, as in the case of data collection for a **pilot study,** or trial run, done in preparation for a major study.

The importance of using a sample becomes obvious in regard to our research question. Suppose there is an urgent need to refine teaching techniques for probing and there is not enough time to adequately assess each second-year dental hygiene student's probing at University X. The researcher may thus decide to use only a portion, or sample, of the first-year class.

If it is decided that a sample of the population is to be used, different techniques are used to choose the sample. There are several types of sampling.

Random sampling. The method of sampling that provides the most external validity, or degree to which the results of the study can be generalized to settings other than the one included, is called **random sampling**. This method provides a sample in which each member of a population has an equal chance of being included and is the procedure of choice because it prevents the possibility of selection bias by the researcher.

As an example, assume that all second-year dental hygiene students at University X have been given a number. There are 50 students in the second-year class, and it is determined that a sample of 10 students will participate in the research. Numbers 1 to 50 would be written on separate slips of paper and placed in a container. From the container a number is drawn. The number is noted as one of the 10 students to be used in this sample. That number is then placed back in the container, and another selection is made until the list of 10 numbers is complete. The importance of placing each number selected back into the container is to preserve a true random selection from 50 numbers. Numbers that are drawn more than once are put on the list only once and are again placed back in the container.

Stratified sampling. What if probing discrepancies are unique to the university's dental hygiene program? A random sample may not accurately assess the problem for all second-year dental hygiene students; it may be necessary to include students from other universities as well in a method called stratified sampling. Subdivisions of a population with similar characteristics, such as second-year dental hygiene students attending different dental hygiene programs, are called strata. The random selection of subjects from two or more strata of the population is another way of defining stratified sampling.

Systematic sampling. Another form of sampling, **systematic sampling,** involves the selection of subjects by including every nth person in a list. For example, if a researcher had a list of second-year dental hygiene students by number and chose every odd-numbered person, he or she would be sampling the population systematically. In this case, unless the list is in random order, not every person may have an equal or random chance of being selected; thus systematic sampling may not be considered a true random sample.

Purposive (judgmental) sampling. If an instructor who most often works with students who are learning probing techniques chooses the sample, it is easy to imagine that a great deal of bias may be introduced into the study. **Purposive,** or **judgmental, sampling** provides a sample, through personal judgment, of subjects who would be most representative of the population.

Convenience sampling. A convenience sample may also introduce bias. Selection of a sample through **convenience sampling** provides a group of individuals who are most readily available to be subjects in the study. For example, a researcher conducting the probing study might enroll only individuals from the researcher's university as subjects.

Experimental and Control Groups and Variables

Experimental and control groups

After the sample population is selected, subjects may be divided randomly into experimental and control groups, which are used to answer a research question posed when an experimental treatment or manipulation is imposed on the research setting. The **experimental group** is the sample group in a study that receives the experimental treatment or intervention. The **control group** is the group in a study that does not receive the experimental treatment or intervention. The control group provides the baseline against which the effects of the intervention on the experimental group can be measured.

For example, let us assume that the study on probing accuracy did find an area of the mouth where inaccuracy predominated. At this point, one might chose to conduct another research study, introducing a new method of probing instruction that would focus on the area of the mouth where most inaccuracies occur. This new method of teaching would be administered to the experimental group, whereas the control group would continue to receive the traditional method of instruction.

Variables

The experimental treatment or intervention that is imposed on the experimental group can also be called the **independent variable.** A **variable** is a characteristic or concept that varies, or is different, within the population under study. The independent variable is controlled or manipulated by the researcher and is believed to cause or influence the **dependent variable.** The dependent variable is thought to depend on or to be caused by the independent variable. It is the outcome variable of interest.

In the case of the research question, which involves teaching a new probing technique to the experimental group, the dependent variable would be probing accuracy. The independent variable would be the probing technique that is being taught. Other variables not related to the purpose of the study are *uncontrolled* variables and may influence the relationship between the independent and dependent variable. To increase *internal validity,* it is important to control for extraneous variables. *Internal validity* refers to the fact that it is the experimental treatment or independent variable that is responsible for the observed effects and that these effects are not due to extraneous variables. A good research study controls for extraneous variables through research design or through statistical procedures.[3] By understanding the previous terms and definitions, one can implement a method of data collection, or the gathering of information, to address a research problem.

Data

Pieces of information, such as numbers collected from measurements and counts obtained during the course of a research study, are known as **data.** Although the concept of data itself may seem fairly straightforward, there are actually several different types of data and ways to measure data:

1. **Discrete data** have only one of a limited set of values and are counted only in whole numbers. Discrete variables may include things like hair color, gender, political preference, and number totals, such as how many times a person brushes his or her teeth or the number of decayed, missing, or filled teeth. These data are considered to be *qualitative* in nature.
2. **Continuous data** are measurements made from a particular value within a defined range. Variables along a continuum, such as temperature, scores on a test, and time, are continuous data. These data are considered to be *quantitative* in nature.

Different scales of measurement are used for discrete and continuous data. Discrete data can use nominal or ordinal scales of measurement. Continuous data use interval and ratio scales of measurements.

Nominal scales of measurement consist of named categories with no order. For example, females may be placed in category A and males in category B.

Ordinal scales of measurement consist of categories of variables in which the categories are in order but there is no equal or defined distance between them. For example, cancer staging for tumors is grouped into four stages designated by Roman numerals I to IV. In general, stage I cancers are small localized cancers that are usually curable, while stage IV usually represents inoperable or metastatic cancer. Stage II and III cancers are usually locally advanced and/or with involvement of local lymph nodes. It is known that type II is worse than type I and that type III is worse than type II, but each type of cancer is slightly different, making it difficult to define precisely for all cancers.[4]

Interval scales of measurement have equal distance between variables, but there is no true zero point (i.e., temperature on a Fahrenheit thermometer).

Ratio scales of measurement have equal intervals between the variables, but there is a meaningful zero point (i.e., height and weight).

As listed next, each scale of measurement takes on the characteristics of the previous one, making ratio the most powerful measurement:

Nominal: named categories only

Ordinal: same as nominal plus categories are in order

Interval: same as ordinal plus equal intervals between categories

Ratio: same as interval plus meaningful or true zero point

After the data have been collected from a chosen population and variables have been defined and measured, it is time to proceed to the next step of the scientific method, presenting and interpreting the data and presenting the results.

Data Analysis and Presentation of Results

Statistics

Statistics is a science that provides a way of processing numbers or analyzing the data that have been collected. Statistics may be used to describe, analyze, and interpret the numbers collected in the data. The purpose of statistical analysis is to make an inference or an assumption about a population.[5] Two types of relevant statistics are as follows:

1. **Descriptive statistics** are used to describe and summarize data. Their objective is to communicate results, without generalizing beyond the sample, to any population. Some ways in which results are communicated are through (a) *measures of central tendency* (mean, median, mode) and (b) *measures of dispersion*.
2. **Inferential statistics** (see later) are used to apply information from the sample to a larger population.

Measures of Central Tendency

Measures of central tendency are used to describe the sample based on the data gathered. They include components such as the mean, median, and mode.

The **mean** is the average of the group. It is a sum of all the values divided by the number (n) of items and is statistically noted as $\bar{x}$. The mean is calculated in the following manner:

$$\text{mean} = \frac{\Sigma \bar{x}}{n}$$

The positive aspect of the mean is that it includes the value of each score; the negative aspect is that it can be affected by any extreme scores and may not give a true average. For example, a test is administered; 10 people in the class score an 85 and 2 people score a 30. The class average becomes approximately 76, which is not a true representation of the class scores.

The **median** represents the exact middle score or value in an ordered distribution of scores; it is the point above and below which 50% of the scores lie. When the total number of scores is even, the sum of the two middle scores, divided by 2, provides the median.

Unlike the mean, extreme scores do not affect the median. In the previous example, the median score would be 85. However, it is not difficult to imagine what would happen if scores were not evenly distributed and the median were used as an example of the middle score. The information provided in this case may not demonstrate a true midpoint for the class.

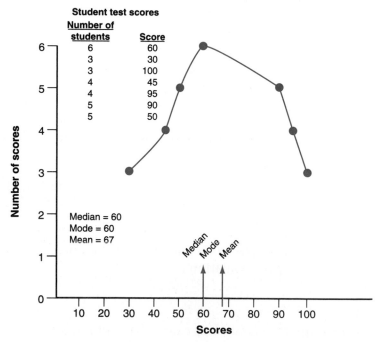

Figure 7-1 Graph of student test scores.

The **mode** is the score or value that occurs most frequently in a distribution of scores. Once again, the mode for the preceding example would be 85. The distribution of scores may be unimodal, bimodal, or multimodal, or there may even be no mode.

Figure 7-1 presents the mean, median, and mode of a group of test scores. Figure 7-2 illustrates a symmetric distribution in which the mean, median, and mode are the same; it also shows skewed curves, where the mean and median are located to the left and right of the mode.

Measures of Dispersion

In addition to the measures of central tendency (mean, median, and mode), measures of dispersion (also known as measures of variation) may also be used to describe data. Measures of central tendency provide a first step in the measure

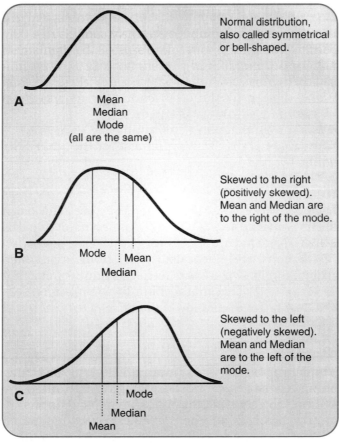

Figure 7-2 **A-C,** Graphing measures of central tendency.

of distributions. Occasionally, however, a measurement is also desired to determine how far scores differ from the mean.

The most obvious way of measuring the dispersion of data is the **range,** which measures the difference between the highest and lowest values in a distribution of scores. If the median is defined as the point where 50% of the scores are lower and 50% of the scores are higher, the location of the 0 and 100th percentile would define the range. More commonly, the value of the range is used to define the 5th and 95th percentiles. These are the points that 5% of the subjects may be below or 95% of the people may be below. If a person has taken a test and is in the 95th percentile, 95% of the people have scored lower than that person has.

Another measure of dispersion, called **variance,** is a method of ascertaining the way individual variables are located around the mean. Variance is most often used to measure interval and ratio variables.

A first step in the calculation of variance is to determine the average deviation, which can be derived through calculating the difference between each point of data and the mean, adding the answers together, and dividing by the total amount of data points. The main problem with calculating the average difference is that there are as many negative data points as positive; this situation ultimately results in an answer of zero.

A way around this problem is to square each data point so that all terms are positive. Therefore the difference between each data point and the mean squared, summed, and divided by the total amount of data points results in the average squared deviation, also known as variance.

Variance is simply a step in determining the **standard deviation (SD)** and is equal to the square of the SD. The formula for the SD is as follows:

$$SD = \sqrt{\frac{\text{sum of (data point - mean)}^2}{\text{No of values}}}$$

It makes sense, then, that the farther away the data points are from the mean, the greater the variance and SD. Box 7-2 presents the calculations to find the range, variance, and SD of student test scores.

Box 7-3 demonstrates the calculations from data collected in a community research project involving unwed teenaged mothers and their knowledge of baby bottle tooth decay. Twelve mothers are in this study group. The mothers' scores from the pretest range from a low score of 25% to a high score of 70%.

Correlation

After we determine the previous information about our data, we may want to next determine whether any **correlation** exists between the variables. Correlation is a statistical method for determining whether a variation in one variable may be related to a variation in another variable. For example, height and weight often show a correlation, because taller people usually have a higher weight than shorter people. Age and periodontal disease may have a correlation, because older people may have higher incidence of periodontal disease than younger people.

Box 7-2 RANGE, VARIANCE, STANDARD DEVIATION OF STUDENT TEST SCORES

Student test scores

Number of students	Score
6	60
3	30
3	100
4	45
4	95
5	90
5	50

Range is the difference between highest and lowest score: $100 - 30 = 70$.
Variance is the average deviation or spread of scores around the mean.
The variance is calculated as (individual score – mean)^2/# of scores.
$(60 - 67)^2 = 49$
$(30 - 67)^2 = 1369$
$(100 - 67)^2 = 1089$
$(45 - 67)^2 = 484$
$(95 - 67)^2 = 784$
$(90 - 67)^2 = 529$
$(50 - 67)^2 = 289$
49×6 (# of scores of 60) = 294
1369×3 (# of scores of 30) = 4107
1089×3 (# of scores of 100) = 3267
484×4 (# of scores of 45) = 1936
784×4 (# of scores of 95) = 3136
529×5 (# of scores of 90) = 2645
289×5 (# of scores of 50) = 1445

All above summed = 16,830

$16830 \div 30$ (total number of scores) = 561
561 is the variance
Standard deviation is the positive square root of the variance: $\sqrt{561}$
The square root of 561 = 23.7 (standard deviation)

The technique used to determine correlation depends on the type of variable being explored. Different techniques are used for discrete or continuous variables. The measurement scale may also influence the technique. For example, nominal, ordinal, interval, and ratio scales of measurement are all calculated slightly differently.

The results of the calculation for correlation show either a negative or positive relationship. When the relationship is *positive,* it is predicted that as the value of one variable increases, the other also increases. Perfect positive correlation is shown by +1.0. An example would be the finding that, in the research with unwed

Box 7-3   Calculations of test scores on baby bottle tooth decay

Subject (mother)	Score	
1	45	
2	45	
3	45	
4	30	
5	35	Median = 45%
6	25	Mode = 45%
7	40	Mean = 48%
8	50	
9	60	Range = 70 – 25
10	65	= 45
11	70	Variance = $\dfrac{\text{sum of (individual scores – mean)}^2}{\text{\# of scores}}$
12	70	= 210
		Standard deviation = $\sqrt{210}$ = 14

mothers, the more time the examiner spends with them on patient education, the greater the increase in the mothers' knowledge. Table 7-1 presents a correlation of increased education with increased knowledge. Figure 7-3 demonstrates a graphic display of the same positive correlation of the two variables.

In contrast, a *negative* correlation shows an inverse relationship between variables. Perfect negative correlation is shown by –1.0. Figure 7-4 shows that a diet including six servings of fruits and vegetables each day *decreases* the incidence of certain cancers.

In review, a perfect positive correlation is noted as +1.0 and a perfect negative correlation showing an inverse relationship is noted as –1.0 Although a perfect positive or perfect negative correlation may occur, it may be possible to find no relationship at all; this instance is noted as 0.0. Some literature states that generally

Table **7-1**   Correlation of test scores and hours of education

Group Number	Group Type and Pretest Scores	Hours of Education	Average Post-Test Score Increase (Points) %
1	Four mothers with an average pretest score of 50	2	60
2	Four mothers with an average pretest score of 50	4	70
3	Four mothers with an average pretest score of 50	6	80
4	Four mothers with an average pretest score of 50	8	90

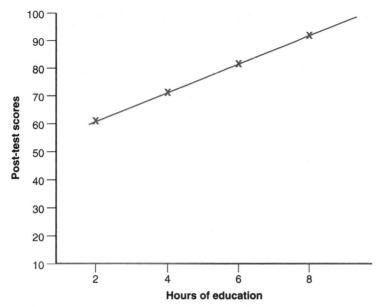

Figure 7-3 Post-test scores and hours of education (positive correlation).

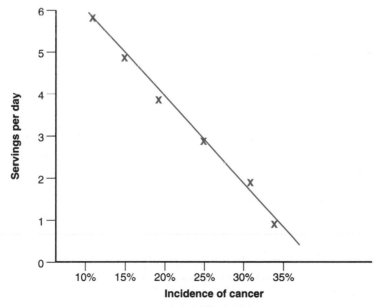

Figure 7-4 Number of fruit and vegetable servings per day related to percent incidence of cancer (negative correlation).

a correlation coefficient above .70 is considered satisfactory.[1] In each study the nature of the variables and the numbers involved in the comparison must also be considered along with the correlation coefficient in determining what is a significant relationship. The closer the relationship is to +1.0 or –1.0, the more perfect, or stronger, the correlation.

Presentation of the Data

In addition to the data displayed in the previous graphs, other types of data display include the following:

A *bar graph* is most often used to display nominal or ordinal data that are discrete in nature. With the use of data that may be gathered from the study on teenaged mothers and baby bottle tooth decay, one can create a bar graph to present the data pictorially (Figure 7-5).

A *frequency polygon* is used to represent data that are continuous in nature. An example from the study with teenaged mothers is depicted in Figure 7-6. The figure contains dots connected to straight lines to present the frequency distribution of the data. In this case the frequency polygon demonstrates how many times per week the mothers brush their children's teeth.

A *histogram,* although a type of bar graph, is used most often to represent interval or ratio scaled variables that are continuous in nature (Figure 7-7). The bars in a histogram are of equal width and touch each other to indicate that the data are being presented on a continuum.

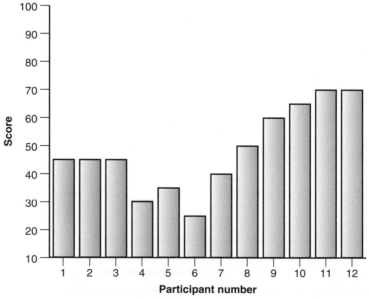

Figure 7-5 Pretest scores of 12 participants as shown in a bar graph.

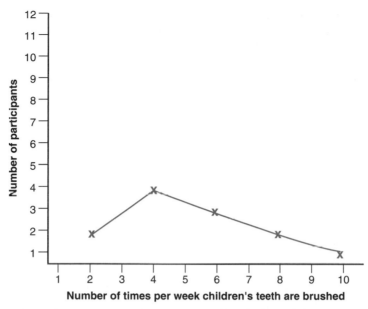

Figure 7-6 Number of times per week participants brush their children's teeth as shown in a frequency polygon.

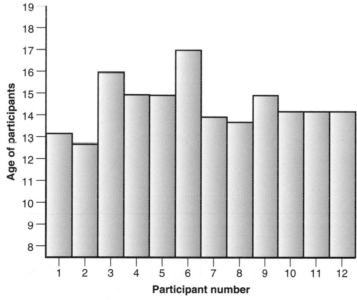

Figure 7-7 Age of 12 participants in the research study as shown in a histogram.

Inferential Statistics

In addition to including descriptive techniques to describe data, inferential statistics may also be used. Whereas descriptive statistics are used to determine information only about the sample being studied, inferential statistics seek to determine a generalization between the sample studied and the actual population. The larger the sample size, therefore, the greater the number of generalizations that can be made regarding the population. Depending on the type of data collected, the use of inferential statistics may include either parametric or nonparametric statistical techniques. Inferential statistics are based on the assumption that sampling is conducted randomly, although that is not always the case.

Parametric Inferential Statistics

Parametric statistics are used when the data include interval or ratio scales of measurement. Parametric techniques work best when the sample is large and randomized and the population from which the sample is taken is normally distributed. In a normal distribution, 50% of the values lie on the left half of the distribution, and 50% lie on the right half. A **normal distribution** assumes that approximately 68% of the population fall within one SD of the mean, approximately 95% fall within two SDs of the mean, and 99% lie within three SDs from the mean.[6] The plotting of these data on a graph results in a bell-shaped curve (Figure 7-8).

t-Test

Parametric statistics are calculated by means of several different methods or tests. One of the most common is the **t-test,** or Student's *t*-test, so named for the man responsible for development of this technique. The *t*-test is used to analyze the difference between two means. It provides the researcher with the difference between treatment and control groups or groups receiving treatment A versus treatment B.

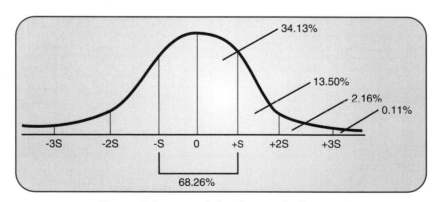

Figure 7-8 Normal distribution (bell curve).

When the test is used on a single group that yields pretreatment and post-treatment scores, it is known as a *t*-test for *dependent samples*. This test analyzes data when only one independent variable is tested. For example, a researcher may want to examine the difference in blood glucose levels of diabetic subjects before and after treatment with a new diet. Assuming that all of the subjects were the same age and had the same degree of disease present, the *t*-test for dependent samples can be used to determine pretreatment and post-treatment scores.

The *independent t*-test determines differences in the mean between two independent groups such as an experimental and control group or males versus females. This test is used when only one or two independent variables are tested. Most often, data involving interval or ratio scales of measurement are statistically analyzed with an independent *t*-test. For example, a study might investigate the effect of a new toothbrushing method on gingivitis. The subjects would be randomized into two groups: (1) a *control* group receiving no instruction and asked to use their normal brushing method and (2) an *experimental* group asked to practice a new method of toothbrushing. The instrument may be a gingival bleeding index that is conducted before the start of the study and again 8 weeks later. The hypothesis is that the new method of toothbrushing will decrease the gingival bleeding index of patients with gingivitis.

Analysis of variance (ANOVA)

Another commonly used test for parametrics is **analysis of variance,** or **ANOVA.** This test allows comparison among more than two sample means and compares interactions among the variability in the multiple sample groups with the variability within the groups.

A simple example is the comparison of the many brands of desensitizing toothpaste. Five brands of toothpaste that claim relief of tooth pain caused by sensitivity have been located. A group of subjects is assembled, and each subject is given a different toothpaste disguised in a plain white tube. Each subject is asked to use this tube and is given other tubes to use until all of the various toothpastes are used. Subjects are asked to rank pain relief from tooth sensitivity on a numeric scale of 1 to 10 for each toothpaste used. The scale may look like the one in Table 7-2.

Table 7-2   Data used in analysis of variance (ANOVA) testing

Patient Number	TP-1	TP-2	TP-3	TP-4	TP-5
1	6.0	5.0	4.0	5.0	2.0
2	5.0	5.0	3.0	4.0	3.0
3	7.0	5.0	4.0	5.0	3.0
4	5.0	4.0	4.0	3.0	4.0
5	6.0	5.0	5.0	4.0	4.0

TP, Toothpaste brands 1 to 5.
Key: 1.0 10 − pain relief (10 is maximum relief).

ANOVA allows the dental hygienist to compare each toothpaste used and the pain relief experienced by the patients. It also allows a comparison of the different responses from each patient for each individual toothpaste brand. ANOVA may yield information about which of the brands is actually more effective and how each brand compares with another. In essence, ANOVA compares variability *within* groups with variability *between* groups.

The *t*-test, or Student's *t*-test, and ANOVA are just two of many tests that may be used in statistical analysis of data. These tests are perhaps the most common parametric inferential statistical techniques.

No matter which technique is chosen, the sample should be randomly and independently selected from normal populations. Although these tests provide more detailed information of the interaction of variables, the research should include means and SDs in the report for accurate assessment of the tests' magnitude.

Nonparametric Inferential Statistics

Besides parametric tests, **nonparametric** inferential statistical techniques may be selected. Nonparametric techniques are most useful for data to be measured on the nominal or ordinal scale. Remember, nominal or ordinal data are "qualitative," and although numbers may be included, these numbers are derived more subjectively than numbers associated with quantitative data. Nonparametric tests involve fewer assumptions about the population. The sample size may be small, and variables are discrete.

The most commonly used nonparametric test is the **chi-squared test.** This test may be used to analyze questionnaire data and to determine whether a relationship exists between two variables. The chi-squared test is used to examine the differences between observed and expected frequencies.

Determining Statistical Significance

Statistical tests provide researchers with an idea of what the data they have collected say about the sample and perhaps what the data imply about the population from which the sample was drawn. An important factor in research is determining the statistical significance of the data. Statistical significance is a way of indicating that the results found in an analysis of data are unlikely to have been caused by chance; more likely, the results have been caused by the independent variable. Using too small or too large a sample may influence the statistical significance. Typically, the use of too small a sample (less than 30) provides too little information to make generalizations about the populations and to create any significance of results.

Power analysis

Determining how many subjects are needed to provide significance is called a **power analysis,** which is calculated according to a specific statistical formula based on what the researcher hopes to observe in most of the subjects. The *power* of a study, or its ability to detect relationships among variables, is directly related to sample size, the definition of the independent variable, and the precision with which the study is planned and conducted.[7] When too large a sample is used, the effects may be statistically significant but clinically of no consequence.

The true importance of determining statistical significance is that the greater the significance, the more statistical inference can be made regarding the population from whom the sample was taken. That is, statistical significance reinforces our ability to generalize the conclusions we make about our study population to a larger population, perhaps even to the "general population."

A major issue in regard to statistical inferences is that every measurement taken from the sample being researched has some degree of error. Researchers may describe the possibility of error or lack of error in various ways.

Confidence intervals

The term *confidence interval* refers to how researchers describe the probability of the statistical results being correct. A confidence interval indicates a range of values within which the parameters of the population have a probability of lying. Researchers usually use a 95% to 99% confidence interval. A 95% confidence interval indicates a probability that the researcher is wrong 5 times in 100. By using a 99% confidence interval, the researcher may be wrong 1% of the time; however, increasing the confidence interval also decreases the specificity of the data. Therefore, when the confidence interval is 95%, there is a 5% chance that the observed results or differences between study and control groups are due purely to chance and not a true difference caused by the independent variable.

P values

Researchers also use **P values** to describe statistical significance. The *P* value states how likely it is that the study could have come to a false scientific conclusion. *P* values are calculated according to the sample size, the difference between the means of the control and experimental group, and the SD of the distribution. The smaller the *P* value, the more significant the findings of the study are considered.

A normally acceptable *P* value is $P < .05$. Results with a *P* value at less than .05 are generally considered statistically significant and provide the basis for rejection of the null hypothesis. $P < .05$ means that the results were due to chance only 5 times in 100. *P* values of approximately .01, .001, and lower increase the significance of the study.

Formulation of a Conclusion and Relationship of Results to the Hypothesis

Based on the statistical results of the data analysis, the researcher determines whether the study shows significance. Whether it shows much, little, or no significance, a conclusion can be formulated. From the results discovered, the researcher decides

Table 7-3   **Null hypothesis**

Null Hypothesis Is Actually...	Null Hypothesis Is Accepted	Null Hypothesis Is Not Accepted
True	No error	Type I α (alpha) error
False	Type II β (beta) error	No error

to either accept or reject the null hypothesis of the study. Occasionally, when formulating a conclusion, a researcher may make an error. Errors within research are of two types:

Type I alpha (α) errors occur when, according to statistical results, the researcher rejects the null hypothesis when it is true. The researcher's conclusion states that a relationship exists when it does not. Most statistical analyses use an α level of .05, which means that there is a 1 in 20 chance that a conclusion will state that a difference exists when there is no difference.

Type II beta (β) errors occur when the null hypothesis is accepted but is actually false. The conclusion states that no relationship exists when one actually does (Table 7-3).

ANALYSIS OF THE LITERATURE

A thorough review of the literature is often completed to begin development of an adequate plan for collecting the data. Being informed and up to date not only are professional responsibilities but also serve a purpose in each of the six contemporary roles of the dental hygienist: Clinician, Educator, Manager, Change Agent, Consumer Advocate, and Researcher.[8] The assimilation of information requires more than listening to colleagues and attending occasional Continuing Education programs. An excellent source of information is dental and other scientific literature.

A literature analysis, besides helping the dental hygienist to develop a data collection plan, provides valuable information about theories, methods, and products that are available. Reviewing the literature is an important step in remaining current within the field of dentistry and provides information used to intelligently answer many questions posed by patients. Scientific literature contains information that can help one to maintain competency and helps to set the exceptional practitioner apart from others in the field of dentistry.

Not all dental hygienists receive regular subscriptions to scientific magazines or have access to Internet services. Although these are the most common ways to obtain information about literature, a trip to a local library with a scientific collection can provide essential information. Becoming skillful at obtaining scientific information is not as easy as might be expected. However, it is a skill worth cultivating because it provides a valuable tool for researchers and for practicing dental hygienists.

The topic described next presents an overview of what is available in the form of written resources, how to choose the best sources of this information, and how to critically review this literature. Although a critical analysis of the scientific literature is ideal, it is best to remain open-minded when inquiring about new products, services, and techniques.[9]

Finally, keeping focused on the research or specific information to be reviewed should help to provide simple yet intelligent answers to the question at hand.

Selection of Literature

To begin a literature review, the dental hygienist or researcher must select appropriate journals. The scientific writing to be reviewed should be comprehensible to the average dental hygienist who is knowledgeable about the topic area. The selection of literature that is pertinent to the field of dental hygiene will allow the researcher to obtain a complete understanding of the research topic while focusing the research on issues important to dental hygiene. Because of the technicality and intricate scientific detail of its topics, the *Journal of Biochemical Research* might not be an ideal place to start looking for information on periodontal host factors, whereas the *Journal of Periodontology* and *Journal of Dental Hygiene* might be preferable choices. Although both journals publish in-depth scientific literature, the material is tailored to the dental field and thus is relevant and understandable to the average oral health researcher.

Equally important is the selection of a reputable journal. Several aspects lend credibility to a reputable source, including an editorial review board that evaluates each contributed article for accuracy, relevancy of content, and issues involving style and method of scientific writing. This is also known as a **"refereed,"** or a *"peer-reviewed"* journal. Individuals who are considered experts on the article's content review the articles submitted with a peer review board. A refereed journal ensures that an article is written in appropriate scientific style and that the data published therein reflect current knowledge. A reputable journal is commonly affiliated with a professional group or society, a specialty group, or a reputable scientific publisher. A reputable scientific journal is not a journal that is a popular magazine or published by a commercial firm.

Examples of poor choices for scientific literature include any of the typical newsstand health and recreation journals and glamour and beauty magazines. Professionals should appreciate the fact that although many attractively presented dental publications exist, many are simply glorified advertising brochures and do not represent an acceptable source of scientific material. When selecting a journal article, the reader should be careful to note that the author has the appropriate qualifications. (An attorney writing an article about orthodontics, for example, might not be the most credible source of information.) Authors should also possess experience or a current relationship with the field about which they are writing. If the written work is a research study, there should be evidence of facilities in which to conduct the research and financial support for the project.

Readers usually find a tremendous amount of available information. Although older information may be considered classic and therefore occasionally useful in conducting a review, most often readers want to research the most current information. One classic study was the Vipeholm study, conducted in Sweden in the 1950s.[10] The study investigated the incidence of decay in relation to sugar intake and is often mentioned in scientific writing. Although the information from this research has proved valuable, this study was conducted in a disadvantaged population and by today's standards would not have received approval because of ethical considerations. One of the most often cited concerns about the Vipeholm study was whether the subjects enlisted possessed the mental capacity to give their consent for the research.

Information is usually considered current if it has been published within the last 3 to 5 years. References cited in journal articles should be carefully screened to validate their relevancy and age. Sometimes only a limited amount of information is available on a given topic, and this is reflected in the article. An example is the lack of true research involving herbal or alternative dental therapies.

Evaluation of the Selected Literature

After a journal and the information relevant to the reader's goals are selected, the reader can pursue a comprehensive evaluation of this literature. Various types of journal articles undergo different types of review. For example, a *review article* may examine an assortment of studies that have already been conducted and provides an overview of the research that has already been done. A review article can help one formulate an idea or a new research question and can help direct the reader to other sources of information through references cited within the article. Validation of a good review article should follow all of the practices stated earlier, including author expertise, accurate and recent references, and review from a refereed journal.

The Primary Research Manuscript

Perhaps the most useful type of journal article and truly the archetypal "research paper" is the primary research manuscript (Box 7-4). A primary research study describes the original research, including its methods, materials, results, and conclusions. When one is considering a primary research article, the practice of checking author expertise, accurate and recent references, and peer review from a refereed journal still applies; additionally, other steps are to be followed. The first step is often an assessment of the paper's abstract.

Abstract

A relevant **abstract** is usually confined to approximately 200 words and concisely defines the study's purpose, methods, materials, and results. The abstract, a brief

Box 7-4   WHAT TO LOOK FOR IN A RESEARCH STUDY MANUSCRIPT

A. Abstract
- Contains 200 words or less.
- Clearly states purpose of study in the first few sentences.
- Includes brief description of the following: population, type of research, overview of statistics, results, and conclusions.

B. Introduction
- Review of the supporting literature.
- Statement of hypothesis (null hypothesis).
- Reason for study.

C. Methods and Materials
- Appropriate selection of instrument.
- Appropriate method of conducting research (i.e., prospective, retrospective, randomized, etc.).
- Descriptive enough that reader can replicate the study.

D. Results
- Appropriate statistical tests.
- Appropriate display of data.
- Clear and understandable presentation of the data.
- Correct interpretation of data.

E. Discussion
- Conclusions are based on fact.
- Results are tied into previous research discussed in introduction.
- Inferences and opinions are stated as such.
- Future plans are included for further research

description of the research, appears at the beginning of the manuscript and is designed to provide the reader with an overview of the study. Although it may present an idea of what the study involved, the abstract may not always paint an accurate picture of the study and the results. The only way to truly assess a scientific article is to read the content within and critically examine each piece for information.

A primary research article begins with a review of the current literature and an introduction to the study. Within this section, an accurate and complete description of the research problem is given and the purpose of the study is clearly stated. The research question can be stated as a hypothesis and may include objectives to be accomplished.

Materials and Methods

The next section of the primary research manuscript, materials and methods, describes the population or sample and the techniques used to gather information about the population studied. One of the primary reasons for disseminating results in peer-reviewed journals (in addition to sharing the results) is so that colleagues might duplicate the experiment to validate the results or might modify it in some respects to further refine the conclusions implied in the study. Toward that end, the materials and methods text should be complete enough so that other readers might reasonably expect to recapitulate the experiment and verify the results.

The reviewer will want to determine whether the researcher has selected an appropriate group to test and whether it is one that is relevant to the reviewer's needs. This necessity for appropriateness applies whether the "group" in question is a population of laboratory animals, human subjects, or tissue culture cells. For example, if reviewers are looking for information regarding nonsurgical periodontal therapy, they should ensure that the study has used a similar population or sample relative to their needs.

The number of subjects in the group is also important. Has the study included enough subjects so that readers can generalize the findings to their group of interest? If the subject is a 35-year-old woman and the research involves men older than 50 years of age, the results may not necessarily be relevant to the reader's cause; if the subject is a 35-year-old woman but only one or two subjects are involved, the information might also be irrelevant.

Ensuring that no author *bias* has been introduced is very important. Bias may be defined as any influence that produces a distortion in the results of a study.[1] Here are some considerations:

- Is the subject a patient of the researcher, who also happens to be the one who developed the new technique?
- Are all variables in the study controlled for (e.g., diet, standard of living, gender, age, dental history)?
- Is there a control group and an experimental group?
- Is one group receiving the standard treatment and the experimental group receiving the new therapy?

An example of a research study may be the evaluation of the efficacy of sealants in caries prevention. The study design may consist of a group of test subjects (the experimental group) who are to receive sealants and are then to be monitored for a number of years to determine the caries rate. Because reference data are essential, a control group (the group without sealants) is compared with the group with sealants.

Readers must also consider the following issues when evaluating research design:

- If an instrument (e.g., a questionnaire) is to be part of the study, have validity and reliability been previously established?

- Are the conditions under which the treatment is accomplished similar and completely described?
- Are both groups monitored for an adequate period of time to assess long-term results of the therapy?

Results

After the methods and materials are described, the results section, including a statistical analysis, follows. The results text should detail how the hypothesis of the study has been tested. Statistical tests should be appropriate for the study and should be described. Tables and graphs may be included to provide a visual representation of the results, but they should be clear and understandable to the reader. The author should justify the statistical method used.

Discussion

Finally, a discussion of the conclusions and the inferences drawn from the results of the research is presented. The conclusions are also used to define outcomes of the research.

The conclusion should clearly state the rejection or acceptance of the null hypothesis. It may discuss facts derived from the research but may also include investigator speculation on what the results mean. The conclusion usually discusses the research study's strengths and weaknesses and may mention further research necessary to obtain the desired results.

Complications observed during the research should also be presented. The results of the study are related to the literature cited. Most important, the conclusions are a direct reflection of the findings. Although speculation may be appropriate, it should be stated as such. It is never appropriate to make statements that are not based on fact or that are not derived from study results.

SUMMARY

This chapter has provided an overview of the basics of research, including the steps in the scientific method, the steps in analyzing the literature, and the components of a primary research manuscript.

Although all research should be conducted according to the scientific method to provide results with a measure of validity and reliability, scientific research remains an inexact science. However, when studies are properly designed and accurately analyzed with the use of the appropriate statistical design, the information obtained not only will be new but also may serve as a springboard for further studies. The inventive and inquisitive practitioner will seek to discover information that both enhances the practice of dental hygiene and all its contemporary roles and keeps the profession moving in a forward direction.

Applying **Your Knowledge**

1. Formulate a research problem based on a question you have that is related to the field of dentistry.
2. Develop a hypothesis and a null hypothesis for the research problem.
3. Considering your research problem, define the following:
   a. Population
   b. Sample
   c. Experimental group
   d. Control group
   e. Independent variable
   f. Dependent variable
4. Determine whether the data collected from your study will be continuous or discrete. Will nominal, ordinal, interval, or ratio scales of measurement be used?
5. Complete a literature review for the research problem formulated in No. 2, and write an abstract for one of the journal articles examined during your literature review.
6. Using data that you have reviewed or collected, determine the mean, median, and mode.
7. Give five examples of positive and negative correlations. Compare variables related to dental hygiene or to data from articles you have read.
8. Using one of the research studies from your literature review, describe the statistical analysis. Were the statistical techniques used appropriate? Were the data displayed in an appropriate manner?
9. Design and complete a research study or community project following the steps listed in Box 7-1 (the scientific method). Complete your study by creating a poster presentation using appropriate displays of data and the description of your study.

DENTAL HYGIENE COMPETENCIES

Reading the material in this chapter and participating in the activities of Applying Your Knowledge will contribute to the student's ability to demonstrate the following competencies:

Core competencies

C.4 Assume responsibility for dental hygiene actions and care based on scientific theories and research as well as the accepted standard of care.

Community involvement

CM.6 Evaluate the outcomes of community-based programs, and plan for future activities.

Patient/client care

PC.1 Systematically collect, analyze, and record data on the general, oral, and psychosocial health status of a variety of patients or clients using methods consistent with medicolegal principles.

PC.3 Collaborate with the patient, client, or other health professionals to formulate a comprehensive dental hygiene care plan that is patient-centered and based on scientific evidence.

Community Case

Allison is a registered dental hygienist who has spent the last 10 years working in a periodontal practice that treats clients referred from several different dental practices in town. Most of the clients present with moderate to advanced periodontal disease. Allison has been intrigued by the different information she has seen in several professional journals regarding the link between periodontal disease and heart disease. Allison is also interested in a nutritional supplementation plan she read about that provides protection from inflammation and facilitates wound healing. Allison remembers that much of the information linking periodontal disease and cardiac health indicates inflammatory factors may be a possible culprit. Allison hypothesizes that she can take the relatively small sample her client population provides and make some generalizations regarding oral health as related to cardiac health. After speaking with her employer and gaining regulatory approval for her project, Allison consents and enrolls 100 subjects into her study. Allison enrolls subjects diagnosed with moderate periodontal disease and randomly assigns half into a group treated with standard therapy and the other half into a group treated with standard therapy plus the nutritional supplement purported to provide anti-inflammatory and wound-healing benefits. Allison hypothesizes that the group treated with standard periodontal therapy plus the nutritional supplemental will present with a lower incidence of cardiac risk at the end of her study. Allison's subjects will be followed over the next 5 years. At the end of the study she plans to compare prestudy laboratory and physical analysis with post-study laboratory and physical analysis to provide information determining whether an increase or decrease in cardiac risk factors occurred in the experimental group. Allison feels she will be able to then generalize her results to other clients in different practice settings who are treated with a similar protocol.

1. The experimental group in this study is:
   a. all the subjects Allison enrolls
   b. the subjects receiving standard care
   c. the subject receiving standard care plus the nutritional supplement
   d. all the subjects Allison attempts to recruit for her study
   e. the clients who will benefit from the study in the future

2. The independent variable in this study is:
   a. subjects with moderate periodontal disease
   b. the standard periodontal therapy provided to each subject
   c. the nutritional supplement
   d. the cardiac status of subjects at the end of the study
   e. the laboratory tests
3. The data that Allison is collecting to perform her analysis include laboratory parameters (hematology and chemistry). An example of one test result would be a cholesterol level valued at 350. The type of data collected and the scale of measurement most applicable to these data would be:
   a. continuous and interval
   b. discrete and nominal
   c. continuous and ratio
   d. discrete and ordinal
   e. none of the above
4. For her data analysis and presentation of results, Allison considers several types of statistical analyses. Allison intends to follow her original plan of applying the information she has collected to patients outside of her study. Which of the following would be the best choice?
   a. Descriptive statistics
   b. Inferential statistics
   c. Nonparametric statistics
   d. Power statistics
   e. There is no specific type of statistical analysis that can provide the information Allison is seeking.
5. Allison finds that her results show that subjects receiving the nutritional supplement (independent variable) plus the standard periodontal care show a much lower incidence of heart disease (dependent variable) at the end of the study in relation to the control group. The information Allison has collected shows:
   a. a positive correlation between the experimental treatment and heart disease.
   b. a negative correlation between the experimental treatment and heart disease.
   c. a positive correlation between the physical exam and the laboratory tests.
   d. both a and b
   e. no correlation at all

REFERENCES

1. Polit D, Hungler B: Nursing Research Principles and Methods, 5th ed. Philadelphia, JB Lippincott, 1995.
2. Monsen E: Research: Successful Approaches. Chicago, American Dietetic Association, 1992.
3. Norman G, Streiner D: PDQ Statistics. Philadelphia, BC Decker, 1986, p 15-18.
4. Cancer Facts and Figures 2004. Cancer Basic Facts: How is Cancer Staged? *Available at http://www.cancer.org* (accessed November 2004).

5. Zarkowski P: Community Oral Health Planning and Practice. In Darby M: Comprehensive Review of Dental Hygiene, 5th ed. St. Louis, Mosby, 2002.
6. Rose L: Overview of biostatistics. In Gluck GM, Morganstein WM (eds): Jong's Community Dental Health, 5th ed. St. Louis, Mosby, 2003.
7. Potter P, Perry A: Research in nursing care. In Contemporary Nursing: Dimensions and Dynamics. St. Louis. Mosby, 1993.
8. Darby M, Walsh M: Dental Hygiene Theory and Practice, 2nd ed. St. Louis, Saunders, 2003.
9. Hittleman E, Afes V: Accessing and Reading Dental Public Health Research: Evidence-based Dental Practice. In Gluck GM, Morganstein WM (eds): Jong's Community Dental Health, 5th ed. St. Louis, Mosby, 2003.
10. Gustafsson BE, Quensel CE, Swenander LL, et al: The Vipeholm Dental Caries Study: The effect of different levels of carbohydrate on caries activity in 436 individuals observed for five years. Acta Odont Scand 11:232-364, 1954.

BIBLIOGRAPHY

Armstrong RL: Hypothesis formulation. In Krampitz SD, Pavlovich N (eds): Readings for Nursing Research. St. Louis, CV Mosby, 1981.
Campbell JP, Draft RL, Hulin CL: What to Study: Generating and Developing Research Questions. Beverly Hills, Calif, Sage Publications, 1982.
Huff D: How to Lie with Statistics. New York, WW Norton, 1954.
Kleinbaum DG, Kupper LL, Morganstern H: Epidemiological Research. Belmont, Calif, Lifetime Learning Publications, 1982.
Kraemer LG: Research and theory development in dental hygiene. In Darby ML, Walsh MM (eds): Dental Hygiene Theory and Practice. Philadelphia, WB Saunders, 1995.
Norman GR, Streiner DL: PDQ Statistics. Philadelphia, BC Decker, 1986.
Polit DF, Hungler BP: Nursing Research: Principles and Methods, 5th ed. Philadelphia, JB Lippincott, 1995.

8

Health Promotion and Health Communication

Beverly Isman, RDH, MPH, ELS

Objectives

Upon completion of this chapter, the student will be able to:

- Apply various health promotion theories to promotion of oral health
- Discuss the distinctions between "generic," "targeted," "personalized," and "tailored" health messages
- Identify strategies for delivering health information to consumer groups by using materials, activities, and evaluation methods that are culturally sensitive and linguistically competent
- Outline the basic components, advantages, and limitations of table clinics, poster presentations, oral papers, and round table discussions as methods for presenting scientific information to health professionals
- List examples of service-learning programs that can increase a dental hygienist's understanding of community dental health issues and approaches
- Identify professional organizations that offer opportunities for personal growth and development in community health and dental public health

Key Terms

Health Promotion	Stages of Change Theory	Social Learning Theory
Theories	Health Belief Model	Community Organization Theory

Diffusion of Innovations
  Theory
Organizational Change:
  Stage Theory
Health Communication
"Framing" Health Messages

"Tailoring" Messages
Focus Groups
Culturally Sensitive
Linguistically Competent
Learning Styles
Quantitative Evaluation

Qualitative Evaluation
Table Clinic
Poster Presentation
Oral Paper
Round Table Discussion
Service-Learning Programs

OPENING STATEMENT

Challenges to Promoting Oral Health

- Despite years of research on prevention of oral diseases, we know very little about how best to promote oral health.

- We need to document more evidence that changes in attitudes and beliefs about oral health lead to improved oral health outcomes.

- Improved knowledge levels alone rarely translate into healthy behaviors.

- Most behavioral change that occurs after oral health education or promotion is short term and is not sustained without periodic reinforcement.

- Despite the lack of evidence of the effectiveness of oral health education and health promotion efforts to improve health, we ethically must disseminate scientific knowledge to the public.[1]

- Today dental hygienists have unique and unlimited opportunities to become involved in community health activities and to contribute to the development of a better understanding of effective oral health promotion efforts.

HEALTH PROMOTION THEORIES

The World Health Organization defines *health* as:

> the extent to which an individual or group is able, on the one hand, to realize aspirations and satisfy needs; and, on the other hand, to change or cope with the environment. Health is, therefore, seen as a resource for everyday life, not the object of living; it is a positive concept emphasizing social and personal resources, as well as physical capabilities.[2]

This view conceptualizes health as a personal resource and a lifestyle that should be promoted and introduces the role of behavior, not just knowledge, into the health equation. This chapter therefore focuses on the concepts of oral health promotion, behavior change, and the dental hygienist's role in communicating health messages to other health professionals and to the public.

Health promotion is a broad concept that refers to the process of enabling people and communities to increase their control over various determinants of health (see Chapter 3) and therefore to improve their own health. Health promotion goes beyond prevention of disease and reduction of health risks. Aspects of health promotion include:

1. Advocacy
2. Efforts to change organizations, policies, and environments
3. Political considerations
4. Ethical responsibilities

Oral health promotion efforts can increase demand for care, use of dental services, and preventive self-care measures. The anticipated outcome of these efforts is a reduced incidence and severity of oral diseases with improved oral health. Yet, as we see in the challenges in the Opening Statement, applied research relating to oral health promotion is still in its infancy and not well integrated or coordinated with research and theories developed by other health disciplines.

In the effort to promote health and prevent disease, **theories** help us to analyze and interpret health problems and then to plan and evaluate interventions. What is a theory?

> A theory is a set of interrelated concepts, definitions, and propositions that present a systematic view of events or situations by specifying relations among variables, in order to explain and predict the events or situations.[3]

A theory is an abstract notion that comes to life only when it is applied to specific topics and problems. Sometimes theories are called *conceptual frameworks* or *models*.

How can you apply theories to dental hygiene practice and public health practice? Every day, dental hygienists face challenging situations that cause oral problems, such as patients who feed their babies cariogenic liquids in baby bottles, athletes who sustain oral injuries because they refuse to wear a mouth guard, and adults who say they are too busy to keep their recall appointment. Theories can help us to analyze these situations and to apply solutions that have been effective in similar circumstances.

Traditionally, dental hygienists have viewed oral health problems primarily as the "patient's" problem and have proceeded to "educate" the patient about how to improve oral health. This approach is doomed to failure because it does not assess or validate the patient's point of view or health beliefs and does not consider the environmental or cultural circumstances that have influenced the person's attitudes, knowledge, or health practices. It is important to analyze oral health problems from more than one perspective and to understand how each perspective affects the others. Behavior that leads to improved oral health can be affected at three levels:

- Intrapersonal (within the individual)
- Interpersonal (between people)
- Community (including institutional or organizational change and public policy)

The following section describes selected health promotion theories that relate to these three levels and that have the most relevance to oral health issues. Each explanation is accompanied by a table that contains key concepts, definitions, and applications of each concept to a problem. For easier reading, the author has included texts that cover overviews of most of the theories in the References instead of citing the original references for the theories.[3,4]

Intrapersonal Level

Stages of Change Theory (transtheoretical model)

Initially developed by Prochaska and DiClemente, the **Stages of Change Theory** views change as a process or cycle that occurs over time rather than as a single event. This theory allows the dental hygienist to assess a person's readiness to change a behavior toward a more healthful lifestyle, for instance, daily brushing to prevent gingivitis. The theory assumes that at any point in time everyone is at a different stage of readiness to make lifestyle changes and that people cycle through the various stages over time, depending on the behavior to be changed. The major stages of this model with definitions and applications are outlined in Table 8-1.

The cycle starts by increasing one's awareness of a problem (e.g., a person has gingivitis) to initiating behavior change (brushing effectively and using antimicrobial rinses) and progresses to maintaining motivation to continue preventive actions (returning in 3 months to check progress). To be effective in changing behavior, health messages and programs should be matched to an individual's current stage of readiness to change.

Table 8-1   Stages of Change Theory (transtheoretical model)

Concept	Definition	Application
Precontemplation	Being unaware of problem; not having thought about change	Increase awareness of need for change; personalize information on risks and benefits
Contemplation	Thinking about change in the near future	Motivate and encourage to make specific plans
Decision/ determination	Making a plan to change	Assist in developing concrete action plans or setting gradual goals
Action	Implementing specific action or plans	Assist with feedback, problem solving, social support, and reinforcement
Maintenance	Continuing desirable actions or repeating periodic recommended steps	Assist in coping, using reminders, finding alternatives, avoiding slips or relapses

Adapted from Glanz K, Rimer BK: Theory at a Glance: A Guide for Health Promotion Practice. Bethesda, Md, National Institutes of Health, 2003. Accessible at http://cancer.gov/cancerinformation/theory-at-a-glance.

Health Belief Model

Originated by Rosenstock and others in the 1970s to explain people's use of preventive health services, the **Health Belief Model** allows us to assess perceptions of how susceptible one is to a health problem and whether one believes that recommended preventive behaviors will result in less susceptibility. For example, does your father think that he is at risk for development of oral cancer because he smokes a pipe? Does he believe that limiting use of the pipe would reduce his oral cancer risk? The model also looks at perceived severity of a disease threat, benefits of taking a health action, and barriers to completing the action. Does your father believe that the effects of quitting pipe smoking are worse than the effects of oral cancer?

One application of the Health Belief Model is to develop messages that are likely to persuade people to make decisions to improve their oral health. The components of the model and some applications are shown in Table 8-2. The primary hypothesis is that increased perception of severity and susceptibility to a disease results in an increased probability of taking action. Perceived ability to take action and cues to action are important factors. Does your father believe he can quit smoking his pipe, and what reminders can you provide to support him?

Table 8-2   Health Belief Model

Concept	Definition	Application
Perceived susceptibility	One's opinion of chances of getting a condition	Define population at risk and risk levels; personalize risk based on a person's features or behavior; heighten perceived susceptibility if too low
Perceived severity	One's opinion of how serious a condition and its sequelae are	Specify consequences of the risk and the condition
Perceived benefits	One's opinion of the efficacy of the advised action to reduce risk or seriousness of impact	Define action to take: how, where, when; clarify the positive effects to be expected
Perceived barriers	One's opinion of the tangible and psychologic costs of the advised action	Identify and reduce barriers through reassurance, incentives, and assistance
Cues to action	Strategies to activate readiness	Provide how-to information; promote awareness, send reminders
Self-efficacy	Confidence in one's ability to take action	Provide training and guidance in performing action

Adapted from Glanz K, Rimer BK: Theory at a Glance: A Guide for Health Promotion Practice. Bethesda, Md, National Institutes of Health, 2003. Accessible at http://cancer.gov/cancerinformation/theory-at-a-glance.

Interpersonal Level

Social Learning Theory

The **Social Learning Theory** posits that people learn primarily in four ways:
1. Direct experience
2. Vicarious experience, such as through the mass media
3. Judgments voiced by others, such as testimony or promotions by experts
4. Inferred knowledge

The basic premise of this theory, developed by Bandera and sometimes known as the Social Cognitive Theory, is that people learn through their own experiences, by observing the actions of others, and by the results of these actions. Behavioral change is accomplished through the interaction of personal factors, environmental influences, and individual behaviors. Self-efficacy and self-confidence are important concepts. Table 8-3 lists the relevant definitions and applications of the major concepts.

An example of applying the Social Learning Theory to oral health is helping a single mother to feel confident about performing toothbrushing for her young child by using techniques such as demonstration, watching a video, providing ongoing encouragement, and giving periodic feedback. When the mother gains some confidence in her skills, she then assists the child care workers and other parents at the

Table 8-3   Social Learning Theory (social cognitive theory)

Concept	Definition	Application
Reciprocal determinism	Behavioral changes result from interaction between the person and the environment; change is bidirectional	Involve the individual and relevant others; work to change the environment, if warranted
Behavioral capability	Knowledge and skills to influence behavior	Provide information and training about action
Expectations	Beliefs about likely results of action	Incorporate information about likely results of action in advance
Self-efficacy	Confidence in ability to take action and to persist in action	Point out strengths; use persuasion and encouragement; approach behavioral change in small steps
Observational learning	Beliefs based on observing others like oneself and/or visible physical results	Point out others' experience and physical changes; identify role models to emulate
Reinforcement	Responses to a person's behavior that increase or decrease the chances of recurrence	Provide incentives, rewards, praise; encourage self-reward; decrease possibility of negative responses that deter positive changes

Adapted from Glanz K, Rimer BK: Theory at a Glance: A Guide for Health Promotion Practice. Bethesda, Md, National Institutes of Health, 2003. Accessible at http://cancer.gov/cancerinformation/theory-at-a-glance.

day care center in learning these skills so that they can support each other and so that oral hygiene care becomes a daily activity for all of the children.

Community Level

Community Organization Theory

> **Community Organization Theory** is the process of involving and activating members of a community or subgroup to identify a common problem or goal, to mobilize resources, to implement strategies, and to evaluate their efforts. People usually refer to this process as *empowerment*. This is a grassroots approach to health promotion, rather than a project that is initiated and conducted by health professionals. Table 8-4 outlines the key components.
>
> To apply an example, consider the role of a church pastor and a congregation in oral health promotion. Church members notice that many of the elders have stopped coming to church suppers because they have lost their teeth and are embarrassed to eat in public. The pastor calls the dental school for help, and the congregation raises money to help defray the cost of examinations and dentures for the elders. Dental and dental hygiene student teams work together to assess each elder's needs and to fabricate and fit the dentures. They also discuss oral health, denture care, and the challenges of eating with dentures. Gradually, the elders begin to become comfortable eating and speaking with the dentures, and they resume their attendance at church suppers. The following year, the church leaders continue to work

Table 8-4   Community Organization Theory

Concept	Definition	Application
Empowerment	Process of gaining mastery and power over oneself or one's community to produce change	Give individuals and communities tools and responsibility for making decisions that affect them
Community competence	Community's ability to engage in effective problem solving	Work with community to identify problems, create consensus, and reach goals
Participation relevance	Learner should be active participant and work starting "where the people are"	Help community set goals within the context of preexisting goals, and encourage active participation
Issue selection	Identifying winnable, simple, and specific concerns as focus of action	Assist community members in examining how they can communicate the concerns and whether success is likely
Critical consciousness	Developing understanding of root causes of problems	Guide consideration of health concerns in broad perspective of social problems

Adapted from Glanz K, Rimer BK: Theory at a Glance: A Guide for Health Promotion Practice. Bethesda, Md, National Institutes of Health, 2003. Accessible at http://cancer.gov/cancerinformation/theory-at-a-glance.

Table 8-5   **Diffusion of Innovations Theory**

Concept	Definition	Application
Relative advantage	The degree to which an innovation is seen as better than the idea, practice, program, or product it replaces	Point out unique benefits: monetary value, convenience, time saving, prestige, etc.
Compatibility	How consistent the innovation is with values, habits, experience, and needs of potential adopters	Tailor innovation to the intended audience's values, norms, or situation
Complexity	How difficult the innovation is to understand or use	Create a program, idea, or product to be easy to use and to understand
Trialability	Extent to which one can experiment with the innovation before a commitment to adopt is required	Provide opportunities to try on a limited basis (e.g., free samples, introductory sessions, money-back guarantee)
Observability	Extent to which the innovation provides tangible or visible results	Ensure visibility of results: feedback or publicity

Adapted from Glanz K, Rimer BK: Theory at a Glance: A Guide for Health Promotion Practice. Bethesda, Md, National Institutes of Health, 2003. Accessible at http://cancer.gov/cancerinformation/theory-at-a-glance.

with the student teams to promote oral health to people of all ages within their parish.

Diffusion of Innovations Theory

Developed by Rogers, the **Diffusion of Innovations Theory** helps us assess how new ideas, products, or services spread within a society or to other groups, that is, how innovations are adopted. During the assessment, attention is directed to the characteristics of the innovation, the communication channels, and the social systems. Table 8-5 displays the components.

Use of dental sealants is a good oral health example. Researchers found that despite numerous clinical trials showing their effectiveness in caries prevention, adoption of sealants by practitioners proceeded slowly. Adoption occurred much sooner in public health clinics, where there was a critical need for effective caries-preventive measures and strong advocacy for the procedure, than in private dental offices, where patients had low caries rates, insurance companies did not reimburse for the service, and practitioners were wedded to the use of amalgams for managing rather than preventing dental caries. Over time, caries rates in occlusal surfaces declined dramatically in children who received regular care at the clinics, whereas caries rates remained stable in the children visiting private dental practices. Major educational efforts, policy changes regarding reimbursement, and advocacy efforts were used to eventually change attitudes and patterns of practice in the private sector, thus resulting in reduced rates of dental caries in all children in the community.

Table 8-6   Organizational Change: Stage Theory

Concept	*Definition*	*Application*
Definition of problem	Problems recognized and analyzed; solutions sought and evaluated	Involve management and other personnel in awareness-raising activities
Initiation of action	Policy or directive formulated; resources for beginning change allocated	Provide process consultation to inform decision makers and implementers of what adoption involves
Implementation of change	Innovation is implemented; reactions and role changes occur	Provide training, technical assistance, and aid in problem solving
Institutionalization of change	Policy or program becomes entrenched in the organization; new goals and values internalized	Identify high-level champion, work to overcome obstacles to institutionalization, and create structures for integration

Adapted from Glanz K, Rimer BK: Theory at a Glance: A Guide for Health Promotion Practice. Bethesda, Md, National Institutes of Health, 2003. Accessible at http://cancer.gov/cancerinformation/theory-at-a-glance.

Organizational Change: Stage Theory

Organizations pass through a series of four stages as they initiate change (Table 8-6). In addition, organizational structures and processes influence workers' behavior and motivation for change.

To apply the **Organizational Change: Stage Theory,** we can consider a situation in which health educators asked the cafeteria staff in the hospital to offer healthier foods. A number of stages were involved in instituting the change (e.g., pricing different food items, looking at sample menus, announcing the new food items). Eventually, a larger percentage of employees began to select the new food options, thus eating healthier lunches. Soon they asked for a larger selection of these foods. The health educator and the cafeteria staff then worked together to distribute health-promoting recipes so that employees also were encouraged to make healthy food choices at home. This process not only resulted in institutional change but also created healthier lifestyles in the employees' families.

ACQUIRING NEW KNOWLEDGE

To use these theories effectively, dental hygienists need to acquire new information for assessing and changing people's health behaviors. In addition, they need to keep abreast of innovative programs occurring in other professions and ways in which other health care systems address health problems. This information guides the approach selected to assess and change people's behaviors (see Guiding Principles).

Guiding Principles

> **Knowledge Needed to Assess and Change People's Behaviors[5]**
> - Factors that are considered a risk for development of oral diseases and those factors that can be modified through preventive efforts at the primary, secondary, and tertiary levels
> - How to assess a person's risk for development of oral diseases and other health problems
> - The level of scientific evidence for and the extent of certainty of the effectiveness of various preventive measures
> - Which categories of interventions yield the desired impact (e.g., personal behaviors, programs, societal and environmental modifications, policies)
> - Effective oral and written communication skills
> - Ways in which innovations are diffused and ways of bringing about organizational change
> - Ways to motivate people to access services and return for continuing care
> - The structure of various health care systems and community-based organizations
> - How to deliver effective services and education
> - How to evaluate efforts (e.g., effectiveness, costs, access, quality, outcomes)

Some of the information may be learned during the dental hygiene educational process, whereas some may be acquired through experience and professional development. Resources for professional development are discussed later in the chapter. Let us now examine how to design health messages, specifically, how to frame and tailor them.

HEALTH COMMUNICATION AS A FIELD

For the first time in the *Healthy People* initiative, **Health Communication** emerged as a separate Focus Area in the national *Healthy People 2010* Objectives. Health communication encompasses the "study and use of communication strategies to inform and influence individual and community decisions that enhance health."[6] One of the challenges in designing health communication programs is to identify the most effective channels, context, and content that will capture people's attention and then motivate them to use health information. Research on strategies to address these challenges is becoming more widespread, sophisticated, and cross-cutting, with results that are applicable to oral health. Figure 8-1 demonstrates the important stages of the health communication process.[7] Keep these in mind as you read the next sections on framing and formatting health messages.

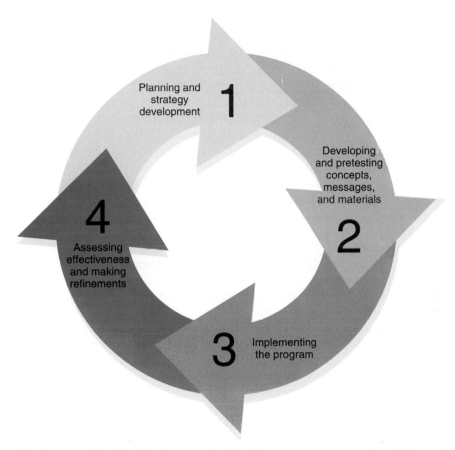

Figure 8-1 Stages of the Health Communication Process. *(From USDHHS, PHS, NIH, NCI: Making Health Communication Programs Work. Bethesda, Md, NCI, 2002.)*

FRAMING HEALTH MESSAGES

Within the past decade, the field of health communication research and media advocacy has increased exponentially.[8] New forms of technology are changing our options for framing, delivering, and evaluating health messages for the public. The concept of **"framing" health messages** relates to the cues (e.g., sounds, symbols, words, pictures) that signal how and what to think about an issue. In the process of framing messages, an attempt is made to connect to people's values, beliefs, knowledge levels, and emotions. **"Tailoring" messages** relates to the specific cues used to make messages meaningful for a specific individual.

A fundamental error in many oral health education efforts is the assumption that increased knowledge will result in changes in behavior. Traditionally, oral health messages have been packaged as "generic" messages that cover a number of concepts and try to appeal to the greatest number of people. A typical brochure would cover brushing and flossing and the use of fluorides, sealants, antimicrobials, and other preventive measures. It might also describe various diagnostic procedures such as radiographs, periodontal probing, and microbial tests. This type of brochure is based on the assumption that dental hygienists should provide as much information as possible and that people will sort through the information to select the pieces that apply to them. Numerous research studies have shown that this assumption is not necessarily valid; the approach is not effective for changing behaviors, particularly in busy people or low-level readers.

With the use of a more focused approach, health professionals began to use "targeted" materials intended to reach a specific subgroup or population, usually based on demographic characteristics (e.g., older adults, African Americans). The assumption that underlies this approach is that a large number of people still can be reached and that homogeneity exists in the group to justify the messages and formats used. Subgroups, however, often represent very heterogeneous groups, thus reducing the effectiveness.

Another approach is to "personalize" messages. Many of these attempts, however, have used personal characteristics on a superficial level (e.g., a person's name), assuming that using a person's name will draw attention to the generic information that is presented. Mail promotions use this technique extensively because lists of consumers and health professionals can be purchased easily. Although this approach initially may have a motivating effect, the appeal soon is lost. A more effective way to personalize information, for instance in a brochure, is to highlight only the information and key messages that apply to the person who receives it.

The most effective way to reach individuals to increase their knowledge or to change behavior is to "tailor" messages.[9] These messages or strategies are intended to reach a specific person on the basis of characteristics unique to that person that were discovered through an assessment process. This is the basis of many computerized risk assessment/risk reduction programs in health care (e.g., heart disease, diabetes.) The technique can be applied to the formation of an individualized oral health plan based on risk assessment and primary prevention measures.[10] The assumption is that tailored messages provide a more meaningful and motivating strategy built on a person's specific input. Unfortunately, professionals sometimes try to tailor messages without going through the essential assessment process, only to find that their messages are ineffective.

EXPANDING COMMUNICATION FORMATS

Health promotion efforts often are viewed with skepticism by dental researchers, who equate them with random distribution of brochures and with no evaluation of behavioral change. As explained earlier in this chapter, health promotion theories go "beyond the brochure" and involve careful needs assessment and evaluation.

Consumer-Oriented Presentations

Before health information is provided to an individual or to a group, an assessment process is crucial. Depending on the audience and topic, a needs assessment can be accomplished through a literature review, informal observations or conversations, surveys, in-depth interviews, or **focus groups.** A needs assessment reveals important cultural beliefs, health practices, and knowledge levels that result in misconceptions, barriers to care, or stumbling blocks to behavioral change. The Surgeon General's "A National Call to Action to Promote Oral Health" emphasizes the need to develop messages that are **culturally sensitive** and **linguistically competent.**[11] This means that language and graphics should be inclusive, not promote stereotypes, and be easy to understand for any level reader or listener. Special considerations are needed when designing or translating materials for non-English speakers.[12] Box 8-1 lists some problems associated with translating materials

BOX 8-1   TRANSLATION BARRIERS AND SUGGESTIONS FOR OVERCOMING THEM

Problems with Translating Materials

- Medical and dental terms may not be understood or may have different meanings, or may not be directly translatable in another language. Even within languages such as Spanish, people from different nations or regions may use different words for a term such as x-ray or baby teeth.
- Literally translating word for word often is confusing because there may be no direct translation or a variety of phrases may be used, depending on the person's age, gender, social standing, or other characteristics. Literal translations without considering local language patterns and word usage may be annoying to the intended audience, causing them to ignore the information or reducing its credibility.
- Some people may speak a language that does not have a written equivalent, or they may speak one language but not be able to read the language.

Suggestions for Overcoming Translation Barriers

- Use materials originally developed in that language or have new materials developed in the target languages rather than translating them from English.
- Field test the materials with a variety of members from the intended audience.
- Some researchers recommend two-way translation—one person translates the text from English to the other language and a second person translates it back to identify any inconsistencies or mistranslations. It is best to use translators who are both bilingual and bicultural.
- Use only trained translators who are familiar with low literacy readers as well as more sophisticated ones.

Some educational materials are produced in a dual language format so that both English and the other language are included. This can be useful for both print and video productions.

and suggestions for preventing or overcoming these problems. These should be considered during any needs assessment and when field testing materials.

The use of focus groups is one effective method of assessment. Group interviews are conducted with 5 to 10 members of the intended target audience and last approximately 30 to 60 minutes. A moderator uses structured questions to guide the discussion. When developing or testing health messages or materials, the moderator can use one or more versions of the materials to ask questions. For example, in field testing a video, you might ask:

- What is one message you remember from the video?
- Were there any messages that were confusing?
- Did you relate to the people in the video? How were they like you? Different from you?
- Was the video too short, just right, or too long?
- Should the video be accompanied by a handout that you can take home to help you remember the information?
- Would this video motivate you to ask about dental sealants for your child's teeth?

Focus groups are particularly useful for determining whether messages are at the appropriate language and literacy levels and whether they are culturally acceptable to the people in the group. Information about the appearance and appeal of materials is particularly important.[7]

A variety of resources are available for dental hygienists to use when designing and evaluating health messages. Examples of formats for presenting information are included in Box 8-2. References in this chapter provide citations describing the benefits and limitations of these various formats.[7,13-15] Some of the formats can be combined to allow for differences in **learning styles** of the audience. Assessing

---

BOX 8-2   FORMATS FOR PRESENTING ORAL HEALTH INFORMATION TO THE PUBLIC

Visual Displays
Posters, flip charts, story boards, bulletin boards, fotonovelas, models

Written Promotions
Newsletters, newspaper articles, model legislation, fact sheets, booklets, storybooks

Audiovisual Materials
Videos, public service announcements, websites, audiotapes, slide shows, multimedia presentations

Interactive Formats
Songs, role playing, storytelling, puzzles or quizzes or games, theater or puppet shows, demonstrations, computerized oral camera, interactive computer programs, science experiments or science fairs, debates, simulations

learning styles of individuals is much easier than planning messages to reach a diverse group of people. As a guide, people usually remember:

- 10% of what they read
- 20% of what they hear
- 30% of what they see
- 70% of what they see and hear
- 90% of what they see, hear, and do

Hands-on, interactive, multimedia formats are usually more effective for retaining knowledge than simply reading or listening to a message. This is true whether one is presenting information to the general public or to other health professionals.

On the basis of the findings from the needs assessment and the methods selected for health promotion activities, an evaluation plan can be designed before any interventions are started. Evaluation plans should be linked directly to the project objectives and should include measures to determine short-term and long-term effectiveness, if possible (see Guiding Principles).

GUIDING PRINCIPLES

Questions to Determine the Effectiveness of Project Objectives[16]

- Has the intervention achieved the desired results? If not, why not?
- Should this intervention be continued in its current form?
- What messages or activities produce the best results?
- How can the intervention be improved?
- Can it be replicated successfully in other settings?
- Are the resources (e.g., people, money, materials) that were used reasonable and cost-effective?

If possible, gain baseline information about knowledge, attitudes, or behaviors before the intervention. Evaluation can occur both during and after the intervention. Measures can be **quantitative** (e.g., *how many* people increased their knowledge of the causes of early childhood caries) or **qualitative** (e.g., *why* did people participate in the activity and *how* do they intend to change their parenting behaviors?) Evaluation plans do not always have to be complicated and do not always have to use sophisticated statistical analysis. The key is to try to evaluate your efforts and document the outcomes. Examples of simple evaluation strategies are listed:

1. Ask five questions to assess parents' knowledge and attitudes about sealants before and after a school-based sealant program.
2. Provide healthy snack recipes to a day care center; follow up after 2 months to determine which snacks have been made for the children and which snacks the children seem to like the best.

3. Survey school soccer coaches before and after initiating an oral injury or mouth guard campaign to determine use of mouth guards during practices and games, changes in policies on athletic equipment, and barriers that have been (or have not been) overcome in the attempt to implement the campaign.
4. Survey members of a community to identify how many heard the radio public service announcement about oral cancer prevention, where and how many times they heard it, and whether they followed any of its recommendations.
5. Use a consumer satisfaction questionnaire in a clinic to determine whether the patients are receiving all of the health information they want and need in formats that answer their questions or concerns in a clear and culturally appropriate manner.

Presentations to Health Professionals

The purpose of professional presentations is to deliver thought-provoking information to a group of health professionals in a short period of time in a clear, concise, and visually appealing format. Presentations generally focus on new research, programs, theories and ideas, clinical techniques, products or materials, career opportunities, educational techniques, policies or legislation, health care systems, or methods for disease prevention or detection. The information covers a specific topic with key messages highlighted and sources well documented.

Specific guidelines for presentations may vary by the sponsoring organization. Various online resources and organizational handouts provide tips.[17] When selecting a topic and format for a presentation, consider the following five questions (see Guiding Principles).

GUIDING PRINCIPLES

Five Questions for Selecting a Topic and Format
- Who will be the audience? How large a group do I want to address?
- What is their level of knowledge or interest in my topic?
- What questions might they ask? Will I be able to learn new information related to my topic from some members of the audience?
- How much time will I need to cover my key points?
- What audiovisual materials will most enhance my key points?

Most presentations follow a sequence, such as:
1. Introduction and Background
2. Methods and Materials

    3. Findings/Results or Key Points
    4. Discussion and Significance
    5. Summary and Conclusions

To apply these principles to the area of community health, consider the following comparison of four common types of presentations at dental or public health meetings.

Presentation for a Table Clinic

Note: The **table clinic** format is not used routinely outside the dental and dental hygiene professions.

Time: 5 to 7 minutes, occasionally 7 to 10 minutes

Format: Oral presentation by one or two people using audiovisuals that are placed on a table; same presentation is repeated a number of times for different groups

Size of Audience: Usually five to eight people per session; number of sessions or total time period is determined by the organization

Appropriate Audiovisuals: A small slide projector with rear projection screen; two to three hinged display panels no more than 3 feet high; samples of models, products, or materials; handout required

Benefits and Limitations: Limited content and very short time frame; same information repeated in a standard format; time for questions

Tips: Practice oral delivery with use of audiovisual materials carefully because time is limited

Presentation for a Poster Display

Note: The **poster presentation** display format (Figure 8-2) is becoming popular because of the number of presentations that can be accommodated in a specified time frame and no audiovisual equipment is needed.

Time: Session lasting 1 to 2 hours; discussion time varies by number and type of questions asked

Format: Presenter discusses visual display with people who stop to look; posters lined up next to each other; poster usually attached by pushpins or double-sided fastening material (e.g., Velcro) to a board or other backing material

Size of Audience: Varies greatly; some people "cruise by" quickly, some just pick up handouts, others stop to read display and discuss topic

Appropriate Audiovisuals: Text, data, artwork, or photos on paper or poster backing or printed on banner; slides and videos not usually allowed, although computer applications can be used; handouts encouraged

Benefits and Limitations: Opportunity to discuss topic, share ideas, and acquire additional ideas; unpredictable attendance (sometimes crowded and noisy but at other times nobody comes by); not appropriate for topics that require videos or other types of media

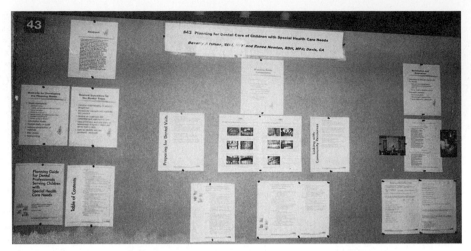

Figure 8-2 Format for poster presentation.

Tips: Use color to attract attention and highlight key points; use large, readable print and catchy title; use outline form; intersperse categories of information with charts, graphics, and photos; consider this format for easy setup and transport; include copy of abstract, which is also printed in the program

Presentation for an Oral Paper

Note: The **oral paper** format usually is part of a session with a theme or a panel.

Time: 10 to 15 minutes, including time for questions

Format: Oral presentation of information (using notes), accompanied by audiovisuals

Size of Audience: Usually more than 30 people but is suitable for hundreds of people

Appropriate Audiovisuals: Slides, overhead transparencies, short videos, computerized presentation

Benefits and Limitations: Large group can be reached; presenter can speak from typed paper or notes; room lighting usually fairly dark; limited interaction with audience; vast array of knowledge in audience

Tips: Try to maintain some eye contact and do not read the paper; use uncomplicated and effective audiovisual materials that highlight important information rather than detract from or repeat information you give orally; practice delivery, timing, and use of audiovisuals before the presentation; decide what information to delete if you are running over time allowance; include transitions between sentences and sections; check audiovisuals and room environment before your session

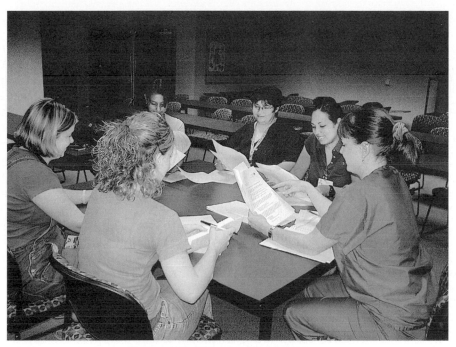

Figure 8-3 Round table discussion.

Presentation for a Round Table Discussion

Note: The **round table discussion** format (Figure 8-3) is gaining in popularity for a more informal presentation.

Time: 30 to 60 minutes, presentation sometimes repeated to a new group

Format: Oral presentation and discussion supplemented by audiovisuals to people seated at a round table or in a circle.

Size of Audience: Usually 8 to 10 people

Appropriate Audiovisuals: Handouts, materials, or products, sometimes a short video

Benefits and Limitations: Format allows interactive discussion; participants can introduce themselves and share information with whole table; good for controversial topics or new ideas and programs; limited number of people hear the topic

Tips: Speak from notes or handouts; you will need facilitation skills and ability to refocus group if discussion is off-track or is monopolized by an individual

Professional presentations can be assessed through the use of course and conference evaluation forms completed by attendees. Evaluation measures usually address the presenter's organization of information, effective use of audiovisuals, relation of theory to practice, knowledge of subject area, and presentation style.

RESOURCES FOR PROFESSIONAL DEVELOPMENT

What avenues are available to dental hygiene students and practitioners to develop skills in health promotion and health presentations? Chapter 7 has outlined the importance of continual review of the scientific literature to keep abreast of new research and trends in dental hygiene research and practice. Because dental public health covers such a broad array of topics, hygienists would benefit by reading literature from other subject areas such as health education/health promotion, health communications, injury prevention, cancer prevention and early detection, maternal and child health, geriatrics, and school health, to name a few. The many Internet sites devoted to health topics facilitate quick perusal of information on any topic and may avoid the limitations of local library systems. Continuing education courses on a variety of topics are now more available online and via CD-ROM.

One excellent way to gain experience in actual community settings is through **service-learning programs** (see Chapter 11). These programs use structured learning experiences designed by faculty and community member teams in which students provide direct services to groups with identified needs.[18] During the process students apply concepts learned in the classroom, increasing their understanding of health care systems and community resources. They observe unique community characteristics that affect disease levels, access to care, and delivery of services. In turn, community members learn to appreciate the roles and skills of dental hygienists while receiving needed education and services in their own environment.

Service-learning settings might include day care centers, Head Start programs, public health or migrant health clinics, schools, group homes, residential care facilities, people's own homes, work sites, hospitals, prisons, homeless shelters, adult activity centers, and health departments. Community members serve as adjunct faculty and learning resources. Although faculty members usually arrange these experiences, dental hygiene students may initiate new sites for programs.

Another avenue for updating knowledge, practicing presentation skills, or networking with other professionals is attendance at professional association meetings. Box 8-3 provides an overview of some of the organizations whose missions include the arena of community dental health. Many of these organizations promote student involvement through reduced membership rates and special contests and awards.

SUMMARY

We live in a multicultural, global society in which some people are bombarded with health information, whereas others are isolated from scientific advances and health information. In the attempt to create a more equitable distribution of resources and information, dental hygienists must broaden their perspectives on how to acquire and provide health information in a credible, appropriate, and effective manner. Ways to accomplish this may include (1) applying well-researched health promotion theories to oral health programs, (2) assessing people's learning styles

Box 8-3   Professional associations as resources for community dental health

---

American Public Health Association   *www.apha.org*

Oral Health Section, Public Health Student Caucus
FT student: $50/yr, Reg: $160/yr
Am J Public Health, Our Nation's Health, Oral Health Section newsletter
Annual meeting in early November

American Association of Public Health Dentistry   *www.aaphd.org*

No separate sections
FT student: $40/yr, Reg: $100/yr
J Public Health Dent, Communique newsletter
Annual National Oral Health Conference in late April/early May

American Dental Education Association   *www.adea.org*

Behavioral Science Section, Community and Preventive Dentistry Section
FT student: $30/yr, Reg: $95/yr
J Dent Educ, Bulletin of Dent Educ
Annual meeting in March

Special Care Dentistry   *www.scdonline.org*

Academy of Dentistry for Persons with Disabilities, American Association of Hospital
Dentists, American Society for Geriatric Dentistry
FT student: $35/yr, Reg: $80/yr
Special Care in Dentistry, Interface newsletter
Annual meeting, usually in March, but may change

International/American Association of Dental Research   *www.dentalresearch.org*

Behavioral Science Group, Oral Health Research Group
FT student: $47.50/yr (online journal + AADR); Reg: $185
J Dent Res, IADR/AADR Reports newsletter
Annual meeting in March

International Federation of Dental Hygienists   *www.ifdh.org*

No sections
Indiv: $75/yr
Int J Dent Hygiene
International Symposium every 3 years

---

and information needs, (3) tailoring information in a culturally and linguistically appropriate manner based on needs assessment data, and (4) evaluating the impact of the activities.

Opportunities for using new communication modalities in a variety of settings outside the traditional clinical private practice setting are endless. Service-learning programs and professional associations can be valuable resources for preparing dental hygienists to meet today's health care challenges.

Applying **Your Knowledge**

1. Create a game based on various health promotion theories. You can use the format of well-known games (e.g., Trivial Pursuit, Jeopardy) or a simple matching or fill-in-the-blank format. Students can also work in groups to design role-playing scenarios based on the types of behaviors described in the theories.
2. Choose a topic and audience for designing an oral health fact sheet. Describe how you would vary the design and frame the messages according to the following types of communication: (a) generic, (b) targeted, (c) personalized, and (d) tailored.
3. Choose an oral health topic for designing a health promotion activity for consumers (non-health professionals). Each student should select a different audience (e.g., age group, ethnicity) for the materials. The assignment is to (a) describe how you would conduct a needs assessment, (b) select an appropriate educational format, and (c) evaluate the impact of your approach.
4. Choose a topic for a 10-minute presentation. Describe how you would present this topic as (a) a table clinic, (b) a scientific poster, (c) an oral paper, and (d) a round table discussion.
5. Brainstorm ideas for service-learning opportunities, and assume that appropriate resources are available. After the session, check off which ones already are offered to students. Now choose one or two of those not offered and discuss which issues should be considered and which resources would be needed to offer these options. (This activity could lead to a class-initiated project to develop and implement a new service-learning opportunity.)
6. Acquire information, copies of journals and newsletters, and agendas of annual meetings from professional associations such as those listed in Box 8-3. Compare the organizations for similarities and differences. Students may wish to interview one of the association officers about the history and current involvement of dental hygienists in the organization.

DENTAL HYGIENE COMPETENCIES

Reading the material within this chapter and participating in the activities of "Applying Your Knowledge" will contribute to the student's ability to demonstrate the following competencies:

Core competencies

C.5 Continuously perform self-assessment for lifelong learning and professional growth.

C.8 Communicate effectively with individuals and groups from diverse populations both verbally and in writing.

Community involvement

CM.4 Facilitate client access to oral health services by influencing individuals and/or organizations for the provision of oral health care.

Health promotion

HP.4 Identify individual and population risk factors, and develop strategies that promote health and quality of life.

Community Case

You are a dental hygienist who has been working in clinical private practice for 3 years and now wants to work part-time in a public health setting. The local health department has hired you to work on a project to help mothers of children ages 0 to 5 years learn about: (1) the relationship between consumption of sugar, including sweetened beverages, and dental caries, (2) how to determine the amount and type of sugar from food labels, (3) how to select food low in refined sugars, and (4) how to use these foods to create healthy snacks for young children.

Your target population is approximately 2000 low-income women whose children are eligible for Medicaid benefits and services from the Women, Infant, and Children (WIC) program, and whose children attend Early Head Start or Head Start programs. According to the most recent health department data, 50% of the women are Caucasian, 25% Hispanic, 10% African American, 10% Asian, and 5% other ethnic background.

1. Your first task is to review the various health promotion theories and determine which one(s) might be useful for this project. You decide that you need to assess whether the women in the target population perceive their children are given food high in sugars and whether that makes them at risk for dental caries. Which one of the following theories might be best to use for this?
   a. Social learning theory
   b. Stages of change theory
   c. Health belief model
   d. Diffusion of innovations theory
   e. Organizational change theory
2. Your next task is to select and frame the health messages you want to include in your health communication approaches. Which one of the following approaches is an example of "tailoring" messages?
   a. Five-page brochure that includes 15 messages covering all of the information
   b. Separate brochures for each ethnic group

    c. Learning modules that focus on the women's roles as mothers

    d. Short learning modules geared to what level of risk for dental decay they perceive their child to be in during the assessment process

    e. Short booklet that leaves a blank place to write the child's name

3. Research shows that people learn in different ways. Which one of the following statements generally is NOT true?

    a. Asking people to demonstrate a skill helps reinforce written instructions.

    b. People usually remember more of what they read than what they see or hear.

    c. Being asked to repeat instructions in their own words helps people remember information.

    d. Hands-on, interactive, multimedia approaches are most effective for retaining knowledge.

    e. People usually remember more of what they see than what they read.

4. You decide that the project materials need to be available in at least English and Spanish. Which of the following approaches is LEAST likely to result in effective and culturally relevant materials?

    a. Use translators who are bilingual and bicultural.

    b. Test the materials in three focus groups: one for English only readers, one for Spanish only readers, and one for women who read some things in both languages.

    c. Do a literal translation from the English version to Spanish.

    d. Create the materials in dual-language format.

    e. Use graphics that are meaningful to mothers in the target groups.

5. During the project you have an opportunity to present information on the project at a statewide public health association meeting. You are most interested in discussing and getting feedback on ways to improve the materials and messages. The presentation format that would allow you the best opportunity to accomplish this is:

    a. Round table discussion

    b. Table clinic

    c. Poster presentation

    d. Oral presentation

    e. Informal networking with individuals.

REFERENCES

1. Kay E, Locker D: Effectiveness of Oral Health Promotion: A Review. London, Health Education Authority, 1999.
2. Robertson A, Minkler M: New health promotion movement: A critical examination. Health Educ Q 21:295-312, 1994.
3. Glanz K, Rimer BK: Theory at a Glance: A Guide for Health Promotion Practice. Bethesda, Md, National Institutes of Health, 2003. Available from *http://cancer.gov/cancerinformation/theory-at-a-glance*.
4. Raczynski JM, DiClemente RJ (eds): Handbook of Health Promotion and Disease Prevention. New York, Kluwer Academic Publishers/Plenum, 1999.

5. An Inventory of Knowledge and Skills Relating to Disease Prevention and Health Promotion. Washington, DC, Association of Teachers of Preventive Medicine, 1994.

6. USDHHS: Chapter 11. Health Communication. In Healthy People 2010, 2nd ed, vol 1. Washington, DC, US Govt Printing Office, 2000.

7. USDHHS, PHS, NIH, NCI: Making Health Communication Programs Work. Bethesda, Md, NCI, 2002.

8. Wallack L, Dorfman L, Jernigan D, et al: Media Advocacy and Public Health: Power for Prevention. London, Sage Publications, 1993.

9. Kreuter M, Farell D, Olevitch, et al: Tailoring Health Messages: Customizing Communication with Computer Technology. London, Lawrence Erlbaum Associates, 2000.

10. Benn DK, Dankel DD, Clark D, et al: Standardizing data collection and decision-making with an expert system. J Dent Educ 61:885-894, 1997.

11. USDHHS: A National Call to Action to Promote Oral Health. Rockville, Md, USDHHS, PHS, CDC and NIH, NIDCR. NIH Publication No 03-5303, 2003.

12. CMS. Writing and Designing Print Materials for Beneficiaries: A Guide for State Medicaid Agencies. DHHS, CMS. Publication No 10145, 1999.

13. CDC: Beyond the Brochure: Alternative Approaches to Effective Health Communication. Atlanta, Centers for Disease Control and Prevention, Publication No PDF-821K, 2000.

14. DeBiase CB: Dental Health Education: Theory and Practice, 2nd ed, Philadelphia, Lea & Febiger, 1991.

15. DeSouza MB, Kressin NR: Dental health education. In Gluck GM, Morganstein WM: Jong's Community Dental Health, 5th ed. St. Louis, Mosby, 2003.

16. Dignan MB, Carr PA: Program Planning for Health Education and Health Promotion, 2nd ed. Philadelphia, Lea & Febiger, 1992.

17. Radel J: Effective Presentations. Available from *www.kumc.edu/SAH/OTEd/jradel/effective.html.*

18. Seifer SD, Conners K: A Guide for Developing Community-Responsive Models in Health Professions Education. San Francisco, Community-Campus Partnerships for Health, 1998.

9

Social Responsibility

Diane Brunson, RDH, MPH

Objectives

Upon completion of this chapter, the student will be able to:

- Define the terms *social responsibility* and *professional ethics*
- Discuss the various opinions surrounding health as a right or a privilege
- Explain how the current delivery of oral health care services affects access
- Identify how the concept of need versus demand affects allocation of resources and the hygienist's role as consumer advocate and educator
- Explain the roles of the dental hygienist as they relate to community education, risk communication, and leadership
- Discuss the responsibility of dental hygienists with respect to cultural competence and their role in providing care to special populations

Key Terms

Social Responsibility	Access	Need
Ethics	Health Security	Demand
Professional Ethics	Pluralistic	Cultural Competence

OPENING STATEMENT

Status and Future of Health Care
- The health care system in the United States is in crisis.

- The public health system in the United States is in disarray.

- Oral health is a component of overall health, and access to health care services should be a right guaranteed to everyone.

- Human rights should be the foundation of public health practice, research, and policy in every country in the world.

- Perceived risks of health care interventions increase when the public receives contradictory opinions from responsible sources.

SOCIAL RESPONSIBILITY AND PROFESSIONAL ETHICS

Social Responsibility

The following questions are often asked in relation to the responsibilities of the dental hygienist:
- What are the hygienist's responsibilities to the profession of dental hygiene, to the patients in the dental practice, and to society as a whole?
- Do these responsibilities entail taking a leadership role in a professional organization?
- Do they include maintaining competency in clinical skills and currency in dental science so as to provide the best possible care for the patient?
- Do they look beyond the patients of record in a practice to individuals and communities that lack access to needed oral health care?
- Do they embrace the art of communication to assure the public that it has the knowledge to improve its own oral health?

Certainly, the responsibilities of the dental hygienist include all of these and more. **Social responsibility** is a broad term that encompasses professionalism, personal and professional ethics, and the role of a profession in the context of the greater society.[1] It includes the concepts of a person's right to health care, the profession's obligation to raise the "dental IQ" of the community, and ensuring the health and well-being of the public. In this chapter, by necessity, more questions are asked than answered, but the stage is set for critical thinking and further discussion about individual and collective hygienists' roles, values, and beliefs. The dental hygienist is encouraged to share thoughts and to discuss personal answers and ideas with colleagues.

Professional Ethics

A term often equated with social responsibility is **ethics,** commonly defined as the general science of right and wrong conduct.[2] Add to this the concept of moral action, and discussions emerge regarding which moral principles should govern a particular action. So intertwined and abstract is this concept that the terms "ethics" and "morals" are often used interchangeably.[3]

Professional ethics, then, is the code by which the profession regulates actions and sets standards for its members, with the recognition that professionals are accountable for their actions.[4] This code serves as a guide to the profession to ensure a high standard of competency, to strengthen the relationships among its members, and to promote the welfare of the entire community.[5] The Code of Ethics of the American Dental Hygienists Association (ADHA) provides this guidance to the dental hygiene profession.

By virtue of the education, the written and clinical board examinations, and subsequent state licensure, dental hygiene is a profession, and dental hygienists are professionals and thus are required to make choices in practice that necessitate ethical decision making. Disagreements occasionally arise from different interpretations of the "proper" roles, responsibilities, and level of decision making of professionals involved in patients' oral care.[6] Often these discussions take precedence over, and are counterproductive to, the larger issues of serving the needs of the public. Examples include whether dental hygienists should be able to (1) determine which teeth would benefit from sealant placement and (2) practice unsupervised in public health settings.

The Code of Ethics and Standards of Professional Conduct, adopted by the American Association of Public Health Dentistry, provides guidance to dental public health professionals through six basic principles, which may be summarized as follows:

Dental public health professionals have the responsibility to:
1. Inform individuals and community organizations about health issues and options available for correcting oral health problems and inequities; facilitate health care decisions; ensure individual patient confidentiality; and respect individual and community customs, beliefs, and other cultural variations (Autonomy).
2. Provide individual and community services in a socially responsible manner while maintaining respect for the value of the services received and conservation of individual, private, and public resources (Nonmaleficence).
3. Provide the best care possible, but with the constraint that care should be equitable, that is, the best possible care that helps the largest number of people for the longest period of time (Beneficence).
4. Not engage in acts of discrimination; but rather, promote policies that ensure equitable distribution of available resources and ensure that spokespersons for the public are included in the health policy development process (Fairness).

5. Abides by his or her written verbal direct, and implied, agreements; respects copyrights; and does not engage in activity in which there is real, or potential for, appearance of conflict of interest (Truthfulness).
6. Participate in professional and community meetings; share knowledge and skills with colleagues and public; and recognize an obligation to protect the public (Professionalism).[8]

Another set of debates arises in the attempt to define the term *public*, for instance:

- Does the word mean only those individuals who seek dental care? Are they the only ones the dental profession has "responsibility" for?
- What is the responsibility of the dental hygienist to the broader group of "public," which includes people without access to oral health care services, culturally diverse populations, and people with special health care needs?
- Do people have a right to receive quality dental health care at a cost they can afford?
- What is a fair, or just, distribution of limited dental health care resources?

It is imperative that these questions be seriously considered, because the dental hygiene profession's commitment to ethical conduct is the foundation of society's trust and confidence.[7]

A SYSTEM IN CRISIS

These questions, to which answers are as diverse as populations themselves, point to the need for a broader look at the general health care system in the United States. Many journals and newspapers report that health care in the nation is in a state of "crisis." Although this statement is resounding in many private and public health circles, it is controversial in the face of the technologic advances in medicine and dentistry that have been responsible for improved health standards not only in the United States but also in many countries of the world. Technology has allowed delivery of advanced surgical and cosmetic dental services to one segment of the population even while significant barriers to accessing even preventive and basic restorative care still exist for others.[9]

It is also apparent that the health care crisis has been recognized, reported, discussed, and debated for more than 50 years, with minimal progress made. The Surgeon General's report on oral health specifically quantifies the disparities in oral health status among underserved populations and the barriers many people face in obtaining care.[10] The health professions, including private and public delivery systems, national and state governments, public apathy, and a general lack of social responsibility on the part of society as a whole all have contributed to the failure of each attempt to render health care accessible to everyone. In one form or another, health reforms have been recommended for several decades; however, these have been implemented with little success, and in most cases oral health care services have not been included. Expecting the public health system to be the sole solution may be problematic, because some believe there is no consensus on what constitutes public health, or what the minimum standards for delivery of services should be.[11]

HEALTH CARE: A PRIVILEGE OR A RIGHT?

Health Care as a Privilege

The crux of the debate is the question of whether health care, including oral health care, is a "right" or a "privilege."[12] Who is responsible for "health?" As one ponders these questions, consider the examples in Guiding Principles.

GUIDING PRINCIPLES

Who Has a Right to Health Care?

- Should the person who smokes have access to the same level of health care as the nonsmoker?
- Should children who are not eligible for Medicaid and who are living in poverty have access to after-hours treatment for ear infections and prescriptions for antibiotics?
- Should the senior citizen on a fixed income have equal access to properly fitting dentures?
- Should the immigrant female of childbearing age have access to culturally appropriate examinations and treatment?

If any of the answers is "yes," who is responsible for delivering the health care and who is responsible for paying for it? Many would argue that it should not be only private providers offering reduced fees or donating their services. Additional publicly funded programs with acceptable reimbursement rates and dollars sufficient to serve the needs of the population are also needed. The following questions relate to whose responsibility it is to provide health care services and to pay for them:

- Should taxes be increased to support these programs or incentives implemented to increase provider participation?
- What is the responsibility of the patient seeking care?
- Should access to health care be a privilege of productive members of society who have the ability to pay for that health care?
- Are rights automatic, or are they "earned" as a reward for being socially responsible?

These questions have no clear answers, and they challenge the individual provider's values and sense of social responsibility.

Health Care as a Right

The United States Constitution does not specifically guarantee a "right to health," because "health" is a dynamic, continually changing state, unique to each individual.[13] One interpretation is that health and access to health care are not so much a legal right; rather, they are a "moral" right and, as such, the obligation of society as a whole is to provide care in response to that right, with providers playing an important role.[2] "The duty to ensure basic oral health for all Americans is a shared duty that includes federal, state, community, public, and private responsibilities. The dental profession . . . as the moral community entrusted by society with knowledge and skill about oral health, has the duty to lead the effort to ensure access for all Americans."[14] Society, however, has not universally accepted that responsibility despite several key events that have attempted to highlight the relationship among individual rights, human dignity, and the human condition.[15]

In 1946, the Constitution of the World Health Organization (WHO) defined health as "a state of complete physical, mental, and social well-being" (see Chapter 1). This was reiterated in the Universal Declaration of Human Rights adopted by the United Nations General Assembly on December 10, 1948 (Article 25):

> Everyone has the right to a standard of living adequate for the health and well-being of himself and of his family, including food, clothing, housing and medical care. . . .[16]

An amendment to the Public Health Service Act, passed by Congress in 1966, states that "promoting and assuring the highest level of health attainable for every person serves the nation's best interests."

The fundamental basis of human rights is the recognition of the equal worth and dignity of everyone and implies that individuals, institutions, and society as a whole should protect and promote health and should ensure that health is neither impaired nor at risk. When the health of people has been left solely to the current health services system, many population groups have been left without access to health care and with little or no constituency advocating for their right to that care. Increasingly, this system has not been able to keep pace with the number of uninsured patients, expanding populations, shifts in demographics, degradation of the environment, and changes in lifestyles and value systems. This discussion becomes pertinent in the field of dental public health, which focuses on the prevention of oral diseases and promotes population-based health activities to ensure the oral health of all people.

ACCESS TO ORAL HEALTH CARE

It is essential to understand the term **access** and its relationship to social responsibility. Access is assuring that conditions are in place for people to obtain the care they need and want.[17] The key word here is "assuring." Many lawmakers and health providers feel that their responsibility is not *to provide* but to make sure that services *are provided* through different means and combinations with other partners. Herrell and Mulholland have termed this latter form of assurance **health security.**[18]

The WHO further defines health security in terms of "the rights and conditions that enable individuals to attain and enjoy their full potential for a healthy life." However, some practitioners and lawmakers do not want the obligation of providing universal and comprehensive health services and do not want any resemblance to "socialized medicine," a system in which the means of funding and distributing health care is centralized, usually with a government entity.

As a result, in the United States a **pluralistic** system has evolved in which numerous, distinct health care delivery systems coexist simultaneously.[12] In dentistry, this translates to private offices, community health centers, Medicaid-only and nonprofit clinics, mobile vans, school-based health centers, and hospital clinics and emergency departments, each with set criteria determining which patients will receive services according to socioeconomic, geographic, age, and cultural variables. In some cases this pluralistic system works well, but it is also easy to see how many populations are confused by the complexity of the system, thus "falling through the cracks" and not receiving any dental services. Oral health professionals, who are members of a society that relies on a moral infrastructure for its existence, are expected to contribute to causes that improve all of society rather than acting only out of self-interest.[14]

DISTRIBUTION OF HEALTH RESOURCES

Shortage of Dental Professionals

The result of the health services system's inability to keep pace with a rapidly changing society is a maldistribution—and, in some instances, a "shortage"—of health care providers; such conditions have a direct impact on access to services. Many might convincingly argue that there has been a shortage of dental hygienists in the 1990s and predict an even greater shortage of dentists and hygienists by the year 2010.

However, the shortage is a complicated phenomenon. It includes the closure of several dental and dental hygiene schools in the last several years, the varied length of time dental professionals remain in clinical practice, and part-time versus full-time employment opportunities. The shortage is particularly evident in the fields of dental education and dental public health, where salaries and benefits have not kept pace with those available in private practice settings.[19] Finally, insufficient numbers of culturally diverse dental professionals are trained and are entering the workforce to provide care to underserved populations.

Need versus Demand

With the ratio of providers to population decreasing, who determines who receives what level of services? The concept of "need versus demand" enters the discussion. Briefly defined, **need** refers to those services deemed by the health professional to be necessary after a variety of assessment and diagnostic tools, and perhaps past experience, have been employed. The disproportionate burden of oral diseases indicates that some population groups are in greater need of oral health care. **Demand** refers to the health care services desired by the individual or community. The extent of oral health disparities among select population groups illustrates that many people in *need* of oral care do not *demand* services.[14]

When tremendous differences exist between need and demand in a community, however, it is imperative that health care providers educate the public and policy makers regarding what is needed to bring public demand as close to what is needed as possible for optimal use of scarce resources. Herein lies a major social responsibility of dental hygienists and other health care providers: education and communication.

As an example, in state Children with Special Health Care Needs (CSHCN) programs, limited funding is available for orthodontic services for low-income children with severe malocclusions. The qualifying malocclusions are usually due to skeletal malformations, resulting in impaired speech and chewing ability, and to facial asymmetry (as in cleft lip and palate) and are not due simply to an overbite or overjet, malalignment of several teeth, or cross-bite. The difference is often difficult for families desiring aesthetically appealing smiles for their children to understand why funds are going to other children for the restoration of functional occlusion. Educating families of children, public health providers, and lawmakers becomes as important as paying for needed services.

An important component and a useful tool in reconciling need and demand is the use of *dental indices* (see Chapter 4). Using Dean's Fluorosis Index, the Community Periodontal Index (CPI), the Decayed, Missing, and Filled Teeth (DMFT) Index, and the WHO Dental Aesthetic Index (DAI) gives health care professionals objective data to use when communicating to policy makers and individuals about the oral health care needs in their community and provides the basis for decisions.

PATIENT RESPONSIBILITY

An earlier question in this chapter concerned the patient's role in accessing health care. In a society where a pluralistic health system exists, greater emphasis is placed on individual responsibility for health; however, when we look at the significant advances in any nation's health to date, personal lifestyle has not been the most important factor.[20] This is particularly true for improvements in overall oral health status, which can certainly be attributed to community water fluoridation, fluoride toothpaste, sealants, and better restorative materials.

Three factors have been associated with health care inequalities and increased burden of disease: (1) education, (2) housing, and (3) nutrition. Each of these factors is recognized by society as primarily the responsibility of government and publicly funded programs.[20] Those in favor of multiple oral health service delivery systems claim that increased patient responsibility would reduce the "demand" for oral health services. This would be easier than manipulating the way in which oral health services are provided, thereby helping to resolve the health care access dilemma.[21] Although prevention would go a long way toward reducing the need for emergency and episodic care, when we consider the 10 greatest public health achievements of the twentieth century (see Chapter 1), very little individual patient responsibility was involved. Some historians point out that most of these significant advances occurred during that century's "infectious disease" era; in today's "information age," however, perhaps increased personal responsibility is appropriate.

Particularly difficult is assigning personal responsibility to children whose dental caries experience, for example, reflects the socioeconomic and educational constraints of their parents and caregivers, or to the elderly, who experience increased periodontal disease, decay, incidence of oral cancer, and tooth loss as income becomes fixed or decreases. Some believe that this type of health status data provides an important indicator of the degree to which human rights are enjoyed or denied as a result of inequity and discrimination. The inequality comes around full circle as declines in dental health and overall health perpetuate the inability to improve socioeconomic status.

This is not to say that individuals should not have responsibility for improving their own oral health and participating in conscientious brushing, flossing, and regular dental visits. According to the results of the Behavioral Risk Factor Surveillance Survey (BRFSS), the primary response adults give for not seeing a dentist in the past year is that they "did not see a reason to go." The dental hygienist, in the role of Educator and Consumer Advocate, is in an ideal position to communicate the importance of regular oral health care and the relationship to general health and systemic disease, not only to patients but to the public as a whole.

RISK COMMUNICATION

Understanding Risk

Another aspect of social and professional responsibility is communication. Not only are health education, oral hygiene instruction, and post-treatment instructions and follow-up of paramount importance; so is the communication of "risk." It is the responsibility of the dental profession, including dental hygienists, to know what the public perceives as risk and to be able to assist in bringing to light peer-reviewed research to reduce public misperceptions.

For example, a segment of the general public perceives inherent risks in radiographs, amalgam restorations, biofilms in dental unit water lines, instrument sterilization techniques, transmission of disease (e.g., human immunodeficiency virus [IIIV] infection, hepatitis) in dental offices, and fluoridation of community water supplies. It is the dental hygienist's responsibility to become knowledgeable about current research regarding these issues for ensuring compliance with recommended protocols, regardless of the practice setting, to minimize these risks. The next task is to communicate pertinent information to the public to reduce the spread of misinformation.

Communication

The messages obtained by the public regarding oral health issues are judged, primarily, not on their content but on whether the person providing the information is someone who inspires trust.[21] As a group, dentists and hygienists are regarded as very trustworthy, but this trust is understandably shaken when a member of the profession openly opposes water fluoridation, advocates removing amalgam fillings for reasons other than recurrent decay or fracture, or blatantly dismisses current infection control guidelines.

Communication is a two-way process, and to fully understand a community's concerns, the professional responsible for communicating risk must take these concerns seriously while providing sound scientific evidence. This is where the hygienist's role in staying abreast of current research and using skills in critically evaluating scientific research and literature not only is important but also is a component of the profession's social responsibility.

Comparative Analysis

Communicating risk is not an easy task. Many professionals use "comparative" risk analyses, which are not always effective and may be a hindrance in conveying trust.[21] Following are a few examples of potential risks in dentistry:

1. For the patient concerned about a full set of radiographs, x-ray exposure is explained as being comparable to 1 hour out in the sun at high altitude.
2. For the patient hesitant to accept amalgam fillings as part of a treatment plan because of the mercury content, the mercury level is considered comparable to that in common foods.
3. For the community resident fearful of 1 part per million (ppm) of fluoride in the water supply, the amount is said to be comparable to one drop of water in a bathtub half full.

Providing these comparisons is not necessarily incorrect, but whether such information can succeed in allaying the concerns of the individual is unpredictable. Herein lies another key point: Scientists and professionals tend to define "risk" in terms of entire populations; laypeople are concerned with the risk to themselves. Each person approaches risk from different frames of reference based on past experience, culture, and the media.

PERCEIVED RISK

In addition to the problems of comparisons, according to Peter Bennett, are "fright factors."[22] Popular antifluoridation arguments and the perceived risks based on these fright factors are outlined in Table 9-1.

Antifluoridation arguments include claims that the presence of fluoride in community water makes consumption of fluoride "involuntary and inescapable" and that some "at-risk" individuals have adverse reactions to fluoride (e.g., allergies, cancer), which remain unsubstantiated; however, adding to the difficulty is the fact that some arguments against fluoridation are true. For instance, fluoride chemicals are a by-product of the fertilizer industry, there is a printed warning on fluoride toothpaste tubes about not swallowing the paste, and the prevalence of dental

Table 9-1   Perceived fluoridation risks

Factors That Heighten Perceived Risk	Popular Antifluoridation Arguments to Illustrate Perceived Risk
1. Exposure is involuntary versus voluntary.	1. Fluoride in community drinking water is unavoidable.
2. Risk is unevenly distributed (some people have problems; others do not).	2. People with suppressed immune systems may be adversely affected by fluoride.
3. Risk is inescapable despite personal precaution.	3. Fluoride is in nearly all foods and beverages.
4. Source is unfamiliar.	4. Fluoride chemicals are a by-product of fertilizer industry.
5. Fluoride is man-made rather than natural.	5. Chemicals used in the process include sodium fluoride, which is different from the calcium fluoride occurring in nature.
6. Hidden and irreversible damage may result.	6. Overexposure in the young results in fluorosis in permanent teeth.
7. Particular danger may be posed to children or pregnant women.	7. Warning on toothpaste tube cautions against swallowing the paste.
8. Illness, injury, or death is possible.	8. Chronic overexposure may result in crippling skeletal fluorosis.
9. Damage occurs to real people, not anonymous victims.	9. Fluoridated water is not used in kidney dialysis because of possible overdosing of fluoride, resulting in death.
10. Fluoridation is poorly understood by science.	10. Caries have decreased in nonfluoridated communities.
11. Statements from responsible sources have been contradictory.	11. Some health professions are opposed to fluoridation.

caries is declining in nonfluoridated communities. However, these statements are used inappropriately and incorrectly when one is discussing fluoridating community water supplies at optimal levels.

The public does not always understand the differences. It is evident why some perceived risks, such as fluoridation, trigger so many more alarms than other health interventions regardless of the scientific basis or evidence to the contrary. The right column of Table 9-1 can easily be changed from "fluoridation" to "amalgam" for another illustration of why perceived risk is a communication challenge.

Responsibility in Communication

Risks not only are dependent on the context in which they are presented but also are intertwined with personal values; thus it becomes difficult to dismiss the antifluoridation arguments as "unreasonable." Attitudes about certain risks are often influenced by how people believe society should be; their relationship with nature;

the benefits and disadvantages of technology; cultural influences; and, occasionally, religious beliefs. Understanding a message regarding health risk is not the same as knowledge. People may understand a message perfectly but still maintain their own opinions.[23] It would be easier if strong beliefs could be altered with presentation of information and education programs. However, people's beliefs change very slowly, even when factual information is presented.[24]

Successful risk communication raises the level of people's understanding of relevant issues and reassures those involved that they are adequately informed within the limits of available knowledge.[25] It is a social responsibility of the dental professional to communicate risk. Successful communication is dependent on respecting beliefs, gathering information consistent with the public's point of view, and then providing a professional account of the evidence underlying sound health decisions and treatment modalities.

SPECIAL POPULATIONS

Cultural Sensitivity

A brief discussion of "special populations" and society's responsibility in ensuring their access to health care is warranted. Special populations include:

- Low-income patients (Medicaid recipients, the working poor, homeless people)
- Patients of various cultures (farm workers, immigrants, Native Americans) who may have different life experiences and backgrounds as well as language barriers
- Patients who are immunocompromised (those with HIV infection/acquired immunodeficiency syndrome [AIDS] and those undergoing chemotherapy or radiation therapy for cancer)
- Women and children in shelters
- Troubled teens
- Nursing home residents
- Patients with Alzheimer's disease
- Mentally and physically disabled persons

Often the traditional dental office setting does not match the needs of the special-population patient. Case managers, social workers, and school nurses are commonly expected to provide education to these populations on how to access the dental office. Look around a dental office or dental hygiene school clinic, and observe how it might welcome a special-population patient. For example:

- Would a Medicaid patient feel comfortable in the waiting room?
- Are written materials, health histories, informed consents, and postoperative instructions translated into other languages and at a literacy level appropriate for the community?
- Is the office or clinic located on a major public transportation route?

- Has someone arranged for a translator (other than a patient's family member) to help the patient understand the diagnosis, treatment, and follow-up instructions?
- Would the people be better served by bringing the dental clinic to them?
- Is the dental staff culturally diverse?

Cultural Competence

These aforementioned considerations fall in the category of **cultural competence** and affect the profession's responsibility in reducing the burden (incidence) of disease. This topic will be discussed at length in Chapter 10. From a social and professional responsibility perspective, oral health professionals may encounter conflicts between an individual's physical well-being and their values.[14]

Special populations typically have a higher burden of oral disease and face many barriers to accessing care.[26] For example, community health centers often employ bilingual or bicultural staff members to encourage access by minority populations. Many populations respond more favorably to health messages from someone of their own culture and language. Health centers serving farm worker populations often have mobile vans that go directly into the fields to provide health education, take blood pressure readings, conduct oral health screenings, and give vaccinations. Patients scheduled for a follow-up appointment are more likely to keep the appointment if someone has reached out to them in a culturally sensitive manner.

Mobile vans and portable equipment also serve low-income populations, as in school-based sealant programs; and mentally and physically disabled persons are served through the National Foundation of Dentistry for the Handicapped's Homebound Dentistry Programs. Native American populations, many served through the Indian Health Service (IHS), often have clinics of their own design and controlled by tribal councils, using IHS or contract providers. Providing culturally competent care is a responsibility of the dental hygienist, requiring attention to technical skill and the individual's personal values.

Alternative Practice Settings

In states where dental hygienists are allowed to practice under general supervision or are allowed to practice unsupervised in public health settings, many hygienists have found rewarding careers providing preventive services using portable equipment in long-term care facilities. Some facilities have set aside rooms with a full dental operatory to make it easier for residents to seek care.

Many states that have school-based health centers (SBHCs) are beginning to research the feasibility of adding dental services to their centers. A few have implemented full dental clinics with paid and volunteer dentists and hygienists, whereas others contract with public and private entities with portable equipment to provide preventive and restorative services. Military personnel (e.g., the National Guard) have also set up portable units in rural and inner-city areas to provide dental care closer to home for underserved populations. Still other communities use state-of-the-art mobile dental clinics to reach rural and frontier areas and special populations.

All of these examples illustrate sensitivity to the increasing cultural diversity of communities and address the needs of special populations by ensuring access to oral health services. Many of these alternative dental delivery systems rely on volunteers and donated services because of limited funding and competing community priorities. By bringing the services *to* special populations in a manner consistent with and comfortable to their culture, dental professionals have been able to provide increased access to services and have helped to improve oral health as well as general health.[27]

PATIENT CONFIDENTIALITY

Besides the dental professional's responsibilities in respecting cultures, maintaining patient confidentiality is paramount. The rights of the patient and maintaining patient confidentiality in private practice settings are emphasized throughout the dental hygiene student's clinical education; however, it is often forgotten that the same principles apply in dental public health practice.

In public health settings, which may include clinics, schools, and health fair screenings, the atmosphere is often less structured and more chaotic at times, thus necessitating greater attention to patient confidentiality. Ensuring a patient's right to privacy during screenings and treatment, protecting records (signed consents and medical histories), and refraining from sharing personal patient information (e.g., HIV status) with school personnel, policy makers, and other patients are part of the social and ethical responsibilities of the dental professional.

Community groups commonly desire to highlight their successful projects by inviting media from newspapers and television to showcase their efforts. However, it is prudent to gain permission from patients if they are going to be in any photographs or film coverage. Many schools require signed permission forms from parents if their child is to be photographed. Inclusion of as many partners in the community as possible in the planning process helps to avoid these social mishaps and ensures program visibility and success.

CHILD ABUSE AND NEGLECT

In the dental hygienist's role in helping to promote the health and well-being of the public, difficult situations sometimes arise that test social and ethical principles and values. In many states the dental hygienist is a mandated reporter of suspected child abuse and neglect. This means that the hygienist is required by law to report to the appropriate authorities any information regarding a child whom the hygienist suspects is a victim of abuse or neglect. PANDA (Prevent Abuse and Neglect through Dental Awareness) programs provide training to dental professionals on recognizing and reporting suspected cases of child abuse and neglect, including dental neglect.[28]

As a mandated reporter, the dental hygienist should be alert for these signs of abuse:

- Bruises, particularly around the areas of the head and neck
- Bruises of various colors, which indicate multiple stages of healing
- Injuries inconsistent with stories of how they occurred
- Inappropriate clothing for the temperature (long-sleeved sweaters in hot, humid climates)
- Unusual shyness or withdrawal or a reaction to oral procedures

These signs should raise questions as to whether abuse may have occurred. Parental disregard of or refusal to follow through on a child's needed dental treatment may be an indication of dental neglect. It is the professional responsibility of hygienists to know the legal requirements in the community, the agency to call to report gathered information, and the steps to take to ensure safety for themselves and for the patient.

LEADERSHIP

For every child without medical insurance, 2.6 children are without dental insurance, and for every adult with medical insurance, 3 adults are without dental insurance.[10] With the increasing number of people without health or dental insurance, continued leadership on the part of dental professionals to eliminate oral health disparities and to ensure access to oral health services for all is needed.

Dental hygiene leadership embraces the following concepts:

- Social responsibility
- Professionalism
- Ethics
- Communication
- Cultural competence (see earlier)

A leader in dental hygiene works within the community to develop consensus on what "oral health care for all" might look like. He or she enables others to see the problem firsthand and to implement solutions and models public health practice by ensuring equal access to care and not tolerating discrimination against any person seeking care. The leader encourages other professionals in the community to participate in health promotion and disease prevention activities and celebrates successes.

The dental hygiene leader challenges "the way things have always been done" and seeks new ways to maximize resources and productivity while remaining mindful of ethical decision-making processes and commitment to quality oral care.[29] The leader respects the other health care providers in the community and forges collaborative relationships in providing total health care for the public.

Finally, the dental hygiene leader works within the profession to ensure continued competency, lifelong learning, and maintenance of quality standards of practice.

SUMMARY

The dental hygienist is a professional. Inherent in the role of the professional is the responsibility of making ethical decisions and choices and opportunities to practice dental hygiene in ways that will increase access to oral health services for all populations. The role requires the leadership to uphold the standards of dental hygiene practice and communication skills to promote optimal oral health for all.

Applying Your Knowledge

1. Conduct a survey of other students on campus, or dental professionals in the community, as to their beliefs of access to health care as a "privilege" or a "right." Present your findings to your class, allowing time for discussion of the various views collected.

2. Choose a dental treatment or preventive measure that is perceived by some members of society as carrying risk. Research two scientific articles in response to one of those perceived risks, and share your expertise with the rest of your class.

3. Invite oral health care professionals in the community who provide services to special populations as the majority of their practice to participate in a panel discussion describing the following:
   a. What they see in terms of the burden of disease among their patients
   b. How they view their role in improving access to care
   c. What they view as their responsibility to the public at large

4. Visit an alternative dental services delivery system (mobile, portable, long-term care, school-based health center), and observe whether the system improves access to oral health services for a special population. Create a poster that compares and contrasts this system with the traditional dental office in terms of:
   a. Access for that population
   b. Dental services provided
   c. Cost per patient
   d. Utilization of auxiliaries

5. Survey local school districts to identify those that have signed contracts with soda companies to place vending machines in their schools as a money-making venture. Prepare an outline for a presentation you might make at a PTA meeting.

DENTAL HYGIENE COMPETENCIES

Reading the material in this chapter and participating in the activities of "Applying Your Knowledge" will contribute to the student's ability to demonstrate the following competencies:

Core competencies

C.1 Apply a professional code of ethics in all endeavors.

C.6 Advance the profession through service activities and affiliations with professional organizations.

C.8 Communicate effectively with individuals and groups from diverse populations, both verbally and in writing.

Health promotion and disease prevention

HP.1 Promote the values of oral and general health and wellness to the public and organizations within and outside the profession.

Community involvement

CM.4 Facilitate client access to oral health care services by influencing individuals and organizations for the provision of oral health care.

Community Case

Jan has been volunteering in a second-grade school-based sealant project operated by the local health department at several elementary schools in the city. Volunteer dentists screen the children to ascertain which teeth are sealable and to prioritize children for urgency of restorative needs. The dental hygienists then apply sealant to the approved teeth, provide one-on-one oral hygiene instruction, and work with school nurses to provide case management and follow-up for restorative needs. One particular child, Joey, has six decayed primary teeth. He is irritable and fearful in the dental chair. Because he is not a legal citizen, Joey does not have insurance and is not eligible for Medicaid.

Upon preparing to place the sealants, Jan notices that teeth Nos. 3, 19, and 30 are approved for sealants. Tooth No. 14 is checked as needing a restoration; however, it is evident to Jan that tooth No. 3 needs the restoration and tooth No. 14 is perhaps sealable, suggesting that the teeth numbers have been switched at screening. Jan does not seal the upper molars until the tooth numbers can be clarified, and she seals the lower molars. She sends a follow-up note home to Joey's parents indicating the findings of the screening and the urgent need for dental care. Jan returns to the school 3 months later to conduct a sealant retention check on the children who had received sealants. She discovers that (1) the status of teeth Nos. 3 and 14 for sealants has not been clarified and (2) Joey has not received the urgent dental treatment. Upon talking with the school nurse, Jan finds that the screening dentist has not been back to rescreen and that the nurse has been unsuccessful in convincing Joey's mother to take him to the dentist and has not found any local dental providers willing to donate the needed dental services.

1. What should Jan have done regarding the apparent switch in teeth numbers for sealants?
   a. Do as she did; do not seal either one, and wait for a rescreening by the dentist.
   b. Note the apparent switch in the child's chart, and seal tooth No. 14.
   c. Call the screening dentist, and explain the situation to try to get verbal approval to seal tooth No. 14.
   d. Indicate in the chart that tooth No. 3 is not sealable, and leave both teeth Nos. 3 and 14 for restorations.

2. What is Jan's responsibility concerning Joey's urgent need for dental care?
   a. She does not have any responsibility. It is up to the child's parents to get him into the dentist.
   b. She needs to work with the school nurse to find dental care for Joey as soon as possible.
   c. She needs to call Social Services to report a suspected case of dental neglect.
   d. She needs to talk to Joey's mother to explain the urgency of the situation.

3. What is Jan's responsibility to the dental professional community at large, in that the school nurse has not been able to find anyone to take Joey?
   a. She does not have any responsibility because dentists can decide whom they want in their practices.
   b. She should file a complaint with the state dental licensing board.
   c. She should make a presentation to local dentists regarding the oral health status of the children and their unmet dental needs.
   d. She should follow the dental professional's lead and try to convince Joey's parents that his dental needs are a priority and that they need to find the resources to pay for it.

REFERENCES

1. Woolfolk MW: The social responsibility model. J Dent Educ 57(5):346-348, 1993.
2. Ozar DT, Love J: Conflicting values in oral health care. J Am Coll Dent 65(3):15-18, 1998.
3. Ozar DT, Sokol DJ: Dental Ethics at Chairside: Professional Principles and Practical Application. St. Louis, Mosby-Year Book, 1994.
4. Gaston MA: Survey of ethical issues in dental hygiene. J Dent Hyg 64(5):217-24, 1990.
5. Frankel MS: Taking ethics seriously: Building a professional community. J Dent Hyg 66(9):386-392, 1992.
6. Weinstein BD: Dental Ethics. Philadelphia, Lea & Febiger, 1993.
7. Christie C, Bowen D, Paarmann C: Curriculum evaluation of ethical reasoning and professional responsibility. J Dent Educ 67(1): 55-63, 2003.
8. Code of Ethics and Standards of Professional Conduct: American Association of Public Health Dentistry. Interim Policy adopted October 16, 1997.

9. Gershen JA: Response to the social responsibility model: The convergence of curriculum and health policy. J Dent Educ 57(5):350-352, 1993.
10. Oral Health in America: A Report of the Surgeon General—Executive Summary. Rockville, Md, U.S. Department of Health and Human Services, National Institute of Dental and Craniofacial Research (NIDCR), National Institutes of Health, 2000.
11. Browning P, von Cube A, Leibrand H: Minimum public health standards as a basis for secure public health funding. J Public Health Management Practice 10(1):19-22, 2004.
12. Stewart GT: Health care in America: Privilege or right? Lancet 2(7737):1305-1306, 1971.
13. Burt BA, Eklund SA: Dentistry, Dental Practice, and the Community, 4th ed. Philadelphia, WB Saunders, 1992.
14. ADEA President's Commission—Improving the oral health status of all Americans: Roles and responsibilities of academic dental institutions. J Dent Educ 67(5):563-581, 2003.
15. Goldsmith MF: Health and human rights inseparable. JAMA 270(5):553, 1993.
16. United Nations: Universal declaration of human rights. Available at http://www.unhchr.ch/udhr/lang/eng.htm.
17. Isman R, Isman B: Oral Health America White Paper: Access to Oral Health Services in the U.S. 1997 and Beyond. Funding from the Robert Wood Johnson Foundation, 1997.
18. Herrell IC, Mulholland CA: Reflections on health in development and human rights. World Health Stat Q 51(1):88-92, 1998.
19. Valacovitch R: Dental education and emerging trends: Challenges for U.S. dental schools. American Academy of Dental Schools, Executive Director's Report to the Legislative Advisory Committee, 2000.
20. Sarll DW: Who is responsible for good oral health? Br Dent J 180(5):164-167, 1996.
21. Bent JP: Health access and social responsibility. Arch Otolaryngol Head Neck Surg 118(3):344, 1992.
22. Bennett P, Calman K: Risk Communication and Public Health. Oxford, UK, University of Oxford Press, 1999.
23. Weinstein N, Sandman P: Some criteria for evaluating risk messages. Risk Analysis 13(1): 103-114, 1993.
24. Slovic P: Informing and educating the public about risk. Risk Analysis 6(4): 403-415, 1986.
25. Deahl ST II, Kromer ME: A taxonomy for lay risk perceptions of dentistry. J Public Health Dent 56(4):213-218, 1996.
26. Warren RC: Oral Health for All: Policy for Available, Accessible, and Acceptable Care. Washington DC, Center for Policy Alternatives, 1999.
27. Jenny J: Basic social values, structural elements in oral health systems and oral health status. Int Dent J 30(3):276-285, 1980.
28. American Academy of Pediatrics/American Academy of Pediatric Dentistry: Oral and dental aspects of child abuse and neglect: Joint statement. Pediatrics 104(2):348-350, 1999.
29. Kouzes JM, Posner BZ: The Leadership Challenge. San Francisco, Jossey-Bass, 1995.

10

Cultural Competency

Magda A. de la Torre, RDH, MPH

Objectives

Upon completion of this chapter, the student will be able to:

- Describe key demographic, social, and cultural shifts and trends influencing oral health among culturally diverse groups in the United States
- Discuss the impact of population trends in oral health and provision of oral health services to individuals and groups
- Define the terms cross-cultural communication, health disparities, and cultural diversity
- Define culture and cultural competence and explain why they are important
- Identify the Oral Health Care Culturally Competent Guidelines (OHCCC Guidelines)
- Discuss the components of the Cultural Competency Continuum Ladder
- Describe the application of strategies and approaches that enhance cross-cultural communication and education in oral health care settings
- Explain and be able to use the LEARN Model
- Explain and be able to use the Explanatory Model
- Discuss the responsibility of the dental hygienist with respect to cultural competence and the role in providing care to special populations

Key Terms

Cultural Diversity	Culture	Cultural Competency
Health Disparity	Ethnocentrism	Cultural Competency Education Model

Self-Exploration

Knowledge

Skill

Cultural Destructiveness

Cultural Incapacity

Cultural Blindness

Cultural Pre-Competence

Cultural Competence

Cultural Proficiency

Cross-Cultural Encounter

Cross-Cultural Communication

OPENING STATEMENT

Status and Future of Oral Health Care

- Closing the gap on health disparities and inequalities among diverse cultures will lead to better health for all Americans and is a responsibility of all health care providers.

- Race, ethnicity, gender, and socioeconomic levels are powerful factors that affect health status, access to health care services, and the quality of health care.

- We must commit ourselves to living in a world and society where respect for human dignity and equality is valued.

- It has been said that the mark of a great community is how well it cares for its most vulnerable citizens.

- There are important variations among and within people from the same country or culture and there may be cultural variations among generations.

- There are noticeable disparities in dental disease by income. Poor children suffer twice as many dental caries than their more affluent peers.

- *Healthy People 2010* goals are to increase the quality and years of healthy life and to eliminate health disparities that are associated with race, ethnicity, and socioeconomic status.[1]

TODAY'S EVOLVING DIVERSE POPULATION

The United States is highly diverse, as evidenced in our neighborhoods, schools, and communities. Diversity extends to integral parts of our existence as human beings such as, race, culture, social and economical status, language, and national origin. Diversity also extends to lifestyles, traditions, personal and family histories, ages, abilities, and other dimensions that constitute who we are and where we come from. In most communities many languages are spoken in schools, workplaces, and homes. All of these components of our being are fundamental in our interpersonal interactions and our community structures. Previously, societies primarily functioned with a monocultural and monolingual perspective. Persons were expected to give up the values, norms, and beliefs of the society they were emigrating from in favor of new opportunities.[2] The United States has lost the image of "melting pot" of racial and ethnic groups. **Cultural diversity** in the American society is more realistically an intricate mosaic consisting of numerous racial and ethnic groups.[3]

Immigrants today are unwilling to passively and submissively assimilate the way that they may have in generations past. People have stopped denying their ethnicity for the sake of being accepted unconditionally into mainstream society. It is now clear that inherent contradiction does not exist between allegiance to someone's own ethnic and cultural heritage and being an American. Instead, these dual identities are complementary and should be respected and promoted.[4]

Today's evolving society is a multiracial, multicultural, and multilingual world (Tables 10-1 and 10-2).[5] The issues of race, ethnicity, and cultural differences have great significance for all who live in the United States. Our society has embraced the concepts of cultural competency, cultural diversity, cultural pluralism, and multi-culturalism. These concepts are being incorporated not only into health care but also business, education, and policies. In health care these concepts have implications on how care is provided for clients and a community that may not share the same culture and language as the provider. The clients may have different beliefs, values, attitudes, and behaviors.

Cultural competency should be a constant pursuit of a health care provider for three reasons: the societal realities of a changing world, the influence of culture and ethnicity on human growth and development, and the challenge of providing effective and quality health care to all people.[4] These reasons depict the need and importance of cultural competency but also the emphasis in developing skills and knowledge to communicate and collaborate with persons of other cultures.

Table 10-1   Ethnicity in the U.S. population, 1990 and 2000 census

Ethnicity	Percentage	
	1990	2000
White/Caucasian	71.3	75.1
Hispanic/Latino	8.9	12.5
Black/African American	12.0	12.3
Asian-American/Pacific Islander	2.9	3.6
American Indian/Alaskan Native	0.7	0.9

U.S. Bureau of the Census (2000) website: http://www.census.gov/.

Table 10-2   Linguistic diversity in the U.S. population

U.S. population (5 years old and older) speaking a language other than English at home	17.9%
Foreign-born U.S. population	11%

U.S. Bureau of the Census (2000) website: http://www.census.gov/.

The 2000 Surgeon General's Report focused on oral health issues and improvements in oral health over the past century. The report reminds us that there are serious challenges for the future and that although oral health has improved in the United States over the last century, disparities in health still exist. Special population groups such as infants and young children, the poor, those living in rural areas, the homeless, persons with disabilities, racial and ethnic minorities, the institutionalized, and the frail elderly experience a greater burden of oral and craniofacial diseases. Great disparities also exist in access to oral health care and use of preventive services, each vital to the establishment and maintenance of optimal health.[6]

CONSIDERING CULTURE

It is understood in the health, medical, and dental communities that there is a critical need to eliminate disparities in health care among the diverse populations in the United States. A **health disparity** is a population-specific difference in the presence of disease, health outcomes, or access to health care.[7] Racial and ethnic groups in the United States continue to experience major disparities in health status. These disparities in heath status are compounded by reduced access to health care services. Although many factors affect health status, the lack of health insurance and other barriers such as transportation, rural settings, and hours of operations of facilities are key components of reduced health care access. Racial and ethnic minorities' use of preventive services and medical treatment are diminished by an inability to obtain health services. Increased use of health services can reduce disease and contribute to improved health status (Figure 10-1).[8]

Health care access problems include several components. Two important components are (1) the influences of race or ethnicity on an individual's perception of a given illness, and (2) the decision to seek health care. A primary requirement in providing culturally sensitive medical care is a basic knowledge of the health status and needs of those groups being served. Health care providers traditionally have their own expectations of how health care should be delivered and how patients are supposed to respond to care. However, if they are to effectively work with a multicultural population, health care providers must alter their traditional ways of treating patients. Historically, many of the health care providers serving ethnic populations have been members of these same ethnic/racial groups themselves. It is imperative that all professionals who provide health care have the knowledge and communication skills that will make them attentive to the cultural differences of their patients.[9]

What is Culture?

Culture is an integrated pattern of human behavior that includes thoughts, communications, languages, practices, beliefs, values, customs, courtesies, rituals, manners

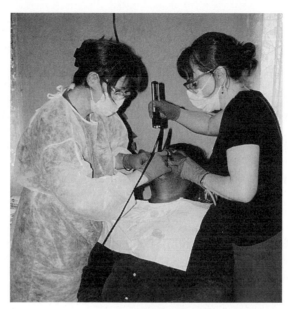

Figure 10-1 Dental hygiene students providing care in a nontraditional setting to address the needs of access to underserved populations.

of interacting and roles, relationships, and expected behaviors of a racial, ethnic, religious or social group, and the ability to transmit the above to succeeding generations.[10] Culture can also be defined as a specific set of social, educational, religious, and professional behaviors, practices, and values that individuals learn and adhere to while participating in or out of groups with whom they usually interact daily.[11] In common terms, culture is what we live every day, our daily interactions at work, school, or in our community. It is the lens that we use to view the world and to form our opinions, thoughts, aspirations, and goals in life. Culture is both inherent and learned; it is a shared way of interpreting the world. Culture is simple yet complex, common yet unique, and constantly evolving based on our life experiences. Several factors influencing culture are listed in Box 10-1.

Box 10-1   FACTORS THAT INFLUENCE CULTURE

• Age	• Socioeconomic status
• Gender	• Educational attainment
• Geography	• Family
• Place of birth	• Length of residency in the United States
• Religious beliefs	• Individual experiences
• Sexual preference	• Power relationships

Why Consider Culture?

Given the wide diversity present in modern societies, cultural competence is a necessary skill, allowing us to provide appropriate services to all citizens. Given our modern technologies, it is also a skill we need for global survival. Historically, the challenges of insufficient cultural competence for cross-cultural collaboration go back to the earliest beginnings of humanity. Every human culture teaches its members to value their beliefs, morals, and views of reality as the best, as the ideal; in some cases cultures teach that their beliefs are the ONLY acceptable way to be or think. The resulting lack of cultural interchange and adaptation could be called **ethnocentrism**—judging other cultures by your own standards consistent with your values, not theirs.[12]

Reasons to incorporate culture in your daily activities include:
- To understand the values, attitudes, and behaviors of others
- To avoid stereotypes and biases that can undermine efforts
- To develop and deliver services responsive to the needs of the patients
- To focus on commonalities, not differences (Figure 10-2)

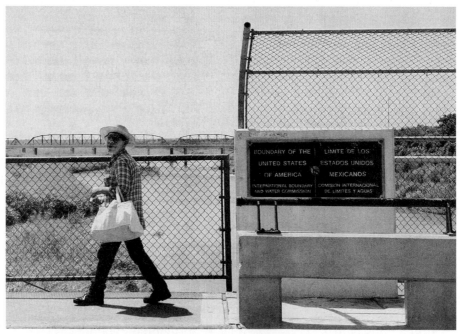

Figure 10-2 Cultural competency should be an integral part of quality oral health care to the population on the U.S.–Mexico border.

CULTURAL COMPETENCY

Cultural competency in health care describes the ability to provide care to patients with diverse values, beliefs, and behaviors.[13] Included in cultural competency is the adaptation of oral health promotion and disease prevention and clinical dental hygiene services to meet the patient's social, cultural, and linguistic needs. Individuals who must be treated in a culturally competent manner include children, the elderly, and people with disabilities. Cultural competency is a developmental process that evolves over an extended period of time. Effective cultural competency needs to be implemented on an individual, organizational, and community level. All three entities can be at various stages of awareness, knowledge, and skills and attitudes along the cultural competence continuum (Figure 10-3).[14]

Cultural Competency Models, Frameworks, and Strategies

Models exist that enable us to acquire the skills for self-assessment, to determine implementation of cultural competency in organizations and systems, and to

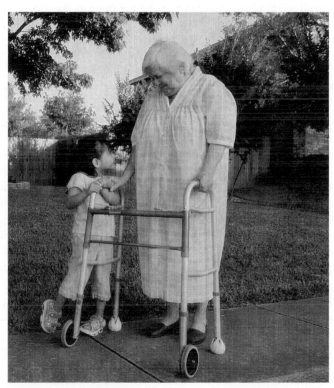

Figure 10-3 Individuals who must be treated in a culturally competent manner include children, the elderly, and the disabled.

Box 10-2   Oral Health Care Culturally Competent Guidelines (OHCCC)

- Develop the capacity for cultural self-assessment
- Value diversity among peers and clients
- Understand the dynamics of the interactions between and within cultures
- Institutionalize and implement cultural knowledge in a nonjudgmental manner
- Adapt preventive and clinical oral health service with an understanding, acceptance, appreciation, and respect of cultural diversity
- Be creative in finding ways to communicate with population groups that have limited English-speaking proficiency
- Understand cultural competency is continually evolving and a long-term developmental process

evaluate effectiveness of appropriate community outreach. Following are examples of models that can be implemented in various settings and cross-cultural encounters to ensure that culturally competent attitudes, knowledge, and behaviors are implemented when providing oral health care in either a clinical or community setting. Box 10-2 outlines guidelines for culturally competent oral health care.

HRSA's Health Disparities Substrategies

As the United States grows in diversity, both in rural and urban areas, health care providers and services are increasingly challenged to understand and address the linguistic and cultural needs of diverse clients. The Health Resources and Services Administration (HRSA), which is under the U.S. Department of Health and Human Services (USDHHS), has had a long-standing interest in cultural competency because many of its grantees provide care and services to traditionally underserved populations that include culturally and linguistically diverse communities. Figure 10-4 depicts the HRSA's strategy to eliminate health disparities through a number of substrategies. In particular, substrategy No. 4, diversify the health care workforce, acknowledges the patient-provider relationship is enhanced by ethnic, cultural, and linguistic concordance. In addition, emphasis is made for the need to support increased numbers of health care providers who are people of color and/or are multilingual. In substrategy No. 5, increase the cultural competence of the health care workforce, it is HRSA's goal to implement a plan to incorporate cultural competence principles throughout their programs, practices, and policies with a focus on targeted clinical areas and populations.[7]

Cultural Competency Education Model

The **Cultural Competency Education Model** is a conceptual model that focuses on the process of developing cultural competency in health care practices. This

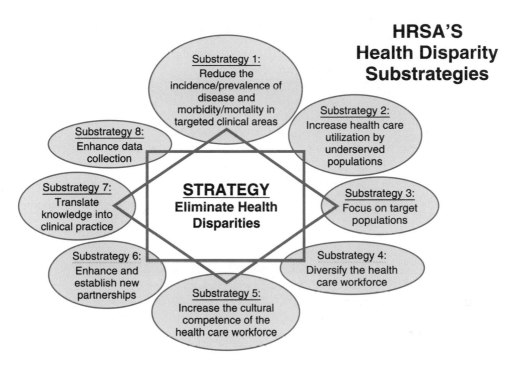

Figure 10-4 HRSA's Health Disparities Substrategies. *(From Health Resources and Service Administration, Substrategies to Eliminate Health Disparities, 2000.)*

model is designed to foster understanding, acceptance, knowledge, and constructive relations between persons of various cultures. The model is designed as a tool for developing the knowledge and skills that health care providers will need to provide quality care.[4] The model is framed on three areas of intervention: self-exploration or awareness, knowledge, and skills (Figure 10-5).

Self-Exploration: Awareness of one's own cultural heritage and increased acceptance of different values, attitudes, and beliefs

Knowledge: To understand that no one culture is intrinsically superior to another and to recognize individual and group differences and similarities

Skill: To master appropriate and sensitive strategies and skills in communicating and interacting with persons from different cultures and to seek information about various cultures within a society

It is through the development of self-exploration/awareness and skill that behaviors are adapted and implemented. The development of skills and knowledge creates the perception that is formed about and by people of diverse cultures. Attitude is explored, enhanced, and broadened by the growth of an individuals' self-exploration/awareness and the gaining of knowledge about diversity and the importance of culture to our daily life.

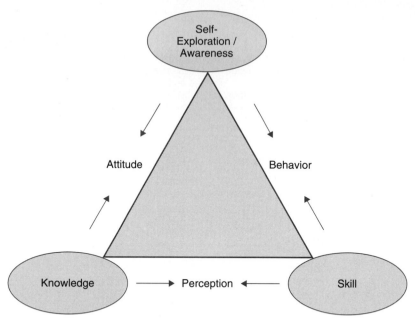

Figure 10-5 Cultural Competency Education Model. *(Adapted from Wells SA, Black RM: Cultural Competency For Health Professionals. Albany, NY: American Occupational Therapy Association, 2000.)*

Cultural Competency Continuum

The Cultural Competency Continuum is extensively referred to in cultural competency literature and training programs. It can serve as a guide to determine the functional competency or organizational activities and philosophies and also as a guide to personal development and expansion on becoming a culturally competent oral health care provider. The continuum has been described as a ladder where an individual can self-assess, plan to move to another step, and then progress in the personal and professional development of cultural competence. The six stages/steps are defined below and are illustrated in Figure 10-6.

Cultural Destructiveness: The most negative end of the continuum. It is represented by attitudes, policies, and practices that are destructive to culture, communities, and individuals. The most extreme example of cultural destructiveness is actively participating in cultural genocide, which is the purposeful destruction of a culture.

Cultural Incapacity: The next step is one in which systems, agencies, or individuals do not intentionally seek to be culturally destructive but lack the capacity to help clients or communities of diverse backgrounds. The systems remain extremely biased and believe in racial superiority.

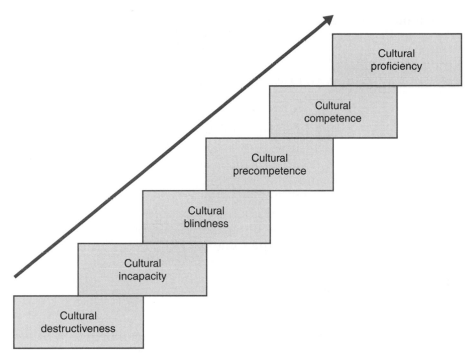

Figure 10-6 Cultural Competency Continuum.

Cultural Blindness: At the midpoint of the continuum, systems, agencies, or individuals provide services with the philosophy of being unbiased. It is believed that cultures make no difference and that all people are the same. This is a well-intended philosophy; however, the consequences of such a belief are to make services ethnocentric and therefore only useful for the most assimilated. People of diverse cultures are anticipated to meet the needs and expectations of the dominant group.

Cultural Pre-Competence: This step is on the positive end of the scale, awareness of some sensitivity but not sure what to do or "what is right." A system, agency, or individual recognizes its weaknesses in serving clients of cultural diversity and attempts to improve. Care must be taken at this level so that a false sense of accomplishment does not prevent the movement along the continuum.

Cultural Competence: Culturally competent systems, agencies, or individuals are characterized by acceptance and respect for difference. There is ongoing self-assessment regarding culture, expansion of knowledge, and adaptation of service models to better meet the needs of specific populations.

Cultural Proficiency: This is the most positive end of the continuum, advanced cultural competency. Culture is held in high self-esteem, and there is high regard in adding to the knowledge base of culturally competent practices, services, research, and approaches. Cultural proficiency indicates advocating for cultural competence through all systems and improves relations between cultures throughout society.[15-17]

COMMUNITY AND ORGANIZATIONAL CULTURAL COMPETENCE

Organizations must have the capacity to value diversity, conduct self-assessment, manage the dynamics of differences, acquire and institutionalize cultural knowledge, and adapt to diversity in the cultural contexts of the community they serve.[10] In addition, organizations must incorporate cultural competency principles in all aspects of policy making, administration, practice, and service delivery and systematically involve clients, stakeholders, and the communities they will serve. Training to increase cultural competence must be incorporated into our national and local infrastructures.[18] Efforts must be made with schools, the media, politicians, and administrators to emphasize the value of cultural competency. Current and future leaders need specific training to increase their cultural competence. It is important for public health agencies to include training and education to ensure that both service providers and clinical providers communicate in a culturally competent manner with every person during health care encounters and in a variety of settings with diverse communities. Several models have been described in the literature that are effective in cross-cultural encounters in health settings including the LEARN Model and Explanatory Model. Both models are best used in one-to-one clinical encounters for communication with clients in community and organizational systems. The LEARN Model (Box 10-3) applies behaviors and attitudes during **cross-cultural encounters**. These encounters or interactions can provide us with opportunities for personal growth, often challenging us in situations that are unfamiliar to our daily living and our beliefs about how things are or should be. The Explana-

Box 10-3   L-E-A-R-N Model of cross-cultural encounter guidelines for health practitioners[19]

Listen with sympathy and understanding to the patient's perception of the problem

Explain your perceptions of the problem and your strategy for treatment

Acknowledge and discuss the differences and similarities between these perceptions

Recommend treatment while remembering the patient's cultural parameters

Negotiate agreement. It is important to understand the patient's explanatory model so that the treatment fits in their cultural framework.

BOX 10-4 EXPLANATORY MODEL

> Kleinman's Explanatory Model to Elicit Health Beliefs in Clinical Encounters provides a sensitive approach to asking about health problems.[20]
> - What do you call your problem? What name does it have?
> - What do you think caused your problem?
> - Why do you think it started when it did?
> - What does your sickness do to you? How does it work?
> - How severe is it? Will it have a short or long course?
> - What do you fear most about your disorder?
> - What are the chief problems that your sickness has caused for you?
> - What kind of treatment do you think you should receive?
> - What are the most important results you hope to receive from the treatment?

tory Model (Box 10-4) assists with the gathering of information by asking the client questions. Questions of *what, why, how,* and *who* are asked to understand and implement individualized health care encounters. These models foster our creativity when interacting with clients or communities of diverse populations.

EFFECTIVE CROSS-CULTURAL COMMUNICATION

Cross-cultural communication is effectively communicating with someone of a different culture. It is important to learn all that you can about the individual or the community's way of life. Two important points to remember:
1. Do not expect to ever completely understand a culture that is not your own. For example, no matter how much you study the Italian culture, you will never be an Italian or share the experiences of growing up in Italy or with an Italian family rich in traditions.
2. Do not fall into the stereotyping or overgeneralization trap. Do not look at people stereotypically and then never move beyond that point. The skill of cultural competency is to learn useful general information and at the same time be aware of and open to variations and individual differences.

Identifying communication strategies that positively influence basic lifestyle behaviors has become increasingly important for improving the health of millions of Americans.[21] Some skills to assist and produce effective cross-cultural communication are listed in the Guiding Principles.

GUIDING PRINCIPLES

Skills That Foster Effective Cross-Cultural Communication
- Communicate in a language that is clear and at the client's level of understanding; send clear messages
- Define any dental terminology; avoid jargon
- Listen well to the client's questions and stories
- Carefully observe the client's body language
- Look beyond the superficial
- Be patient, persistent, and most important, flexible
- Recognize your own cultural biases
- Emphasize common grounds; do not focus on differences, instead focus on similarities
- Withhold judgment; accept others' differences
- Empathize; treat each person as an individual
- Do not assume understanding; ask for clarification
- Always communicate in a respectful manner
- Increase your knowledge and skills of cultural competence

Culturally and Linguistically Appropriate Services (CLAS)

The Office of Minority Health (OMH), U.S. Department of Health and Human Services, published the final recommendations on National Standards for Culturally and Linguistically Appropriate Services (CLAS) in health care. "Federal and state health agencies, policy makers, and national organizations now have a blueprint to follow for building culturally competent heath care organizations and workers."[22,23] There are 14 National Recommended Standards to inform, guide, and facilitate implementation of CLAS (Box 10-5).

The standards are organized by three themes:
1. Culturally Competent Care (Standards 1-3)
2. Language Access Services (Standards 4-7)
3. Organizational Supports for Cultural Competence (Standards 8-14)

THE CULTURE OF HEALTH

Cultural competence integrates health beliefs and cultural values, disease prevalence and incidence, and treatment efficacy.
- Health is culture-bound.
- Culture influences approaches and definitions of health and healthy living.
- The conceptions and expressions of health are culturally determined and vary both between and within cultural groups.

Box 10-5   CLAS STANDARDS FROM THE OFFICE OF MINORITY HEALTH

1. Patients and consumers receive effective, understandable, and respectful health care.
2. Recruitment, retention, and promotion of diverse staff and leadership.
3. All staff receive ongoing education and training.
4. Language assistance services, including bilingual staff and interpreters, must be offered at no cost to the patient.
5. Patients and consumers must be informed of their right to language assistance services.
6. Health organizations must ensure the competence of language assistance provided by interpreters/bilingual staff.
7. Availability of easily understood patient materials and applicable signage posted.
8. Written strategic plan with clear goals, policies, and accountability mechanisms.
9. Conduct initial and ongoing organizational self-assessments, and integrate cultural and linguistic competence measures into overall program activities.
10. Patient data collection to include: race, ethnicity, and spoken and written language.
11. Maintain current demographic, cultural, and epidemiologic community profiles, and conduct needs assessment on cultural and linguistic characteristics of the service area.
12. Participatory, collaborative partnerships to facilitate community and patient/consumer involvement.
13. Ensure that conflict and grievance resolution processes are culturally and linguistically sensitive.
14. Keep the public informed about progress and successful innovations in implementing the CLAS standards.

From U.S. Department of Health and Human Services, Office of Minority Health. Closing the Gap: National Standards for Culturally and Linguistically Appropriate Services. Rockville, Md, March 2001. http://www.omhrc.gov/clas/.

How an individual or community perceives health, illness, and a disability is influenced by culture. Also influenced are attitudes toward health care providers and facilities and how health information is communicated. Culture can even have an impact on health-seeking behaviors, preferences for traditional versus non-traditional approaches to heath care, and perceptions regarding the role of family in health care.[24] It is important to know that individual beliefs about health and illness affect the delivery and provision of health care. Why groups are affected differently is also important, but this is sometimes more challenging to differentiate. Some cultural factors to consider include:

- Self-treatment strategies
- Body image

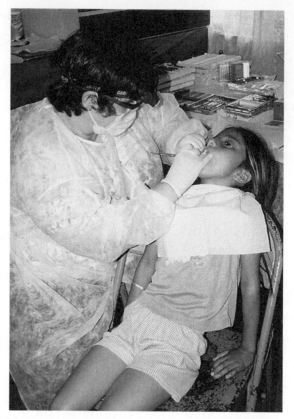

Figure 10-7 A dental hygiene student providing culturally competent oral health care to a patient.

- Social networks and social support
- Family rituals
- Crisis management
- Dietary patterns
- Child-rearing practices
- Gender roles
- Beliefs about origins of disease
- Folklore
- Traditional healing beliefs and folk medicine

Why do we need to consider these cultural factors when working with clients and communities if, as health care providers, we are taught to treat everyone the same? Because what people want is to have their differences acknowledged and respected. By incorporating individualized care in the context of everyone's own culture, a higher quality of care is achieved (Figure 10-7).[25]

A cross-cultural approach to health care and healing does not eliminate the foundation of Western medical methods. Instead, it expands and enhances ways that assess and deliver health care services by acknowledging, appreciating, and incorporating the beliefs, values, rituals, symbols, and standards of conduct that belong to the community we work with that may also affect its health status. The cross-cultural approach combines medical science and social science for the most effective outcomes.[25]

SUMMARY

To become a culturally competent oral health care provider, it is important to pursue broad efforts at all levels of oral health promotion and disease prevention. Cultural competency needs to be incorporated into all levels: personal, educational, community, organizational, administration, programs, and policies. It is up to the dental hygienist: the clinician, the health educator and wellness promoter, the consultant, the advocate, the researcher, and the administrator to value, implement, support, and foster cultural competency in every encounter made with a client. As oral health care providers we should appreciate the key role culture plays in our ability to influence behavior in our clients in both one-on-one and community settings. We cannot afford to let cultural barriers limit our ability to meet the oral health needs of our patients or reduce the opportunities to benefit from the services we can provide.

APPLYING **YOUR KNOWLEDGE**

1. Team up with two other students and list 10 examples of slang or idioms (in your own language) that would probably be misunderstood or misrepresented during an oral health encounter with someone from a culture other than yours. Next to each example, use other words you may use to convey the same message. Do the alternatives mean exactly the same as the slang or idiom?

2. Differences in gender, age, and physical abilities contribute to the diversity of clients. Every dental hygiene cross-cultural encounter with a client should be culturally competent. Working with a classmate, role play a dental hygiene care appointment in which:
   a. A woman in a community health fair is receiving oral hygiene education by a male dental hygienist.
   b. An older person at a nursing home is being treated for periodontal disease by a dental hygienist.
   c. A person using a wheelchair is at your community/migrant health center and you need to provide dental hygiene services.
   How did differences between the client and the dental hygienist influence the encounter? What can you do to improve culturally competent care for your clients?

3. For more effective culturally competent dental hygiene care to occur, it is vital to be aware of your own culture (self-assessment). Write a brief (three to four paragraphs) description of your own culture, including the role that

culture has on your daily life, your family traditions, your values, and your view on health.

4. Suppose you are moving to another geographic part of the country to practice dental hygiene. The community you will be working with is highly diverse and of different ethnic backgrounds than the community you worked with previously. Make a list of things you may need to know to provide culturally competent care to your clients.

5. Encourage, facilitate, and create a formal format for an open discussion of cultural customs among dental hygiene students of diverse cultures so that differences will not seem strange or unexplainable. Students may also share experiences of various cross-cultural experiences while on community rotations or service learning experiences.

DENTAL HYGIENE COMPETENCIES

Reading the material in this chapter and participating in the activities of "Applying Your Knowledge" will contribute to the student's abilities to demonstrate the following competencies:

Core competencies

C.8 Communicate effectively with individuals in groups from diverse populations both verbally and in writing.

C.10 Provide care to all clients with the use of an individualized approach that is humane, empathetic, and caring.

Health promotion and disease prevention

HP.2 Respect the goals, values, beliefs, and preferences of the patient or client while promoting optimal oral and general health.

HP.4 Identify individual and population risk factors and develop strategies that promote quality of life.

HP.5 Evaluate factors that can be used to promote patient or client adherence to disease prevention or health maintenance strategies.

Community involvement

CM.3 Provide community oral health services in a variety of settings.

Patient and client care

PC.1 Systematically collect, analyze, and record data on the general oral and psychosocial health status of a variety of patients or clients using methods consistent with medical legal principles.

PC.3 Collaborate with the patient or client or other health professionals to formulate a comprehensive dental hygiene care plan that is patient-centered or client-centered and based on current scientific evidence.

Community Case

You are the dental hygienist in a Community/Migrant Health Center. As a dental hygienist you have been asked by the Health Center Director to participate in applying for a grant to fund an interdisciplinary project for the elderly Asian clients of the Health Center. The grant will focus on health promotion and disease prevention.

1. All of the following are important factors to learn about the community to enhance the cultural competency of the proposed grant EXCEPT?
   a. Social network and social support
   b. Tooth loss
   c. Dietary patterns
   d. Beliefs about origin of disease
   e. Traditional healing beliefs and folk medicine

2. Select a cultural competency model that can be implemented into the grant that would meet the goals of the proposed grant, the community, and the researchers, especially in six stages of personal development and expansion of becoming a culturally competent health care provider:
   a. HRSA's Health Disparities Substrategies
   b. Cultural Competency Education Model
   c. Cultural Competency Continuum
   d. LEARN Model
   e. Oral Health Care Culturally Competent Guidelines

3. You are planning interdisciplinary service trainings for all of the health professionals that will be gathering and recording the data collected for the project. All of the following are skills to include in the training that will enhance cross-cultural communication EXCEPT?
   a. Treat each client as an individual
   b. Be patient and flexible
   c. Observe the client's body language
   d. Demonstrate your professional knowledge by incorporating your discipline's terminology
   e. Listen well to the client's questions and stories

4. Health care providers working with a multicultural population do not need to alter their traditional ways of treating patients. It is understood in the health, medical, and dental communities that there is critical need to eliminate health disparities.
   a. The first statement is true, the second statement is false.
   b. The first statement is false, the second statement is true.
   c. Both statements are true.
   d. Both statements are false.

5. For the grant proposal the interdisciplinary team will be developing appropriate educational materials for the clients. Utilizing the Oral Health

Care Culturally Competent Guidelines (OHCCC), which is the *most* relevant for this task?

a. Value diversity among peers and clients.
b. Adapt preventive and clinical oral health services with an understanding, acceptance, appreciation, and respect of cultural diversity.
c. Be creative in finding ways to communicate with population groups that have limited English-speaking proficiency.
d. Develop the capacity for cultural self-assessment.
e. Understand the dynamics of the interactions between and within cultures.

Resources: Cultural Competency

DHHS Initiative to Eliminate Racial and Ethnic Disparities in Health
   http://www.raceandhealth.hhs.gov/
HRSA
   http://www.hrsa.gov/
ETHNOMED
   http://www.hslib.washington.edu/clinical/ethnomed/index.html
Diversity Rx
   http://www.diversityrx.org/
Cross-Cultural Health Care
   http://www.xculture.org/
Bureau of Primary Health Care
   http://bphc.hrsa.gov/
Substance Abuse and Mental Health Services Administration
   http://www.samhsa.gov/
Centers for Medicare and Medicaid Services
   http://www.cms.gov/
National Institutes of Health
   http://www.nih.gov/
Indian Health Service
   http://www.ihs.gov/
Office of Civil Rights
   http://www.hhs.gov.progorg/ocr/ocrhmpg.html
Centers for Disease Control and Prevention
   http://www.cdc.gov/
Bureau of Health Professions Division of Interdisciplinary Community-Based Programs
   http://bhpr.hrsa.gov/interdisciplinary/
National Center for Cultural Competence
   http://www.georgetown.edu/research/gucdc 1-800-788-2066
National Clearinghouse for Alcohol and Drug Information
   1-800-729-6686
National Clearinghouse on Primary Health Care
   1-800-400-2742

Office of Minority Health Resource Center
    1-800-444-6472
A Su Salud! New Haven, Conn: Yale University Press, 2004
    http://www.yale.edu/yup/salud/
Addressing Cultural and Linguistic Competence in the HCH Setting: A Brief Guide
    http://www.nhchc.org/cultural.htm

REFERENCES

1. Healthy People 2010: Understanding and Improving Health (Conference ed, 2 vols). Washington, DC, U.S. Department of Health and Human Services, 2000.
2. Parillo, VN: Strangers To These Shores: Race and Ethnic Relationships in the United States, 5th ed. Boston, Allyn & Bacon, 1997.
3. Morey, DP, Leung, JJ: The multicultural knowledge of registered dental hygienists. J Dent Hygiene 67:4, 1993.
4. Wells SA, Black RM: Cultural Competency For Health Professionals. Albany, NY, Boyd Printing Company, 2000.
5. U.S. Bureau of the Census (2000) Website: http://www.census.gov/
6. U.S. Department of Health and Human Services (DHHS): Oral Health in America: A Report of the Surgeon General. Rockville, Md, DHHS, National Institute of Dental and Craniofacial Research, National Institutes of Health, 2000.
7. Health Resources and Services Administration (HRSA), Eliminating Health Disparities: HRSA's Strategic Directions for Health Disparities. Washington, DC, U.S. Department of Health and Human Services, 2001.
8. UCLA Center for Health Policy Research and Henry J. Kaiser Family Foundation: Racial and Ethnic Disparities in Access to Health Insurance and Health Care, Report #1525, April 2000, 1-800-656-4533 www.healthpolicy.ucla.edu
9. Mutha S, Allen C, Welch M: Toward Culturally Competent Care: A Toolbox for Teaching Communication Strategies. Center for the Health Professions, UCSF. www.futurehealth.ucsf.edu/pdf-files/Ccposter.ppt.
10. National Center for Cultural Competence of Georgetown University Center for Child and Human Development: Conceptual Frameworks, Models, Guiding Values and Principles, 2004. http://www.georgetown.edu/research/gucdc/nccc/framework.html
11. Diversity Rx Website. Supported by the National Conference of State Legislatures (NCSL), Resources for Cross Cultural Health Care (RCCHC), Henry J. Kaiser Family Foundation. http://www.diversityrx.org/HTML/ESGLOS.htm
12. U.S. Department of Health and Human Services (DHHS): Health Care Rx: Access For All Chartbook, Washington, DC, 1998.
13. Bentacourt, JR, Green AR, Carillo JE: Cultural Competence in Health Care: Emerging Frameworks and Practical Approaches. Commonwealth Fund, October 2002.
14. Cross TL, Bazron BJ, Dennis KW, Isaacs MR: Towards a Culturally Competent System of Care: Vol 1. Washington, DC, National Technical Assistance Center for Children's Mental Health, Georgetown University Child Development Center, 1989.
15. Pursuing Organizational and Individual Cultural Competency: An Epistemology of the Journey Toward Cultural Competency. Austin, Texas, Texas Department of Health, 1998.
16. National Alliance of Hispanic Health: Quality Health Services for Hispanics: The Cultural Competency Component. DHHS Publication No. 99-21, 2001. http://www.hispanichealth.org
17. Cohen E, Goode TD: Policy Brief 1: Rationale for Cultural Competence in Primary Health Care. Washington, DC, National Center for Cultural Competence, 1999. Available online at www.dml.georgetown.edu/depts/pediatrics/gucdc/nccc6.html
18. U.S. Department of Health and Human Services, Office of Minority Health: Closing the Gap: Moving Toward Consensus on Cultural Competency in Health Care. Rockville, Md: U.S. Department of Health and Human Services, January 2000. http://www.omhrc.gov/clas/

19. Berlin EA, Fowkes WC, Jr: A teaching framework for cross-cultural application in family practice, in cross-cultural medicine. West J Med 12:139, 93-98, 1983.
20. Kleinman A: Patients and Healers in the Context of Culture. The Regents of the University of California, 1981. http://www.diversityrx.org/HTML/MOCPT3.htm
21. Institute of Medicine (IOM), Committee on Communication for Behavior: Change in the 21st Century: Improving the Health of Diverse Populations: Speaking of Health: Assessing Health Communication Strategies for Diverse Populations. Washington, DC, National Academies Press, 2003.
22. U.S. Department of Health and Human Services, Office of Minority Health: Closing the Gap: Office of Minority Health Publishes Final Standards for Cultural and Linguistic Competence. Rockville, Md, February/March 2001. http://www.omhrc.gov/clas/
23. U.S. Department of Health and Human Services, Office of Minority Health. Closing the Gap: National Standards for Culturally and Linguistically Appropriate Services. Rockville, Md, March 2001. http://www.omhrc.gov/clas/
24. Denoba DL, Bragdon JL, Epstein LG, et al: Reducing health disparities through cultural competence. J Health Educ 29(suppl):5, 1998.
25. Kaiser Permanente, Multicultural Caring: A Guide to Cultural Competence for Kaiser Permanente Health Professionals, 2000.

11

Service-Learning

Sheranita Hemphill, RDH, MPH, MS

Objectives

Upon completion of this chapter, the student will be able to:

- Compare traditional dental hygiene community service outreach efforts with experiential outreach efforts
- Define Service-Learning and list the characteristics that distinguish it from other experiential learning experiences
- Describe essential components of Service-Learning
- List the common experiential learning methods and their unique purposes
- List benefits of Service-Learning for the student, community partner, dental hygiene program, dental hygiene faculty, the academic institution, and the nation's oral health
- Recall methods to manage the challenges associated with Service-Learning
- Use resources to plan and implement Service-Learning

Key Terms

Healthy People 2010
  (HP 2010)
Oral Health in America: A
  Report of the Surgeon
  General (OHARSG)
Essential Public Health
  Services for Oral Health

Association for State and
  Territorial Dental Directors
  (ASTDD)
Experiential Learning
Service-Learning (SL)
Learning Objectives (LO)

Service Objectives (SO)
Service-Learning
  Objectives (SLO)
Collaboration
Orientation

The Health Insurance
  Portability and
  Accountability Act (HIPAA)
Preparation
Reflection

Evaluation
Formative Evaluation
Summative Evaluation
Community Service
Clinical Rotation

Internship
Practicum
Volunteerism
Risk Management

OPENING STATEMENT

Findings of service-learning research in higher education include:
- Service-Learning has a positive effect on student personal development such as a sense of personal efficacy, personal identity, spiritual growth, and moral development.

- Service-Learning has a positive effect on interpersonal development and the ability to work well with others, leadership skills, and communication skills.

- Service-Learning has a positive effect on reducing stereotypes and facilitating cultural and racial understanding.

- Service-Learning has a positive effect on social responsibility and citizenship skills.

- Service-Learning has a positive effect on commitment to service.

- Service-Learning contributes to career development.

- Students and faculty report that Service-Learning improves the students' ability to apply what they have learned in the "real world."

Eyler JS, et al. At A Glance: What We Know about the Effects of Service-Learning on College Students, Faculty, Institutions and Communities, 1993-2000. 3rd ed. Learn and Serve America National Clearinghouse, 2001. Available at http://www.compact.org/resource/aag.pdf.

Recent national health initiatives emphasized the need for community-based strategies to address oral health disparities. Consequentially, the national attention has caused a tremendous increase in interest in the nation's oral health. Oral health conversations at the national, regional, and local sectors have increased and have led to extensive research, comprehensive publications, numerous conferences, and targeted programs focused on treatment and health promotion. The entire dental community has become involved in advancing the public's interest. The increasing national momentum has served to advance "dental" concerns to authentic public health issues and has presented an opportunity for dental hygiene education programs to contribute to the improvement of the oral health of the nation starting right in our neighborhoods.[1-7]

The oral health recommendations found in ***Healthy People 2010*** (HP 2010) (see Chapter 4) and the ***Oral Health in America: A Report of the Surgeon General*** (OHARSG) are a road map for change to the current method of teaching Community Dental Health by dental hygiene education programs. If integrated into the dental hygiene curriculum, the recommendations will positively influence community dental hygiene instruction for students and community outreach dental hygienists. Preparing students for the public health workforce is arguably one of the most important outcomes for today's dental hygiene programs. Ensuring that students acquire the knowledge and skills of the public health worker will contribute to students' career options. These public health initiatives have made it clear that the dental community must respond to broader community issues, and the community dental health curriculum must be positioned to prepare students to work in this changing public health environment.[2,3,6-8]

This chapter focuses on another learning technique through which the existing community-based dental hygiene curriculum can be enhanced to better meet the oral public health needs of the community. In addition, it provides guidance and suggestions designed to prepare dental hygiene students to address oral health disparities in their communities. It challenges students to use their dental hygiene education as the foundation for future public health career opportunities. Integrating the objectives of the nation's health agenda, as outlined in national public health initiatives, into the dental hygiene curriculum will position the dental hygiene profession into the public health arena more decisively and affect the public's oral health positively.

DENTAL HYGIENE COMMUNITY SERVICE OUTREACH EFFORTS

Traditional Outreach Efforts

Historically, dental hygiene students have provided community dental health outreach for diverse populations. The current educational methods used to prepare dental hygiene students to instruct these populations regarding oral health include health education lectures with a focus on lesson plan development and implementation at schools and other settings. The benefits of these methods are excellent in preparing dental hygiene students to deliver appropriate and effective oral health messages.

Further assessment regarding educational methods reveals that the primary benefit of traditional outreach instruction and methodology is the acquisition of technical skills.[9-12] The methods provide a practical experience in organizing a dental health presentation, and they assist dental hygiene students in perfecting their presentation techniques. Preparing dental hygiene students to master the teaching skills and delivery methods with confidence usually occurs in a short period within the community oral health course. As a result, the traditional approaches of preparing dental students to deliver health education, lectures, and lesson plan development are prone to be one-shot short-term projects, rendering the aim to favorably affect oral health behavior as insufficient.

Once students have mastered the traditional methods of oral health outreach, they are then ready to move to the next level, which involves changing health behaviors. Long-term teaching strategies are needed to improve the oral health behavior of populations for lifelong benefits. It is also important for the dental hygiene program to cultivate permanent relationships with various populations in the community. Continuing partnerships with a variety of populations will also pave the way for the dental hygiene students to gain diverse and repetitive experiences in applying health behavior principles for the purpose of helping populations improve their oral health behaviors.

Behavioral change is an integral component of effective oral health promotion strategies (see Chapter 8). Students often complain that their patients do not follow their oral health instructions. Practicing dental hygienists are all too familiar with this sentiment. However, once the experienced hygienist realizes that oral health "instructions," delivered in one appointment, do not translate into better oral health behaviors, they eventually start treating their patients as individuals.

They design oral health education messages that are spread out over time, and they ensure that the messages are individually tailored to the language, reading level, and cultural perspective. They stop assuming that everyone values oral health as much as they do; instead, they ask the patients what is important to them. Experienced hygienists begin to incorporate the assistance of the patients' significant others for support, and they integrate cultural specific information so that the patients can perceive benefits for themselves (see Chapter 10). In effect, they use theories of health education to motivate, educate, and empower their patients.

Health education theories are equally beneficial for community dental health education projects. The use of planned strategies, grounded in theory, to promote individual and community healthy behaviors requires continuing commitment. To positively affect health behavior, dental hygiene students must acquire knowledge of the principles of health promotion, and they must design and implement ongoing projects using them.[8,13,14] Short-term community outreach provides little opportunity for community members to become empowered with the skills and knowledge they need to sustain the intended goals of the program. Likewise, short-term community dental health outreach provides inadequate opportunity for dental hygiene students to become proficient in applying theoretic concepts and for investigating public health career options in depth. And last, short-term community dental health outreach efforts inhibit the development of a collective national oral health agenda for the dental hygiene programs in the country.[3,4,8,15,16]

Dental hygiene students can contribute to the national oral health agenda. Imagine the oral health benefits if the more than 250 dental hygiene programs in the United States adopted a standard approach of instructing students in community dental health outreach efforts. What would be the impact if all the programs used the HP 2010 objectives in developing durable community dental health projects? Likewise, imagine the possibility of comparing oral health outcomes across the country.

Adopting a standard teaching method for implementing community dental health outreach would permit the dental hygiene programs to consistently evaluate and measure the impact of their collective public health efforts. The oral health promotional efforts and results of dental hygiene students could then move beyond the anecdotal; their efforts could have a lasting impact on the nation's oral health.

The traditional approaches to planning and implementing community dental health outreach projects make it difficult to compare oral health findings and chart progress. HP 2010, with its baseline data and targets for improvements, is instructive in preparing dental hygiene students to affect oral public health. Students will be able to compare their findings with other states and with those of the nation. This in turn will contribute constructively to the nation's oral health agenda.

Essential Public Health Services For Oral Health

The hygienist of the future must be capable of responding to the disparities in oral health. Dental hygiene students will need to gain a working knowledge of the role of public health dentistry (PHD) in the overall public health infrastructure. Questions that must be addressed while learning about dentistry's role in public health matters include: What is the function of PHD in responding to the oral needs of the public? In addition to state health departments, are there additional levels of response to oral health needs? Is there a place for dental education programs, like dental hygiene programs, to contribute to the oral public health services?

The **Essential Public Health Services For Oral Health** represents the **Association for State and Territorial Dental Directors (ASTDD)** recommended services for state oral health programs. These services challenge the PHD community, including the dental hygiene students, to join the collective efforts of state and local oral health improvement strategies. The core functions and suggestions for integration in community dental health outreach programs can be examined in Table 11-1.

Table **11-1**   **Examples of essential public health services for oral health**

Core Function	Essential Public Health Service	Oral Health Illustrations
Assessment	Monitor oral health status of the community	Dental hygiene students will annually assess the tobacco use of the community, analyze the data, and report the findings to the community
Policy development	Mobilize the community to help solve the underage smoking in the community	Dental hygiene students will research the state's tobacco policies and laws regarding the sale of tobacco to minors
Assurance	Enforce laws and regulations to protect health and safety of the community	Dental hygiene students will develop training material for neighborhood store clerks to improve compliance of state tobacco policies

ASTDD is one of many resources that support efforts aimed at improving the oral health of the public. One of ASTDD's purposes in developing the Essential Public Health Services For Oral Health was ". . . to provide a working document for guidance to health agency officials and public health administrators in the development and operation of oral health programs at the state level."[17] These guidelines, in addition to the HP 2010 and the SGROH, can also be used in the strategic preparation of dental hygiene community outreach programs across the country.

Experiential Outreach Efforts

Increasing access to oral health involves a variety of participants: the federal government, consumer health advocates, coalitions, philanthropists, and professional organizations. Dental hygiene programs are also positioned to increase access. Specifically, the community dental health course can be adapted to meet the academic goals of students while addressing various community access issues. The combination of classroom learning and practical learning, such as community outreach programs, provides students the opportunity to (1) apply public health concepts, (2) reinforce academic knowledge and skills, (3) increase community awareness, and (4) address real community needs.[1-3]

Experiential learning, commonly referred to as "practical learning" or "real-world learning," originated from the grassroots research of such theorists as John Dewey, Kurt Lewin, Jean Piaget, and Carl Rogers. Experiential learning is an umbrella term that references various models of learning in which experience governs the learning process.

Experiential learning theory is different from cognitive learning theory. In the cognitive approach, theorists see learning as primarily a mental process in which the learner is able to recall acquired facts and figures. Unlike cognitive learning, experiential learning incorporates personal experiences. It involves the application of new skills in an environment in which it is acceptable to construct knowledge while using a known concept. For instance, here is a case where personal experience is incorporated in the learning. A service-learning team of dental hygiene students meets to plan oral health activities for a youth group. Only one of the dental hygiene students has previous experience working with this population and quickly mobilizes the dental hygiene team into action. Experiential learning outcomes are beneficial to student growth and professional development.

Cognitive knowledge is very important in experiential learning, but it should be used in conjunction with experiential methods for increased proficiency in interpreting situations and acting appropriately. If, for instance, a dental hygiene student finds that the caregivers in a long-term facility are reluctant to provide frequent oral health care to the patients, the student's efforts may be better spent by having the group of caregivers brainstorm for a decision regarding what is reasonable in their circumstances. In this instance, although the student is fully aware of what the literature says regarding the removal of prostheses during the

GUIDING PRINCIPLES

Outcomes of Experiential Learning
- Connects classroom learning with authentic situations
- Continuously reinforces learned knowledge and skills through practical experience
- Challenges the student to think critically in addressing real needs
- Increases aptitude for teaching various populations
- Enhances the skills of the dental hygiene workforce

---

night, they are also able to interpret the fact that the habits of the staff are not going to be changed quickly, but gradually.

Experiential learning takes place in authentic situations. A Women, Infant, and Children's (WIC) facility is a good example of an SL setting in which an appropriate learning context for dental hygiene students is provided. In the community oral health course, students are learning about the social determinants of oral health. That a woman is visiting the WIC public health facility may signify more than the fact that she is receiving nutritional provisions and medical care for her family. In assisting this woman, the student will have to use his or her learned skills to "see" beyond the obvious. The dental hygiene student will need to apply cognitive skills such as the recall of facts regarding the public health facility and pediatric dentistry, but he or she will also need to construe other oral health needs that the mother and her family may have. In this case the dental hygiene students will learn more because they construct the strategies that they will use to assist this family. In essence, they are learning through experience. Experiential learning links genuine learning opportunities to the classroom and the textbook material.

A specific example of experiential learning is when first-year dental hygiene students enrolled in a didactic dental radiology course are learning how to interpret radiographic findings. Thus far, the instructor and the dental hygiene students are not pleased with the retention and comprehension of the content. The dental radiology course instructor and a secondary education teacher decide to collaborate for mutual benefit by providing an environment where experience is dominant in the learning process. The dental hygiene students will connect their didactic training with the real need of the high school teacher's objectives for her students through experiential learning. The dental hygiene students have to design age-appropriate activities and present on radiographic findings to the group of high school students. Experiential learning changes the focus of learning, shifting it from the classroom to the community. Classroom learning is supplemented with purposeful work-based learning opportunities within the community, and to ensure that the course objectives are being met, the students apply their program planning skills with guidance from their faculty and from the community partner.

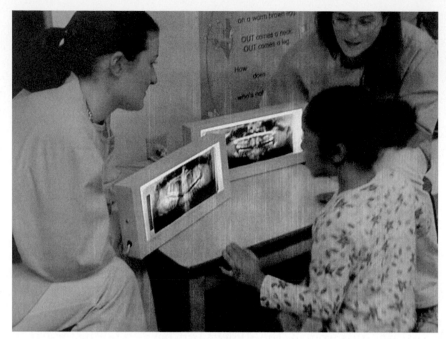

Figure 11-1 First-year students reinforcing their acquired radiographic interpretation skills through teaching.

Experiential outreach efforts should place emphasis on tasks that contribute to the students' knowledge base (Figure 11-1).

SERVICE-LEARNING AND ITS DISTINGUISHING CHARACTERISTICS

Service-Learning Defined

Service-Learning (SL) is an example of an experiential learning method. SL is a jointly structured learning experience in which the course **learning objectives (LO)** and the community partner's **service objectives (SO)** are deliberately combined for mutual benefit. The outcome of combining the LO and the SO is known as **SL objectives (SLO)**. Box 11-1 summarizes each of the three objectives. SL is experiential because it is applied pedagogy.

For example, when students are learning about the socioeconomic status of the underserved, the faculty may rely on the textbook to convey background information about the subject. In addition to specific reading assignments, students may also watch a video or read a journal article to supplement the textbook material. Additional details may be gathered from the media and through classroom lectures. SL can further supplement student learning by placing the student in a setting in which the relative class objectives can be met. SL is not a substitute for traditional classroom instruction; instead, SL enhances traditional methods of instruction.

BOX 11-1   SERVICE-LEARNING OBJECTIVES DEFINED

Service Objectives (SO)	Learning Objectives (LO)	Service-Learning Objectives (SLO)
The SO is a written statement of need provided by the agency. Through this process, dental hygiene students are positioned to provide a needed service as opposed to what they think is needed.	This is the course LO. Note that not all LO are appropriate for Service-Learning (SL) programs. LO that require higher-level thinking (e.g., exploring barriers to oral health access) are best for SL experiences.	The SLO is the result of combining the LO with the SO. Ideally, the community partner should work with the students to combine the objectives. If this is not possible, the partner should be given the chance to modify the SLO.

Continuing with this scenario, students may design a survey to assess the types of dental insurance found in the population of interest. They may wish to determine the frequency of dental visits and then compare findings with that of state and national data. In this instance the National Oral Health Surveillance System (NOHSS) database (see Chapter 4) would serve as an excellent oral health resource for comparing oral health findings among states. NOHSS's website address can be located in the list web resources found at the end of this chapter. In this case students would be using and reinforcing skills and knowledge they learned in concurrent or previous classes such as community dental health and biostatistics.

GUIDING PRINCIPLES

Ideas That Can Be Integrated into Service-Learning Projects
- Develop a brochure listing dental public health resources including Safety Net facilities
- Plan and conduct a Basic Screening Survey and issue oral health "report cards"
- Identify public and private dental facilities that are currently accepting public health insurance (Medicaid) and assist families in finding dental homes
- Assist the school nurse in following up with dental referrals
- Collaborate with local law enforcement/students to promote child safety by performing bite impressions for use in identification of children
- Assist the community in assessing the adequacy of their community water fluoridation
- Develop and implement oral health lesson plans for allied health students and/or other health professionals (e.g., medical doctors, nurses)

The Service-Learning objectives (SLO) have characteristics that distinguish SL from other community-based experiences. The equal weighing of the SO and the LO is a classic feature of SL that emphasizes the fact that both the students and the recipients of the service are equally important in the educational process. Note that even the configuration of the very word "Service-Learning" illustrates the fact that both the service and the learning are equivalent. The "S" in service and the "L" in learning are always written in identical fashion, either capitalized or in lower-case letters.[12,16,18] Also note that, in this chapter, a hyphen is used to emphasize that the service and the learning are "connected." The service is a community task and the learning is the academic goal.[11,12,16]

Definitions of SL may vary, but they all imply equality between the service activities and the learning activities. For example, the Community Campus Partnership for Health (CCPH), a nationally recognized organization whose mission is, in part, to improve the health of the public by promoting collaboration between communities and educational institutions, emphasizes the fact that both the service and the learning occur equally. Sarena Seifer, MD, the executive director of CCPH, defines SL in the following manner:

> Service-Learning is a structured learning experience that combines community service with preparation and reflection. Students engaged in Service-Learning provide community service in response to community-identified concerns and learn about the context in which service is provided, the connection between their service and their academic coursework, and their roles as citizens. (Seifer, 1998)[18]

Like the CCPH, the Center for Healthy Communities (CHC), a nationally known academic-community partnership in Ohio, defines SL in terms that also emphasize the reciprocal benefits of SL. The CHC has many years of experience in preparing multidisciplinary health professional students, including dental hygiene students, for practice, and they have acknowledged SL as a practical model for preparing students to meet the needs of the public. In a recent pre-post survey of multiprofessional health professions students, the CHC found that after an SL experience, students reported better knowledge of health care concepts and issues, and that they were more willing to work in nontraditional health care settings. See Box 11-2 for a listing of those areas that resulted in statistically significant changes.[10,19]

Service-Learning can improve a traditional classroom assignment in several ways. The "rules" of SL require students to become active in the learning process. Students are expected to bring their personal experiences into the situation, and they are expected to apply their experiences and their knowledge of current events and social situations to the assignment. In this way, students are actually constructing their own learning.

In an example of how SL can modify a traditional classroom assignment, the community health instructor presents a written case study that asks students, among other things, to identify oral health resources for the individuals in the case. Students also have to present a two-page report. The level of skill required to accomplish this task is minimum and requires very little active involvement.

Box 11-2   Pre-post Service-Learning survey results

Reports of Better Knowledge

Community resources
Health care delivery systems
Health care needs of community
Barriers to receiving care
Impact of socioeconomic status on health

Willingness to Work in Diverse Settings

Work on a multiprofessional team
Work in a rural setting
Volunteer their time
Feeling better prepared to work in community settings
Feeling more comfortable working with diverse patient populations
Greater commitment to work in health professions shortage areas and with
  diverse patient populations

Service-Learning can enhance this experience by engaging the student in the assignment. If, for instance, students are asked to implement this assignment for an actual population, they must become active participants. Critical thinking will be required, team processes will be tested, previous experiences may assist the process, and a sense of accomplishment will prevail. As a result of the active learning that will take place, their cognitive knowledge will increase. For instance, though they may have read about oral health resources such as the NOHSS, ASTDD, Centers for Disease Control and Prevention Oral Health Resources, National Maternal and Child Oral Health Resource Center, and the OHARSG, now they will actually use the data sources.

GUIDING PRINCIPLES

Service-Learning Contributions to Classroom Learning

- Students become active learners as they construct much of the learning experience
- Exposure to oral public health becomes a reality as SL projects require action such as the utilization of national and local public health resources
- Course content is relevant and timely as the national and local oral public health issues are firmly linked to the curriculum
- Students see the big picture; their professional roles are clearly linked to the national health issues identified in HP 2010 (the nation's health objectives)

Students in this case will also find that their local and/or state health department has a wealth of useful information. Likewise, students will find that organizations outside of dentistry, such as social service agencies, are very helpful in their search for health and social service resources. SL promotes access to oral health by ensuring that dental hygiene students are exposed to issues of public health in a broad sense. In summary, dental hygiene students who engaged in SL provide community service in response to community-identified needs, and in the process they learn more about the circumstances of the community, they apply and test learned material, and they provide a public health service.

ESSENTIAL COMPONENTS OF SERVICE-LEARNING

Service-Learning is distinguished from other teaching and learning methods by the equal emphasis that it places on the recipients (service component) and the students (learning component). This is a characteristic that is not only unique to SL instruction but is also essential. Founding principles of SL serve to protect the integrity of SL as a teaching method.

The CHC developed principles of SL that are used extensively as a model for developing SL programs throughout the United States. Their model, known as the Service Learning Protocol for Health Professions Schools (SLPHPS), consists of seven guidelines that are discussed below. These guidelines serve to enhance SL partnerships. Additional models can be located by referring to the web resources listed at the end of this chapter. In summary, guiding principles list the essential characteristics of SL, without which SL is ill defined.*

Community Partner Collaboration

Collaboration means working together to accomplish a goal. Other words that may come to mind when thinking about collaboration include "joint effort," "teamwork," or "partnership." In SL projects the outreach program is jointly planned by the course instructor, the community partner, and the students. The parties collaborate to ensure that the needs of the community partner, student, and faculty are met. The faculty is interested in making sure that student LO are attended to, the community partner is interested in ensuring that its organization's needs are met, and the dental hygiene students are interested in applying their health education knowledge and skills.

Traditionally, the dental hygiene faculty initiated the communications leading to a community service experience for the dental hygiene students. The faculty would contact an agency representative and inform them that they wanted to place dental hygiene students in their organization to gain community experience. With

---

*References 8, 11, 12, 16, 18, 19.

the SL teaching and learning method, the faculty, community partner, or student can initiate the conversation. The community agency can contact the faculty to request the services of the dental hygiene students, and likewise, the student can initiate the discussion by contacting an agency to discuss the possibility of developing a mutually beneficial project. In this latter instance, the students must identify the appropriate LO from the course syllabus, and they must work with the agency representative to identify their needs or service objectives.

Mutual Objective Formation

The needs of the community partner are referred to as SO, and they are developed from their mission statements. Student course objectives are referred to as LO, and they originate from the guidelines of the Commission on Dental Accreditation (CODA) Standards for Dental Hygiene Education Programs and the dental hygiene competencies developed by the Section on Dental Hygiene Education of the American Dental Education Association (ADEA).

Standard 2 of CODA addresses the requirements for dental hygiene educational programs, and these standards serve as the model for all dental hygiene programs. Direction is provided for all aspects of the program development and maintenance including the instruction, the curriculum content, and the patient care competencies. ADEA's competencies detail the level of skill expected of the entry level dental hygienist, and each program is encouraged to use them to guide their program development and/or improvement.[20,21]

It is important for the students, the agency, and the faculty to become acquainted with each other's mission and/or assignment. Communication is the best approach to gaining insight to the different perspectives, after which they can jointly determine how their objectives may be combined for mutual benefit.

In an example of mutual objective formation, a team of dental hygiene students have been assigned to find "dental homes" for a public elementary school. The faculty is satisfied because this task meets the needs of the curriculum in that the dental hygiene students will assist patients who have public insurance obtain dental care. This assignment also meets the needs of the school board in that it satisfies their desire to have healthy children in the classroom. The dental hygiene students are also satisfied because they finally get the opportunity to apply their program planning skills.

This SL project represents the third year of an ongoing partnership between the elementary school and the dental hygiene program. The school nurse informs the dental hygiene team that the service need for this year's project is securing dental homes for children needing immediate care. After considering the service objectives, the students decide which of the course's LO will work best with the school's need. They may choose one course LO, or they may select several LO. After informing the school nurse of their LO, the students and the school nurse jointly combine their respective objectives, which are then presented to the faculty for assessment. The planning for the SL program can now proceed.

Orientation

A formal **orientation** provides an opportunity for all parties to get acquainted, to become familiar with each other's facilities, and to plan the SL experience. A formal orientation provides a forum for the agency representative to become more familiar with the level of student expertise, the course objectives, and the history of the students' community service exposure. Similarly, students become familiar with the agency, its staff, and the population. The smallest of details is addressed.

The agenda for the orientation should include a community partner presentation, which will provide an overview of their organization and their needs. The overview is often accomplished through an oral presentation supplemented with informational pamphlets and followed by a question and answer session. Ideally, the orientation should occur in two steps; one should take place at the dental hygiene program site, and the other should occur at the community agency's site. Orientations serve several purposes, including increasing the familiarity of all stakeholders with each location. A few of the purposes of orientation are listed below, and many more can be found by searching through the list of web resources listed at the end of this chapter.

- Risk management and relevant policy and procedures guidelines can be discussed
- The **Health Insurance Portability and Accountability Act (HIPAA)** regulations can be reviewed
- Appropriate attire, including protective wear, can be determined
- The expectations of the community partner and those of the students can be discussed
- Issues of transportation, directions, and parking can be assessed
- Work space for student workers may not be available, yet may be needed
- Determining the availability of lockers for students' personal belongings can be assessed

A formal orientation minimizes disruptions to the SL program. It ensures the appropriateness of the facilities, and it provides an occasion for all parties to discuss concerns and resolve issues for the success of the SL program.

Preparation

Preparation involves program planning skills that have been presented in another chapter in this textbook. With the use of previously learned team-building skills, activities are brainstormed, roles are identified, action plans and contingency plans are developed, and timelines are set. Student leadership skills evolve as each student takes responsibility for the success of the program outcomes.

In a scenario illustrating preparation, an urban child development program partnered with a dental hygiene program to expand oral health access for the children in three of the public elementary schools. Ms. Kane, the director of a local children's program, and the three principals participated in the orientation phase. Ms. Kane presented background information using oral presentation and a multimedia CD that depicted captivating scenes from each of the schools.

The principals introduced themselves and provided an overview of their school's history, demographics, and economic status of the families. The dental hygiene students were divided into three teams, and each team was assigned to one of the three schools. The students then met with the respective principal and began the process of team building.

Each team developed an overall goal for their SL project, uniquely tailored for the particular school's needs. Using relative course objectives from the syllabus and the service objective articulated by the principals, the teams developed SL objectives using the SL grid template as a guide, and they also developed evaluation measures. Everyone took an active role in the program planning, and this contributed to the overall success of the SL program.

Service-Learning Experience

At this point the program is implemented. Previously developed lesson plans and evaluation tools are used in this phase of the SL project. Refer to Figure 11-2 to view an SL lesson plan template.

Reflection

Reflection involves critical thinking and critical expressions about the SL experience and the specific encounters. The aim of reflection is to draw meaning from the experience. Whether the meaning is in the form of self-appraisal or societal appraisal, the goal for the dental hygiene student is to grow in understanding regarding the surrounding social, cultural, and economic events that have contributed to the shape of the situation.

Reflection is not intended to be a condemning session aimed at the "system"; its purpose is to assist in the formation of knowledge by permitting the dental hygiene students to consider course content in relation to the multiple sociologic factors affecting the situation.[8,11,22] Theoretic content has been applied in the community, and reflective activities permit the students to process the experiences encountered and place them in the context of the course objectives. Ideally, dental hygiene students should first consider the SL experience introspectively and then share their findings through dialogue with the other students, the instructor, and the community partner.

In reflective activities the processes used in the SL experience and the end-product are carefully considered. Some researchers liken the hyphen in SL to the idea of reflection. In this instance the hyphen forces the dental hygiene student to pause and consider the implications of the SL project. Students should entertain critical questions regarding the benefit of the experience to them and to the community they served. The hyphen symbolizes the importance of processing the SL experience.

Deliberate reflection that is tied to the curriculum and community-based service is a key component of SL and community-based dental education. Reflection facilitates critical thinking skills and helps students see the connection between dental

SERVICE-LEARNING LESSON PLAN

Student Hygienist's Name _____

Date _____

Agency _____

Contact Person _____

Address _____ Phone _____ FAX _____

Email _____

Audience _____ Age _____

Service Objective	Learner Objective	Service-Learning Objective

Concepts	Strategies	Time
1	1	1
2	2	2

Material Needed	Resources Used

EVALUATION

Basic Questions: What went well? What will I change in the future? What additional materials or resources were needed?

Formative Measures:

Summative Measures:

Figure 11-2 Service-Learning lesson plan template.

Box 11-3   REFLECTION METHODS

- Have the community partners facilitate prepared and impromptu discussion sessions
- Present a poster session and invite the entire college and community
- Organize round table discussions where the senior students present their findings to the junior students
- Incorporate audiovisual into any reflection method
- Guided journaling that addresses the connection, challenges, context, and continuity of the Service-Learning (SL) experience
- Create a website that highlights the continuous nature of the SL efforts of your school
- Develop an evaluation instrument for implementing in future SL programs
- Publish an article in a dental hygiene newsletter or journal

---

public health and the sociocultural environment. Reflection also provides an opportunity for faculty to assess and evaluate student learning. Review Box 11-3 for reflection ideas. Specific formats for conducting reflective sessions offer additional guidance and can be located by researching the web resources located at the end of this chapter. Questions, poster presentations, round table discussions, audiovisual presentations, and keeping journals all offer opportunities for students to consider the quality of the process and the outcome.

Evaluation

Implementation of the evaluation phase begins with initiation of the program planning. **Evaluation** also presents an opportunity for the program coordinators and students to continuously assess the success of the SL program. To evaluate the program, standards by which the objectives are rated must be determined, and the degree of satisfaction that is sought must be explicit. The task of developing standards to judge program outcomes is very important.[5,11,16]

The oral health chapter in the HP 2010 publication provides a common standard for meeting the oral health objectives of the nation. Baseline data and targets for improvement of oral health diseases for a variety of populations are included. This standard can be modified for use in community outreach programs that occur in dental hygiene programs across the country. Use of the HP 2010 baseline and targets as the evaluation norm will add a dimension of consistency to community dental health programs, and it will assist everyone in assessing the success of the community dental health program objectives.[3,4,16,18]

Evaluation that occurs during the planning and execution of the program is called **formative evaluation.** Accordingly, students, faculty, and the community partners should assemble assessment measures during planning of the program, and

Table 11-2   Formative and summative evaluation measures

Category of Evaluation	Service-Learning Objective	Example Measures
Summative	At the end of this program, the dental hygiene students will be able to conduct an oral health family assessment to determine and incorporate the resources, priorities, and concerns of the family	Increase in skill development (interviewing skill), awareness (cultural awareness), knowledge (knowledge of resources), and outlook (socioeconomic perspective)
Formative	At the end of this program, the dental hygiene students will be able to use national data sources to compile appropriate oral health information from different ethnic and racial populations	Number of resources used, adequacy of materials, scope of resources, and accuracy of measurement

these should be inserted throughout the program phases. The key to mastering formative evaluation is to recognize that the purpose of it is to improve the program while it is in progress. If the evaluation results indicate that the program is not effective or if it is determined that a component should be modified, corrective measures can be implemented right away. Formative evaluation is a dynamic process that is very constructive in increasing the potential for program success.

Evaluation that occurs at the end of the program is called **summative evaluation**, and it can be thought of as an end-report that summarizes the outcomes of the entire program and informs all parties regarding the impact of the program. Summative evaluation measures serve as the document that future programs will be based upon. Conversely, it can be used to determine whether future programs will even be continued. Both summative and formative evaluations operate by measuring the outcomes of the program, and both serve to improve the program. Refer to Table 11-2 for example formative and summative evaluation measures.

THE ARRAY OF EXPERIENTIAL LEARNING METHODS

The spectrum of experiential learning methods in health professions education is broad, and the decision regarding which method to use is determined by the intended goal. As such, care must be taken in choosing methods that are reflective of the goal. It is not unusual for multiple experiential methods to be used in health professions education. Refer to Box 11-4 for a list of common experiential methods and their unique purposes.

GUIDING PRINCIPLES

Essential Components of Service-Learning (SL)

- Collaborate: all parties should be included in the planning of the SL project
- Mutual Objective Formation: work with the agency in combining the objectives
- Orientation: formal opportunities must occur to ensure that all issues are discussed
- Preparation: planning the project requires participation and leadership from all students
- Experience: a well-constructed lesson plan will assist in the success of the SL project
- Reflection: forces consideration of the SL activity to self and to the public's health
- Evaluation: formative and summative evaluation should be planned and implemented

---

BOX 11-4   EXPERIENTIAL LEARNING SPECTRUM

Community Service: Students provide a service to the community and the primary focus is on the community's needs. This activity may or may not have a curriculum connection. The student may provide the service for reasons other than a classroom assignment (e.g., club requirement, religious obligation)

Clinical Rotation: This curriculum-based activity is not necessarily associated with a service outcome and is designed primarily to benefit the student learning. Students are assigned rotation through clinical experiences so that their skills, knowledge, and expertise are enhanced.

Practicum/Internship: This activity is typically longer than a clinical rotation and is designed to benefit the student. In this instance the student may be assigned to work in a particular specialty area for an entire academic quarter or semester. An example of practicum/internship is when a dental hygiene bachelor's completion program assigns senior students to various public health agencies, higher education institutions, and governmental agencies for the practical experience of on-the-job exposure and training.

Volunteerism: Students provide a service to the community and the major benefit is for the community. This activity is not necessarily associated with an academic course. Examples include assisting at the concession stands at an athletic event and/or participating in a secondary tutoring program.

BENEFITS OF SERVICE-LEARNING

Student Benefits

Service-Learning can foster leadership, cultural competency, lifelong learning, and a commitment to caring for the underserved. SL involvement may ultimately contribute to increased civic responsibility. SL projects can increase students' awareness of the social and political topics and processes, and it may encourage students to become actively involved in civic responsibilities.[1,11,22]

In SL projects, dental hygiene students are exposed to multiple aspects of diversity, which can foster a healthy appreciation for the differences they experience and thereby reduce stereotypical ideas and behaviors. These opportunities include exposure to different populations, different religions, various neighborhoods, different levels of wellness, and mental and physical abilities. When students reflect about the social determinants of health that are known factors in health and wellness conditions, they are challenged to view the community's endurance in a non-stereotypical manner, perhaps even as an asset. They are able to explore sensitive issues in the secure environment of the classroom, before they encounter such instances in the world of work.

Personal contact with community members that are different from "you" encourages personal growth, broadens horizons, decreases the tendency to stereotype, and increases interpersonal skills. Many health profession students have never cared for or spoken to someone of a different culture or race, and understandably the first time may be uncomfortable. But when placed into perspective, it is much simpler to gain this exposure in the comfort of an SL experience. In this instance faculty guidance, community partnering mentoring, and multiple opportunities for reflection can make a great difference in personal and professional growth.[10,16,18,19,22]

As dental hygiene students become acquainted with the local resources in their communities, the practical implications become clearer. Students can apply this knowledge to the patients that they care for in the clinical dental hygiene settings. SL turns the theoretic into the practical when concepts that were once considered complex and ambiguous become clearer to students who put them into practice. In summary, students engaged in SL are more likely to make the connection between their service and their academic coursework because they provide community service in response to community-identified concerns, and they learn in the context of the service provided.

Community Partner Benefits

A major benefit to the community partner is the opportunity to create long-term community-campus relationships. Activities to foster retention of the community partners are essential, and they are specific to the needs of the community partner. The dental hygiene faculty can invite a particularly supportive community partner to serve on the dental hygiene department's advisory committee. Or, the dental hygiene faculty could provide the agency's staff with an oral health continuing education session during an academic term in which the dental hygiene students are not available to participate in an SL project. Thus the continued contact with the community partner serves to minimize the disruption of the established SL program, and the continuity of the SL project is maintained. Other community partner benefits include:

Increased access to expertise: Relationships with academic faculty are beneficial. Faculty and/or the institution's research and planning office may be able to collaborate with the agency, for instance in grant writing, professional presentations, research, data analysis, and program evaluation.

Affirmation of the agency's mission: Community agencies provide much assistance for the public, yet too often their contributions go unnoticed. SL experiences will permit both the students and faculty to experience the strengths of the agency.

Opportunity to shape health professions education: SL is a way to extend the community teaching perspective. Agency professionals are experts in their area, and based upon the principle of partnership, they should anticipate the role of teaching or share their expertise with the students.

Extended service delivery: In addition to providing oral health instruction, dental hygiene students can assist the agency in a number of ways such as

- Develop and implement a survey
- Create evaluation tools
- Data entry and basic analysis of descriptive statistics
- Design and develop oral health column or newsletter

Dental Hygiene Program Benefits

The integration of SL into the dental hygiene curriculum can increase the quality and quantity of extramural training sites for dental hygiene students. As dental hygiene programs become more involved in the surrounding neighborhoods, the service mission of the academic institution is likely to be sustained through SL. As a result of SL involvement, dental hygiene faculty are more likely to serve on community health organizations, demonstrating that dental hygiene programs that are actively engaged in SL are more responsive to the communities they serve.

Dental Hygiene Faculty Benefits

Service-Learning permits faculty to work with the experts in the field. Community partners possess the expertise to assist faculty in integrating community-based experiences into the dental hygiene curriculum. Continuous faculty development is essential to pedagogic excellence. SL increases the growth opportunities, quality, and perspective of the dental hygiene faculty.

Academic Institution Benefits

Service-Learning can serve to assist academic institutions in fulfilling their community objectives. Academic institutions are under increasing pressure to demonstrate accountability to the stakeholders, or those who have a "stake" in the institution.

Funding and enrollment are, in many cases, dependent upon federal, state, and sometimes the local community. Long-term SL projects demonstrate the institution's commitment to the community. SL supports the mission of many higher education institutions.

Benefits for the Nation's Oral Health Agenda

The *Surgeon General's Report on Oral Health* (SGROH) has clearly articulated the public health benefit of expanding the services provided by dental hygienists. SL, while rapidly evolving as a teaching and learning development, has also shown promise in its ability to assist health profession students meet the health objectives that are outlined in the nation's health agenda. In addition to placing dental hygiene students into the customary sites for dental health education, students can also be placed in long-term community-based settings. Long-term SL projects provide for expanded access, continuity of care, curriculum integration, outcomes assessment, and evaluation.[6,7,18]

Issues of access to health care are challenging, and nationally health profession schools are moving towards sustained community-based partnerships. As such, the dental health professions need to actively investigate effective means to instruct our students to participate fully in these partnerships. Service-Learning has tremendous potential to reduce the unmet dental needs of the underinsured, uninsured, underserved, and underrepresented. Box 11-5 presents a summary of the SL benefits for the various stakeholders.

CHALLENGES OF SERVICE-LEARNING

Service-Learning challenges are encountered by all of the stakeholders: students, faculty, and academic partners. However, the approaches to managing the issues encountered with SL are unique in that they vary depending upon the SL project. However, SL challenges are embraced as a valuable element in experiential learning. Refer to Table 11-3 for a partial listing of the challenges facing students, faculty, and the community partner.

Program planning does not occur in a space devoid of situational challenges. **Risk management** is a phase that suggests that risks can be managed with organizational influence. Academic institutions and community organizations are likely to have their very own risk management department. Thus guidance in formulating risk management procedures for the purpose of implementing SL experiences should be readily available. The academic institution may have an affiliation agreement that they require the community partner to sign, and likewise, the community partner may have a similar agreement for the faculty and a policy document for the students to sign.

Leaders in the field of experiential learning suggest that all stakeholders involved in the planning and implementing of SL projects should also be involved in

Box 11-5   SUMMARY OF SERVICE-LEARNING BENEFITS

Students	Agency	Faculty
Exposure to multiple aspects of diversity	Partnering in educating future health professions students	Increases the training sites
Practical application of team skills and didactic content	Lasting community-campus relationships	Course enrichment
Secure environment for discussing sensitive issues	Real needs addressed	Increased awareness of community needs, resources, and strengths
Enhance self-confidence, interpersonal and leadership skills	Continuous community-campus relationships	Support the mission of the institution
Preparation for leadership role in dental hygiene organizations	Increased visibility of agency and its mission	Enhancement of scholarship and professional growth
Potential for interdisciplinary learning and collaboration	Increased networking opportunity	Meets core educational requirements
Cross-cultural skill development	Continuing education	Work experience with experts in the field
Explore career options	Use of academic resources such as Institutional Planning and Research	Meeting of academic goals of service, scholarship, and teaching

planning for risk management. The issue of risks involving the students, the faculty, the academic institution, the community agency, and the community members should be discussed openly, and strategies should be developed and distributed to all parties. Contingency planning, documentation, and review are prudent components of experiential learning opportunities.[14,23] A few of the issues that will need to be considered for inclusion in risk management discussions include those found in Box 11-6.

SUMMARY

Traditional methods of familiarizing dental hygiene students with community-based outreach methods such as community service, volunteerism, clinical rotations, and/or field experiences, though limited in scope, are useful in the dental hygiene curriculum. The dental hygiene community outreach efforts can be enhanced with SL, an underused instructional method.

Table 11-3   **Challenges facing students, faculty, and the community partner**

Student Challenges	Suggestions
Indifference	Provide Service-Learning (SL) training
	Link the experience to future employment options
	Include students in the planning
Optional status in curriculum	Integrate SL into the curriculum
	Course credit should be awarded
Dilemmas	Develop contingency plans for unexpected occurrences
	Develop the objectives with the agency partner

Community Agency Challenges	Suggestions
Previous negative experience with faculty and/or students	Get to know each other's programs, services, and needs
	Develop a mutual mission statement
	Plan the SL experience together
	Emphasize team planning, shared responsibility, and individual accountability
	Provide SL training session
Lack of continuity of service	Provide agency staff with professional development sessions in the nonacademic quarters
Lack of real authority	Reference the partner as "community faculty"
	Partner participation in reflection and evaluation
Time	Advance planning is critical
	Heavy workload initially, but diminishes with time

Faculty Challenges	Suggestions
Hidden agendas	Conduct research jointly with the agency
Time	Advance planning is critical
	Heavy workload initially, but diminishes with time
	Secure grants to support your service outreach
	Get a faculty mentor
Promotion	Document your work using portfolios, publications, and presentations
	Examine the institution's mission for service statements. Serve on the promotion and tenure committees to ensure a voice at the table
Colleagues' acceptance	Advocate for the inclusion of SL as a topic at conferences
Assumptions	What is obvious to faculty is not the case for students
	Do the work required to get students to perceive the obvious

Service-Learning has the potential to enhance the students' educational experience and to affect the oral health of the public in a positive fashion. SL emphasizes partnership stability. This, in turn, results in continuity of services, which contributes to the success of SL programs. SL challenges students and compels them to become more active in their learning. In addition to listening to lectures, participating

Box 11-6   Risk management considerations

• Service-Learning (SL) agreement	• Travel and transportation
• Special insurance policies	• Record of SL placements
• Policies/procedures	• Approved lesson plan
• Contact information	• Storage of personal items
• Emergency procedures	• Orientation checklist
• HIPAA compliance	• Evaluation documentation
• Background checks	• Scope of practice
• Student misconduct	• Attendance policies

in classroom discussions, and completing other assignments, students can tailor their own learning opportunities so that they improve in areas that are important to them. SL transforms the learning experiences for dental hygiene students and the oral health of the community.[11,12]

APPLYING **YOUR KNOWLEDGE**

Service-Learning Objectives Writing Exercise

The ideal time to combine objectives is during the orientation phase. The community partner's needs are more likely to be met when they take an active role in forming the SLO. Table 11-4 provides examples of SO, LO, and SLO to facilitate skill development in writing objectives. A few of the examples have been intentionally left blank for you to practice the objectives. Your job is to complete the service-learning objectives for the blank examples and compare your results with those of your classmates.

Table **11-4**   **Service-Learning grid exercise**

	Service Objective	*Learning Objective*	*Service-Learning Objective*
Example 1	The dental hygiene students will support the school nurse with follow-up and referral dental services, including the identification of resources.	Dental hygiene students will demonstrate knowledge of health and non-health barriers to dental hygiene services.	Dental hygiene students will learn about the health and non-health barriers to dental hygiene services by assisting the school nurse with follow-up and dental referrals.
Example 2	Children and parents will receive age-appropriate and culturally sensitive dental health education.	Dental hygiene students will prepare dental health education lessons for children in inner-city public schools.	Dental hygiene students will prepare and present age-appropriate and culturally sensitive dental health education to families.

Continued

Table 11-4   Service-Learning grid exercise—*continued*

	Service Objective	Learning Objective	Service-Learning Objective
Example 3	Adolescents will be able to list the oral health consequences of a diet high in sugar.	Dental hygiene students will demonstrate skills in communicating effectively with adolescents.	
Example 4	Adolescent minority youth at the Jefferson House will be encouraged to consider careers in dental hygiene.	First- and second-year dental hygiene students will demonstrate an understanding of basic principles of adolescent learning, including behavior management.	
Example 5	School teachers will learn basic pediatric oral health information that will assist them to recognize the need for urgent dental treatment.	Dental hygiene students will be able to demonstrate effective skills and knowledge when communicating with school teaching.	
Example 6	The adults will receive a confirmation of oral findings.	Dental hygiene students will demonstrate knowledge and skills in collecting and analyzing the results of an adult Basic Screening Survey.	
Example 7	The participants will receive a dental health report card that illustrates the results of a screening.	Dental hygiene students will develop a reporting instrument for a longitudinal study that will convey the results of an oral screening.	

DENTAL HYGIENE COMPETENCIES

At the end of this chapter the student should be able to demonstrate success in the following competencies:

Health promotion and disease prevention

HP.1 Promote the values of oral and general health and wellness to the public and organizations within and outside the profession.

HP.4 Identify individual and population risk factors and develop strategies that promote health-related quality of life.

Community involvement

CM.1 Assess the oral health needs of the community and the quality and availability of resources and services.

CM.3 Provide community oral health services in a variety of settings.

CM.4 Facilitate client access to oral health services by influencing individuals and organization for the provision of oral health care.

CM.6 Evaluate the outcomes of community-based programs, and plan for future activities.

Professional growth and development

PGD.1 Identify alternative career options within health care, industry, education, and research, and evaluate the feasibility of pursing dental hygiene opportunities.

PGD.3 Access professional and social networks and resources to assist entrepreneurial initiatives.

Community Case

The local dental society and the local dental hygiene program collaborated on the Give Kids a Smile Day (GKSD) national event. The dental hygiene department at Your Community College (YCC) and volunteers from the dental society conducted a massive oral screening on area underserved children. The results revealed that 60% of the 250 children aged 7 to 13 had an urgent need for dental treatment, and 75% had never visited the dentist.

The dental hygiene faculty, community dentists, and dental hygiene students want to provide dental services for this group of children. You are a student in the dental hygiene program, and you have agreed to serve as a member of the planning committee. The committee members consist of community members, agency members, dental hygiene faculty, dental hygiene advisory board members, and dentists from the local dental society.

1. Which national data source can be used as a model for the formation of program objectives?
   a. *Healthy People 2010*
   b. *Surgeon General's Report on Oral Health*
   c. Association for State and Territorial Dental Directors
   d. Basic Screening Survey
   e. Essential Public Health Services for Oral Health
2. Which of the following teaching methods provides concentrated benefit to the recipients of service and to the learner?
   a. Community service
   b. Volunteering

    c. Service learning

    d. Clinical rotations

    e. Practicum

3. In the development of this community dental program, which category of evaluation is it that allows the planners to assess the program while it is in progress so that modifications, if necessary, can be instituted?

    a. Summative evaluation

    b. Formative evaluation

    c. Normative evaluation

4. Which of the following core functions is addressed in the screening phase?

    a. Assessment

    b. Policy development

    c. Assurance

5. What type of objective is the following?

    "Students will be able to identify the five major sources of public health financing for oral health services."

    a. Service objective

    b. Learning objective

    c. SL objective

Resources: Service-Learning

Community-Campus Partnership for Health

    http://depts.washington.edu/ccph/

Learn and Serve America: Corporation for National Service

    http://www.learnandserve.org/

National Oral Health Surveillance System

    http://www.cdc.gov/nohss/

National Service Learning Clearinghouse

    http://www.servicelearning.org/

Service Learning Clearinghouse Project

    http://www.gseis.ucla.edu/slc/

Service Learning Home on the Web

    http://csf.colorado.edu/sl/

Service Learning and Risk Management Center for SL

    http://www2.sjsu.edu/csl/fac-topics_risk.html

REFERENCES

1. Haden NK, Catalanotto FA, Alexander CJ, et al: Improving the oral health status of all Americans: Roles and responsibilities of academic dental institutions. J Dent Educ 67(5):563-583, 2003.

2. Hemphill SL: Curriculum as intervention: Transforming a dental hygiene community dental health course into a service-learning course [Newsletter]. American Public Health Association Oral Health Section, 2003. http://www.apha.org/private/newsletters/oralhealthwinter2003.htm.

3. Hemphill SL: Public health advocacy and access through education [Newsletter]. American Public Health Association Oral Health Section Newsletter, 2003. http://www.apha.org/private/newsletters/oralhealthwinter2003.htm#anchor1475749.

4. Rice A: Interdisciplinary collaboration in health care: Education, practice and research. National Academies of Practice Forum 2(1):59-73, 2000.

5. U.S. Department of Health and Human Services: Healthy People 2010, 2nd ed. Understanding and Improving Health and Objectives for Improving Health (2 vols). Washington, DC, U.S. Government Printing Office, November 2000.

6. U.S. Department of Health and Human Services, Public Health Service: National Call to Action to Promote Oral Health. National Institutes of Health, National Institute of Dental and Craniofacial Research. NIH Publication No. 03-5303, Rockville, Md, 2003.

7. U.S. Department of Health and Human Services. Oral Health in America: A Report of the Surgeon General, Executive Summary. National Institutes of Health, National Institute of Dental and Craniofacial Research, Rockville, Md, 2000.

8. Kolb DA, Boyatzis RE, Mainemelis C: Experiential learning theory: Previous research and new directions. In Sternberg RJ, Zhang LF (eds): Perspectives on Cognitive, Learning, and Thinking Styles. Mahwah, New Jersey, Lawrence Erlbaum, 2000.

9. Bailey TR, Hughes KL, Moore DT: Working Knowledge: Work-Based Learning and Education Reform. New York, RoutledgeFalmer, 2004.

10. Canfield A, Clasen C, Dobbins J, et al: Service-Learning in Health Professions: Education: A Multiprofessional Example. Academic Exchange, Winter, 102-108, 2000.

11. Eyler J, Giles DE: Where's the Learning in Service-Learning? San Francisco, Jossey-Bass, 1999.

12. Furco A: Service-Learning: A balanced approach to experiential learning. In Expanding Boundaries: Service and Learning. Columbia, Md, Cooperative Education Association, 1996.

13. Bensley LB: Using theory and ethics to guide method selection and application. In Bensley RJ, Brookins-Fisher J, (eds): Community Health Education Methods, 2nd ed. Sudbury, Mass, Jones and Bartlett, pp 1-130, 2003.

14. Bringle RG, Hatcher JA: Institutionalization of service-learning in higher education. J Higher Educ 71(3):273-288, 2000.

15. McKenzie JF, Pinger RR, Kotecki JE: An introduction to community health, 4th ed. Boston, Jones and Bartlett, 2002.

16. Rice C, Brown JR: Transforming educational curriculum and service learning. J Experiential Educ 12(3):140-146, 1998.

17. Guidelines for State and Territorial Oral Health Programs. (Revised July 2001). Association of State and Territorial Dental Directors. [Electronic version]. Retrieved June 30, 2004. http://www.astdd.org/docs/ASTDD_Guidelines.PDF

18. Seifer SD: Service-learning: Community-campus partnerships for health professions education. Acad Med 73(3):273-277, 1998.

19. Cauley K, Canfield A, Clasen C, et al: Service-Learning: Integrating student learning and community service. Educ Health 14(2):173-181, 2001.

20. Strass R, Mofidi M, Sandler ES, et al: Reflective learning in community-based dental education. J Dent Educ 67(11):1234-1242, 2003.

21. Reams P: Service learning in health care higher education: Risk or not to risk. Education for Health: Change in Learning & Practice 16(2):145-154, 2003.

22. Commission on Dental Accreditation: Accreditation standards for dental hygiene education programs. Chicago, American Dental Association, 1998. [Electronic version]. Retrieved on August 7, 2004. http://www.ada.org/prof/ed/accred/standards/dh.pdf

23. American Association of Dental Schools (ADDS): Competencies for Entry into the Profession of Dental Hygiene: Washington, DC, AADS Section on Dental Hygiene Education; approved March 1999.

12

Test-Taking Strategies and Community Cases

Kathy Voigt Geurink, RDH, MA

Objectives

Upon completion of this chapter, the student will be able to:

- Develop an overview of the National Board Dental Hygiene Examination
- Develop guidelines for answering multiple-choice test items and community testlets
- Identify tips for examination preparation
- Take a practice examination on community cases
- Increase his or her confidence level in preparing for the examination

Key Terms

Community Health Activities

Community Cases

Multiple-Choice

Questions

Critical Thinking

OVERVIEW OF THE EXAMINATION

The National Board Dental Hygiene Examination (NBDHE) is written and administered by the Joint Commission on National Dental Examinations of the American Dental Association. The purpose of the examination is to determine professional competency in the various subject areas that are taught in the schools of dental hygiene.

According to the NBDHE Candidate Guide, the examination consists of 350 multiple-choice questions and is administered during 1 full day consisting of two 4-hour periods. Component A (4 hours in the morning) contains approximately 200 multiple-choice questions; Component B (4 hours in the afternoon) contains 150 questions based on 12 to 15 dental hygiene cases. Component A is composed of the following three major areas:

- Scientific basis for dental hygiene practice
- Provision of clinical dental hygiene services
- **Community health activities**

In the community health activities area, approximately four **community cases** are presented with a series of **multiple-choice questions** related to the situation described. The community cases are simulated situations that might occur in the community. They usually involve the dental hygienist's participation in a community oral health activity. Multiple-choice questions following the community cases require that the dental hygiene student apply information, such as that within this textbook, to select the correct answer. The community cases and the related questions are referred to as *testlets* within the examination.

MULTIPLE-CHOICE QUESTIONS

Multiple-choice questions are used to test the student's knowledge and understanding of content. A multiple-choice test item consists of a *stem*, which poses a problem that is followed by a list of answers. The stem is presented either as a question or as an incomplete statement. A choice of four or five answers is given per question. Only one of the answers is correct or best. The other answers are called *distracters*. Following are some suggestions:

1. When answering multiple test questions, use your time wisely. Look over the test initially to determine how many questions are presented, and calculate approximately how much time you will need to answer them.
2. Read directions and questions carefully.
3. Attempt to answer every question; if you are unsure of an answer, mark that question to enable you to return to it later if time permits.
4. Actively reason through each question, and read all the answers before making your choice.

Here are some tips that may help you in answering the questions. Look for the following within the questions and answers:

- Logical clues that help you select the correct answer
- A repeated word or concept in both the question and answer
- Length of the correct response: often the longest answer
- A similarity in or a direct opposite of responses; you can eliminate contradictory answers or complete opposites to the question

Examples of Multiple-Choice Questions

The following multiple-choice test questions relate to information in Chapter 8 and demonstrate how to answer multiple-choice questions using the clues already presented. Answer the following questions using your knowledge and these clues.

1. Which choice describes the Stages of Change Theory?
   a. It is an example of ways to effect changes in public policy
   b. It assesses a person's readiness to change and adopt behaviors that lead to a healthy lifestyle
   c. It includes key concepts such as reciprocal determination, observational learning, and reinforcement
   d. It directly assesses how susceptible a patient perceives oneself to be to periodontitis
2. An example of the tailoring technique that is used in formulating an individual's oral health plan is:
   a. Highlighting one or two messages that might apply to your patient
   b. Using photographs of American Indian women for posters in the Indian Health Service clinic
   c. Providing three individualized recommendations based on risk factors identified during a personal risk assessment
   d. Asking a group whether they prefer a video, slides, or a demonstration
3. You have developed a new program to promote oral health to teenaged mothers. You would like to discuss your ideas with other health professionals at an upcoming public health conference. Which of the following formats would be best for presenting your information?
   a. Round table discussion
   b. Oral presentation
   c. Research poster presentation
   d. Table clinic
4. Which of the following formats would you use to ensure the highest retention of information about oral cancer in a group of adults?
   a. Reading a booklet about oral cancer
   b. Using a multimedia presentation
   c. Demonstrating an oral examination, followed by a discussion and a return demonstration of how to perform the oral cancer examination
   d. Watching a video

The answers to these questions are provided here using clues versus a knowledge rationale. See Chapter 8 for a knowledge review.

1. **b.** This is the *logical* answer because Chapter 8 is on health promotion and behavioral change. Although a. has the word *change,* the topic is not relevant. Answers c. and d. have no wording similar to that of the question.
2. **c.** This answer uses a *similar* idea—the concept of individualization—even if one does not connect risk with tailoring. Answers b. and d. can be eliminated because they are opposites of the question, referring to groups rather than

an individual. Answer a. uses the vague term *might,* which makes it a less viable answer than c.

3. a. This answer uses *repetition* of the term *discuss,* which gives the clue to the best answer. The other three answers are ways to present the information, but a. is the best answer.

4. c. This answer has *length,* and it is logical that you will retain information better when you involve more of your senses.

ANSWERING COMMUNITY CASE QUESTIONS (TESTLETS)

When answering the community cases, you must change your train of thought from thinking about private practice to thinking community. Recall the definitions from within this text and the comparisons of private practice and community oral health practice. Your selection of the correct answer must be in relation to what is best for the community as a whole. You will be applying the information you have learned in your community course to a simulated situation in the community.

In most dental hygiene schools, students have an opportunity to apply the information that they have learned in the community course by conducting projects in the community. These projects require **critical thinking** skills to determine the best way to achieve maximum oral health for the population the student chooses to work with. Studying the "Applying Your Knowledge" features at the end of each chapter in this textbook is a good way for students to practice their critical thinking skills. Testing with cases requires students not only to retrieve knowledge, as in the stand-alone multiple-choice questions, but also to use their knowledge and critical thinking skills to make choices. Your critical thinking skills are just that—thinking about what you know. The NBDHE measures your ability to solve problems and to make decisions based on the knowledge you have acquired in your coursework.

Once you are in a community frame of mind, read carefully through the community situation. Then start on the multiple-choice questions; remember that the questions refer to the case presented. Some of the questions can probably be answered on a stand-alone basis, but they are intended to relate only to the case presented. The best answer is the one related to the information in the case.

If time permits, rereading through the case one more time after answering the questions allows you to catch any incorrect answer you may have selected without recalling important information from within the case. The community cases are located in the test in the latter half of the morning. If you do better with case-type questions early in a 4-hour period, consider answering the cases first and then the other multiple-choice questions in this section.

In your general preparation for the examination, try to identify your weak areas and concentrate your review on them. Do not cram for an examination of this magnitude. Set aside scheduled time for review, possibly using a calendar to set aside hours weekly to use for study. Some people study well in groups. Group studying can be beneficial because you learn other students' ideas and ways to recall information. Other students do better alone. It is your choice, but perhaps you can try a little of both.

Previous examination questions give you practice in test taking and often cover material that never changes. Alternate your review periods with practice examinations. Staying calm is important to your psyche. Remember, you won't know everything. A positive attitude always helps!

Examples of Critical Thinking: Community Oral Health Practice Testlets

The following four testlets and community cases are compiled as a practice test in community oral health. The number and type of questions are similar to what you will encounter on the NBDHE in this area. You should complete these questions in less than 40 minutes so that you will still have about 1 minute per question on the other multiple-choice questions in the morning section. There are four testlets with five questions each.

Testlet No. 1

You practice dental hygiene in a low-socioeconomic-level, multicultural city with a population of 1.5 million. The office you work in, however, serves a relatively higher socioeconomic population of the city. The city water supply is not fluoridated; consequently, dental decay is prevalent in the mouths of children residing in the poorer sections of the city. Most families in the city are of Hispanic descent. You recently assisted the public health dental hygienist in conducting a screening on the children in a local elementary school to document their oral health status. Fluoridation was defeated 10 years ago because of a strong antifluoridation campaign. Fluoridation will be on the ballot again in 8 months. The following questions relate to this situation:

1. What would be the best thing for you, as a private practice dental hygienist, to do to help get the fluoride referendum passed?
   a. Continue educating your patients on the benefits of fluoride as you have been doing
   b. Start calling community leaders
   c. Make a financial contribution to the cause
   d. Wait and see what happens; you do not want to stir up the antifluoridationists
   e. Check with your local dental hygiene component to determine whether a unified plan of action has been developed and how you might help
2. The following political tactics will be beneficial in ensuring that the fluoridation referendum will pass except one:
   a. Public debate with the antifluoridationists
   b. Analysis of the referendum of 10 years ago
   c. Securing of an expert consultant to work with the professionals
   d. Endorsements by community leaders
   e. Distribution of literature in Spanish and English throughout the community

3. The best index to use to determine the decay rate in the elementary school-aged children would be:
   a. DMFT
   b. CPI
   c. OHI
   d. PDI
   e. GI
4. To make sure that your data will be reliable before you conduct the screening, you should:
   a. Contact the parents of the children
   b. Inform the children about oral hygiene
   c. Calibrate the examiners
   d. Plan how many children will be included
   e. Choose a stratified sample
5. If the fluoridation referendum fails to pass once again, which alternative plan would be the most effective?
   a. Sending letters to parents requesting them to take their children to the dentist for treatment and fluoride
   b. Giving oral hygiene lessons in the classrooms
   c. Initiating a school fluoride mouth rinse program
   d. Getting the children to participate in a sealant program
   e. Sending letters to parents about the benefits of fluoride

Testlet No. 2

You have recently been employed as a public health dental hygienist in a local health department. You have been asked to plan, implement, and evaluate a school-based educational and preventive program for selected elementary schools located in your school district. The program is to be based on the *Healthy People 2010* oral health objectives. Your plan includes classroom education and the use of a mobile dental van to provide cleanings, sealants, and fluorides. The following questions relate to the formation of this program.

1. All of the following are *Healthy People 2010* objectives that will be affected by your program except:
   a. Increasing the proportion of health departments that have an oral health component
   b. Increasing the proportion of children who receive sealants
   c. Increasing the proportion of children who are provided with topical fluoride
   d. Reducing the incidence of dental caries in children
   e. Reducing the incidence of periodontitis and gingivitis in children
2. Your planning includes collecting data using the DMFT Index. This tool of measurement will be helpful in assessing which of the following?
   a. The demand for services from your oral health program

    b. The amount of gingivitis and periodontitis in children's teeth

    c. The need for services from your oral health program

    d. The children's risk of contracting other health diseases

    e. The need for more dentists in your school district

3. In the evaluation phase of your program, you plan to measure the children's performance skills in the area of oral hygiene. Which method would be best to accomplish this?

    a. A written pretest and post-test

    b. A demonstration of the procedures by the children

    c. An oral survey of the children's attitudes on oral health

    d. A surprise index at the school after lunch

    e. A questionnaire for parents reporting on their children's brushing habits

4. On the dental van, you want to assess the needs of the children and make appropriate referrals for treatment. Which of the following methods would be best to relay to the parents the overall needs of their children after the screening?

    a. Sending the DMFT Index numbers home with the children

    b. Mailing literature on the importance of oral health to the parents

    c. Phoning the parents and reporting on the findings

    d. Sending a list of local dentists home with the children who need treatment

    e. Using the Basic Screening Survey (BSS) and sending the results home with a list of local community clinics

5. All of the these programs would be resources for payment in treating the children's teeth at the dentists' offices except:

    a. Medicare

    b. Medicaid

    c. State Children's Health Insurance Program (CHIP)

    d. Private insurance

    e. Head Start

Testlet No. 3

One of your private practice patients is a nursing home administrator. She requests your assistance in providing an oral health care program for the patients with Alzheimer's disease who reside at the Manor Care. The program is to include education, screening, and referral. The residents are from a lower socioeconomic group and have complex health histories. The social worker has consents for dental treatment, if needed, and a vehicle for transportation.

1. What would the first step be in planning this program?

    a. Arranging a time for an in-service for the nursing home staff

    b. Assessing survey attitudes of the residents to determine what is needed

    c. Arranging a meeting of the people to be involved to assess the needs and to determine goals and objectives for the program

     d. Determining which residents are receiving Medicare payments

     e. Planning an educational session for the residents

2. Which activity would be most beneficial to the goal of improving the residents' oral hygiene?

     a. Providing toothbrushes for the staff

     b. Purchasing electric toothbrushes for the residents

     c. Educating the staff on the importance of good oral hygiene self-care

     d. Educating the residents on oral diseases

     e. Showing the residents how to perform an oral cancer check

3. The screening indicates that there is a need for better oral hygiene and dental restorative work. All of the following are possibilities for dental care for the patients who are mobile except:

     a. Taking the elderly residents to a private practice dentist who accepts Medicare patients, since Medicare pays for dental treatment

     b. Checking with the nearby dental school for arranging to transport residents to their clinic for care on a reduced-fee or no-cost basis

     c. Taking the residents to a community clinic that bases its fees on a sliding scale

     d. Asking the dentist and hygienist in your community who use portable equipment to include Manor Care on their list of nursing homes to visit

     e. Discussing the problem with the local dental society to determine whether the members would be willing to participate in a community program to help the elderly receive dental care

4. The Gingival Index (GI) was performed on the residents with natural teeth. The following scores were recorded: 2.5, 2.7, 2.8, 3.0, 2.5, 2.4, and 2.9. Which score represents the mean GI score of the residents?

     a. 2.50

     b. 2.55

     c. 2.61

     d. 2.63

     e. 2.69

5. In analyzing the assessment data, the dental hygienist found the correlation between age and oral cancer to be +.80. This relationship could be described as:

     a. Weak

     b. Negative

     c. Strong

     d. Moderate

     e. Not significant

Testlet No. 4

You reside in a small town and work in a community clinic. The regional public heath dental hygienist asks for your assistance in assessing, planning, and implementing oral health programs in your town. She is especially concerned about the elderly population and about developing a tobacco awareness program in the middle school.

1. You perform an assessment of the community's needs, including a description by age, gender, and socioeconomic status. This assessment is referred to as the:
   a. Design of your plan
   b. Community profile
   c. List of priorities
   d. Needs assessment
   e. Problem definition

2. You decide to collect some baseline data to document the needs of the adults in the community and, possibly, to secure funds for program development. You want to measure healthy gingiva, presence or absence of bleeding, supragingival or subgingival calculus, and periodontal pockets. Which index would you use to screen the adults who visit your clinic?
   a. OHI
   b. DMFT
   c. PDI
   d. CPI
   e. RCI

3. You intend to survey the middle school students to assess their perception of how susceptible they are to addiction and to cancer caused by tobacco products. In your prevention program, you will present the benefits of not smoking or chewing and will discuss the results of their decisions. Which model of health promotion are you using?
   a. Stages of Change Theory
   b. Social Learning Theory
   c. Community Organization Theory
   d. Health Belief Model
   e. Diffusion of Innovations Theory

4. Upon completion of your tobacco awareness program, you intend to present the results to other health care professionals at a health promotions meeting. Which strategy would you choose if you wish to reach a large number of people, have time for interaction, and do not intend to use audiovisual equipment?
   a. Poster presentation
   b. Round table discussion
   c. Oral paper
   d. Table clinic
   e. Written handout with your e-mail address on it

5. You bring your tobacco awareness program to the state public health dental hygienist. In attempting to follow the essential services of the public health core functions, the state dental hygienist wants to support and implement

programs at all levels of prevention. At which level of prevention is your tobacco program?
a. Primary
b. Secondary
c. Tertiary
d. Planning
e. Implementing

Answers and rationales to the questions are presented next. Also see the chapters in which the information can be retrieved from within the text.

ANSWERS AND RATIONALES

The answers, rationales for each answer, and chapter cross-references are presented next.

Testlet No. 1

1. e.   A unified plan of action is the best defense against a strong antifluoridation group. Answers a., b., and c. are also possibilities of things you can do, but e. is best and foremost (see Chapter 6).

2. a.   A public debate with antifluoridationists only provides them with an opportunity to reach more people with their scare tactics (see Chapter 6).

3. a.   The DMFT Index is used to determine the decay rate in children (see Chapter 4).

4. c.   Calibration of examiners is the best way to make sure that the data that you are collecting are reproducible or reliable (see Chapter 7).

5. c.   A school fluoride mouth rinse program would be the next choice because it is inexpensive and would benefit all the children in reducing dental decay. Sealants are more expensive, and education does not guarantee a reduction in decay. These programs should be used in conjunction with fluoride (see Chapter 6).

Testlet No. 2

1. e.   Reducing the incidence of periodontitis and gingivitis in children is not an objective of *Healthy People 2010;* all the other choices are objectives (see Chapter 5).

2. c.   An assessment such as that conducted using the DMFT Index determines the *need* for oral health services. Answers b. and d. would not be appropriate because the DMFT Index is an assessment tool for determining decay. Although e. might be a conclusion, through critical thinking you can determine that this one single service probably is not the best solution (see Chapters 4 and 9).

3. b.   Evaluation of performance is best conducted with an activity or demonstration by the person being evaluated (see Chapters 6 and 8).

4.   e.   The Basic Screening Survey is an easy tool to let parents know whether the child needs emergency care, whether treatment is necessary, or whether routine care is recommended. Local community clinics provide the best fee for service for low-income patients. It is difficult to reach people by phone, and the follow-up list for referral is very important to the screening process (see Chapters 2 and 4).

5.   a.   Medicare is a program for elderly people, and it does not cover dental services. All of the other programs offer oral health treatment for children (see Chapter 6).

Testlet No. 3

1.   c.   Assessment of needs is always the first step in program planning (see Chapters 3 and 8).

2.   c.   The residents in nursing homes rely on the staff or caregivers to assist them with oral hygiene. Therefore the staff must be educated on the importance of their own oral health first (see Chapters 2, 6, and 8).

3.   a.   All of these ideas would work except a., since Medicare does not offer dental benefits (see Chapter 6).

4.   e.   To find the mean, add the scores and divide by the total number of scores (see Chapter 7).

5.   c.   In comparing two variables, if the correlation is .7 or higher, the relationship is strong (see Chapter 7).

Testlet No. 4

1.   b.   "Community profile" is the term used to describe the community, including gender, age, and socioeconomic status (see Chapter 3).

2.   d.   The Community Periodontal Index (CPI) entails gathering data in all the areas described. It is a modification of the Community Periodontal Index of Treatment Needs (CPITN) and is more readily used. The other indexes are too specific and not as inclusive. The PDI is not widely used anymore. (see Chapter 4).

3.   d.   The Health Belief Model is the only one listed that includes information on the people's perceptions or beliefs about oral health (see Chapter 8).

4.   a.   The poster presentation allows for the most interaction with the largest number of people. This is a popular presentation method at health promotion meetings. Audiovisual equipment is not used, and personal interaction is foremost (see Chapter 8).

5.   a.   Preventive services, such as a tobacco awareness program, are at the primary prevention level; they prevent the disease before it occurs. Secondary prevention reduces or eliminates disease in the early stages. Tertiary prevention limits disability from disease in later stages. Planning and implementing are phases of program development (see Chapters 1, 2, and 6).

APPENDIX
A

Website/Community Resource List*

Academy of General Dentistry
http://www.agd.org
American Academy of Pediatric Dentistry
http://www.aapd.org
American Association of Endodontists
http://www.aae.org
American Association of Orthodontists
http://www.aaortho.org
American Association of Public Health Dentistry
http://www.aaphd.org
American Dental Assistants Association
http://www.dentalassistant.org
American Dental Association
http://www.ada.org
American Dental Hygienists Association
http://www.adha.org; http://www.adha.org/governmental_affairs
American Medical Association
http://www.ama-assn.org
American Public Health Association
http://www.apha.org
Association of State and Territorial Dental Directors
http://www.astd.org
Block Drug Company
http://www.blockdrug.com

---

*Updated URLs for these resources and more can be found on this book's Evolve site.

Centers for Disease Control and Prevention, Oral Health Division
http://www.cdc.gov/nccdphp/oh
Centers for Medicare and Medicaid Services (CMS)
http://www.cms.hhs.gov
Colgate Company
http://www.colgate.com
Federation Dentaire Internationale (FDI) World Dental Federation
http://www.fdiworldental.org
Government Grants
http://www.grants.gov
Health Resources and Services Administration
http://www.hrsa.gov
International and American Associations for Dental Research
http://www.iadr.com
National Institute of Dental and Craniofacial Research
http://www.nidcr.nih.gov
National Maternal and Child Oral Health Resource Center
http://www.ncemch.org/oralhealth
National Oral Health Information Clearinghouse
http://www.nohic.nidcr.nih.gov
Occupational Safety and Health Administration (OSHA)
http://www.osha.gov
Oral Health America
http://www.oralhealthamerica.org
Procter & Gamble
http://www.dentalcare.com
Synopsis of State Dental Public Health Programs
http://www.2.cdc.gov/nccdphp/doh/synopses/index.asp
The American Academy of Periodontology
http://www.perio.org
The American College of Prosthodontists
http://www.prosthodontics.org/acpros/index.html
U.S. Department of Health and Human Services
http://www.dhhs.gov
U.S. Department of Health and Human Services Oral Health Initiatives
http://www.hrsa.gov/OralHealth.cfm
World Health Organization
http://www.who.ch

Dental Hygiene Competencies*

According to the "Competencies for Entry into the Profession of Dental Hygiene" approved and adopted by the ADEA House of Delegates in 2003, the dental hygienist must exhibit competencies in the five following domains:

1. The dental hygienist must possess, first, the **Core Competencies (C),** the ethics, values, skills, and knowledge integral to all aspects of the profession. These core competencies are foundational to all of the roles of the dental hygienist.

2. Second, inasmuch as **Health Promotion (HP)** and Disease Prevention is a key component of health care, changes within the health care environment require the dental hygienist to have a general knowledge of wellness, health determinants, and characteristics of various patient/client communities. The hygienist needs to emphasize both prevention of disease and effective health care delivery.

3. Third is the dental hygienist's complex role in the **Community (CM).** Dental hygienists must appreciate their role as health professionals at the local, state, and national levels. This role requires the graduate dental hygienist to assess, plan, and implement programs and activities to benefit the general population. In this role, the dental hygienist must be prepared to influence others to facilitate access to care and services.

4. Fourth is **Patient/Client Care (PC),** requiring competencies described here in ADPIE format. Because the dental hygienist's role in patient/client care is ever changing, yet central to the maintenance of health, dental hygiene graduates must use their skills to assess, diagnose, plan, implement, and evaluate treatment.

---

*Also available on this book's Evolve website.

5. Fifth, like other health professionals, dental hygienists must be aware of a variety of opportunities for **Professional Growth and Development (PGD).** Some opportunities may increase clients' access to dental hygiene; others may offer ways to influence the profession and the changing health care environment. A dental hygienist must possess transferable skills (e.g., in communication, problem solving, and critical thinking) to take advantage of these opportunities.

Core Competencies

C.1 Apply a professional code of ethics in all endeavors.

C.2 Adhere to state and federal laws, recommendations, and regulations in the provision of dental hygiene care.

C.3 Provide dental hygiene care to promote patient/client health and wellness using critical thinking and problem solving in the provision of evidenced-based practice.

C.4 Assume responsibility for dental hygiene actions and care based on accepted scientific theories and research as well as the accepted standard of care.

C.5 Continuously perform self-assessment for lifelong learning and professional growth.

C.6 Advance the profession through service activities and affiliations with professional organizations.

C.7 Provide quality assurance mechanisms for health services.

C.8 Communicate effectively with individuals and groups from diverse populations both verbally and in writing.

C.9 Provide accurate, consistent, and complete documentation for assessment, diagnosis, planning, implementation, and evaluation of dental hygiene services.

C.10 Provide care to all clients using an individualized approach that is humane, empathetic, and caring.

Health Promotion and Disease Prevention

HP.1 Promote the values of oral and general health and wellness to the public and organizations within and outside the profession.

HP.2 Respect the goals, values, beliefs, and preferences of the patient or client while promoting optimal oral and general health.

HP.3 Refer patients or clients who may have a physiologic, psychologic, or social problem for comprehensive patient and client evaluation.

HP.4 Identify individual and population risk factors and develop strategies that promote health-related quality of life.

HP.5 Evaluate factors that can be used to promote patient or client adherence to disease prevention or health maintenance strategies.

HP.6 Evaluate and use methods to ensure the health and safety of the patient or client and the dental hygienist in the delivery of dental hygiene.

Community Involvement

CM.1 Assess the oral health needs of the community and the quality and availability of resources and services.

CM.2 Provide screening, referral, and educational services that allow clients to access the resources of the health care system.

CM.3 Provide community oral health services in a variety of settings.

CM.4 Facilitate client access to oral health services by influencing individuals and organizations for the provision of oral health care.

CM.5 Evaluate reimbursement mechanisms and their impact on the patient or client's access to oral health care.

CM.6 Evaluate the outcomes of community-based programs and plan for future activities.

Patient and Client Care

Assessment

PC.1 Systematically collect, analyze, and record data on the general, oral, and psychosocial health status of a variety of patients or clients using methods consistent with medicolegal principles.

This competency includes the following steps:
a. Select, obtain, and interpret diagnostic information, recognizing its advantages and limitations.
b. Recognize predisposing and etiologic risk factors that require intervention to prevent disease.
c. Obtain, review, and update a complete medical, family, social, and dental history.
d. Recognize health conditions and medications that affect overall patient or client care.
e. Identify patients or clients at risk for a medical emergency, and manage the patient or client care in a manner that prevents an emergency.
f. Perform a comprehensive examination using clinical, radiographic, periodontal, dental charting, and other data collection procedures to assess the patient's or client's needs.

Diagnosis

PC.2 Use critical decision-making skills to reach conclusions about the patient's or client's dental hygiene needs based on all available assessment data.

This competency includes the following steps:
a. Use assessment findings, etiologic factors, and clinical data in determining a dental hygiene diagnosis.
b. Identify patient or client needs and significant findings that affect the delivery of dental hygiene services.
c. Obtain consultations as indicated.

Planning

PC.3 Collaborate with the patient or client or other health professionals to formulate a comprehensive dental hygiene care plan that is patient-centered or client-centered and based on current scientific evidence.

This competency includes the following steps:

a. Prioritize the care plan based on the health status and the actual and potential problems of the individual to facilitate optimal oral health.
b. Establish a planned sequence of care (educational, clinical, and evaluation) based on the dental hygiene diagnosis; identified oral conditions; potential problems; etiologic and risk factors; and available treatment modalities.
c. Establish a collaborative relationship with the patient or client in the planned care to include etiology, prognosis, and treatment alternatives.
d. Make referrals to other health care professionals.
e. Obtain the patient's or client's informed consent based on a thorough case presentation.

Implementation

PC.4 Provide specialized treatment that includes preventive and therapeutic services designed to achieve and maintain oral health. Assist in achieving oral health goals formulated in collaboration with the patient/client.

This competency includes the following steps:

a. Perform dental hygiene interventions to eliminate or control local etiologic factors to prevent and control caries, periodontal disease, and other oral conditions.
b. Control pain and anxiety during treatment through the use of accepted clinical and behavioral techniques.
c. Provide life support measures to manage medical emergencies in the patient or client care environment.

Evaluation

PC.5 Evaluate the effectiveness of the implemented clinical, preventive, and educational services, and modify as needed.

This competency includes the following steps:

a. Determine the outcomes of dental hygiene interventions using indexes, instruments, examination techniques, and the patient or client self-report.
b. Evaluate the patient's or client's satisfaction with the oral health care received and the oral health status achieved.
c. Provide subsequent treatment or referrals based on evaluation findings.
d. Develop and maintain a health maintenance program.

Professional Growth and Development

PGD.1 Identify alternative career options within health care, industry, education, and research and evaluate the feasibility of pursuing dental hygiene opportunities.
PGD.2 Develop management and marketing strategies to be used in non-traditional health care settings.
PGD.3 Access professional and social networks and resources to assist entrepreneurial initiatives.

The American Association of Dental Schools (now called the American Dental Education Association) drafted these competency statements. Representation was provided from both baccalaureate and associate degree dental hygiene programs. It also included representation from dental hygiene, clinical, social, and basic sciences and the American Dental Hygienists Association. A separate committee, the Dental Hygiene Education Competency Draft Review Committee, further reviewed and provided feedback on the document. The competency statements were presented for public comment at the 1998 AADS Annual Session, the 1998 Dental Hygiene Directors conference, and the Section on Dental Hygiene Education home page on the World Wide Web, and went into effect in January 2000.

BIBLIOGRAPHY

American Dental Education Association (ADEA): Competencies for Entry into the Profession of Dental Hygiene: ADEA Section on Dental Hygiene Education (approved March 2003 House of Delegates).

C

Community Partnerships for Oral Health

APPENDIX C-1 POTENTIAL COMMUNITY PARTNERS

Patients, Clients, and Consumers of Services

- Patients and clients
- Parents and family representatives
- Consumers of services
- Public representatives

Government Agencies and Programs

- State and tribal departments of health (e.g., administrators and staff)
- State and tribal human service agency staff and administrators (e.g., programs for individuals with mental illness and mental retardation, state/tribal hospitals and institutions, programs for individuals with special health care needs [e.g., blind, deaf], departments of correction)
- Regional council of governments
- Area agencies on aging
- County extension agencies

- Local health departments (e.g., county and/or city health officials—oral health, Maternal and Child Health, WIC, primary health care, family planning, rural health, health disparities, minority health, HIV, chronic diseases, etc.)
- Local human service agency administrators and staff
- Representatives such as county and/or city officials working with child care, youth services, literacy, elderly and disabled services, public transportation, public housing, workforce development, etc.
- Environmental health—community water supervisors or managers related to community water fluoridation

Policymakers and Organizations

- U.S. Congress—state senators and representatives
- Local government elected officials—county judges, mayors, city councilors, and county commissioners, etc.

- Policy advocates (e.g., Legal Aid, League of United Latin American Citizens [LULAC], National Association for the Advancement of Colored Persons [NAACP])
- Policy institutes

Community Organizations

- Advocates for clients and consumers of services
- Advocates for children and adults with disabilities, HIV, cancer, homeless children, and adults, etc.
- United Way, American Cancer Society, Diabetes Association, March of Dimes, Easter Seals, Mental Health Association, Success by 6, Healthy Mothers/ Healthy Babies Coalition, League of Women Voters, Association for Retarded Citizens (ARC), United Cerebral Palsy, American Red Cross, Urban League, American Association of Retired Persons (AARP), etc.
- Community action agencies
- Senior nutrition services and sites
- Early-childhood intervention organizations
- Community information and resource centers (e.g., 311 programs—state and local area information centers [AIC]/ information and resource [I&R] networks)
- Representatives of consumer and regional advisory groups
- Community coalitions, collaborations, initiatives

- Faith-based organizations (e.g., Catholic Charities, Salvation Army)
- Local representatives active in collaborative service programs with health and human service agencies that specifically address key issues (e.g., community planning)
- Service organizations for vulnerable population groups (e.g., literacy, elderly and disabled services, youth services, veterans, women, migrant and seasonal farm workers, public transportation, public housing, workforce development, child care, food banks, homeless shelters)
- Americorps, City Year, etc.
- Community foundations
- Community centers and neighborhood associations
- Business leaders/Chamber of Commerce (e.g., Women Chamber of Commerce, Hispanic Chamber of Commerce)
- Unions
- Civic organizations—Junior League, Rotary International, Kiwanis Lions Club, Elks
- Youth Groups—Boys and Girls Clubs, YMCA, YWCA, Big Brothers/ Big Sisters, Special Olympics

- Medicaid and CHIP Outreach Coalitions outreach staff and community-based organizations, Insure-A-Kid school outreach grantees, Covering Kids & Families grantees, etc.
- Foundations
- Local media—newspapers, television, radio, etc.

Education-Related Organizations and Groups

- Regional education service centers
- Local school districts and boards— superintendents, principals, teachers, school nurses, school social workers, parent liaisons
- Local child development/child care grantees and Head Start grantees (e.g., Head Start executive directors, Head Start health coordinators)
- Parent-Teacher associations/organizations
- Parenting education programs
- Adult education and literacy programs
- Home school programs
- Employment and vocational education
- Education-related unions
- Fraternities and sororities

Health and Human Service Providers, Groups, Organizations, and Associations

- Health systems and hospitals (e.g., rural and community, public, nonprofit, private, children's hospitals, Department of Veterans Affairs Hospitals and Clinics, county hospital districts)
- Community health centers
- Safety net health and dental programs—community dental clinics, nonprofit dental clinics
- Maternal and child health programs
- State and local health professional associations
- Dentists, dental hygienists, and dental assistants
- Physicians, pediatricians, family physicians, physician assistants, etc.
- Nurses, nurse practitioners, nurse midwives, etc.
- Speech pathologists
- Dieticians
- Nursing home administrators
- Early childhood intervention providers
- Social workers

Third-Party Payers

- Health plans
- Dental insurers
- Employers providing dental insurance coverage

- Managed care organizations
- Health maintenance organizations (HMOs)
- Medicaid

- Employers not providing dental insurance coverage

Higher and Professional Education

- Universities and colleges
- Dental and dental hygiene schools
- Nursing schools
- Medical schools
- Allied health schools
- Schools of public health

- Schools of social work
- Schools of public policy and health administration
- Schools for speech pathology
- Schools for dietetics

Business Organizations and Retail Outlets

- Airlines
- Banks
- Beauty and barber shops
- Chambers of commerce
- Computer companies and stores
- Grocery stores

- Delicatessens, specialty and ethnic food stores
- Health clubs
- Insurance companies
- Shopping malls
- Maternity stores
- Movie theaters

BIBLIOGRAPHY

Association of State and Territorial Dental Directors. Best Practice Approaches for State and Community Oral Health Programs: State Oral Health Coalitions and Collaborative Partnerships, 2003.

Centers for Disease Control and Prevention, Division of Oral Health. Infrastructure Development Tools: Oral Health Coalition Framework, 2002.

Seven Days of Immunizations: National Infant Immunization Week, U.S. Department of Health and Human Services, Public Health Service, Atlanta, Ga: Centers for Disease Control and Prevention, 1995.

Steffensen JEM. Guide for Oral Health Listening Sessions: Activation of a Collaborative Oral Health Plan in Texas, San Antonio, Texas: Department of Community Dentistry, University of Texas Health Science Center at San Antonio, Dental School, 2004.

Washington State Oral Health Coalition. Community Roots for Oral Health: Guidelines for Successful Coalitions.

APPENDIX C-2   ORAL HEALTH COALITION FRAMEWORK

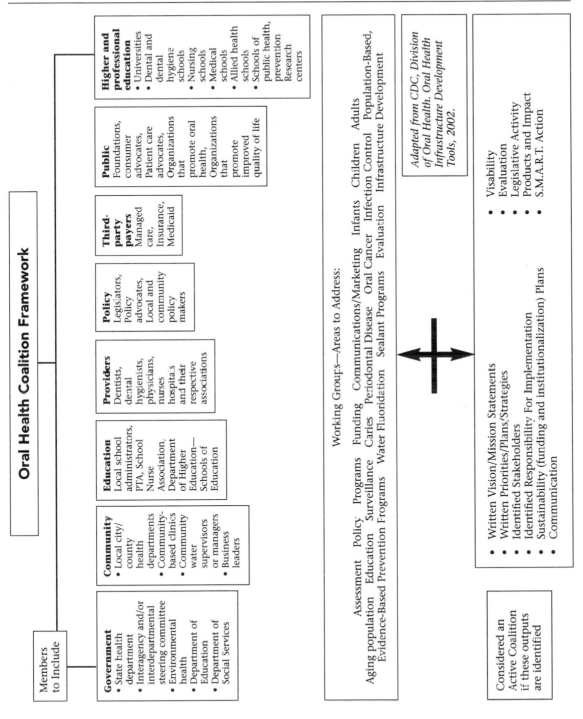

Oral Health Coalition Framework

Members to Include

Government
- State health department
- Interagency and/or interdepartmental steering committee
- Environmental health
- Department of Education
- Department of Social Services

Community
- Local city/county health departments
- Community-based clinics
- Community water supervisors or managers
- Business leaders

Education
Local school administrators, PTA, School Nurse Association, Department of Higher Education—Schools of Education

Providers
Dentists, dental hygienists, physicians, nurses hospitals and their respective associations

Policy
Legislators, Policy advocates, Local and community policy makers

Third-party payers
Managed care, Insurance, Medicaid

Public
Foundations, consumer advocates, Patient care advocates, Organizations that promote oral health, Organizations that promote improved quality of life

Higher and professional education
- Universities
- Dental and dental hygiene schools
- Nursing schools
- Medical schools
- Allied health schools
- Schools of public health, prevention Research centers

Working Groups—Areas to Address:

Assessment Policy Programs Funding Communications/Marketing Infants Children Adults Aging population Education Surveillance Caries Periodontal Disease Oral Cancer Infection Control Population-Based, Evidence-Based Prevention Programs Water Fluoridation Sealant Programs Evaluation Infrastructure Development

- Written Vision/Mission Statements
- Written Priorities/Plans/Strategies
- Identified Stakeholders
- Identified Responsibility For Implementation
- Sustainability (funding and institutionalization) Plans
- Communication

- Visability
- Evaluation
- Legislative Activity
- Products and Impact
- S.M.A.R.T. Action

Adapted from CDC, Division of Oral Health. Oral Health Infrastructure Development Tools, 2002.

Considered an Active Coalition if these outputs are identified

Resources for Community Health Assessment

APPENDIX D-1   EXAMPLES OF INFORMATION FOR A COMMUNITY PROFILE

Physical and Spatial Characteristics

Geopolitical boundaries, community-designated boundaries, geographic size, community location description, population size, population density, community type, general physical environment, geographic isolation, physical conditions of neighborhoods, community assets, people-made environment, layout of the community, residential neighborhoods, business districts, buildings, greenspace, parks, transportation routes, roads, traffic, congestion, environmental conditions, air quality, water supply, water quality, community infrastructure, education resources and facilities, location and characteristics of local institutions, landmarks, art, media, playgrounds, recreation facilities and resources, libraries, public commons and informal gathering places, number of places of worship, religious denominations, local economy and types of industry, signs of development or decay in community areas, patterns of day-to-day activities, and everyday human interactions.

Community Inventory

History of community, community traditions, dominant values, significant beliefs, events that have occurred in the community with a short- or long-term effect on the health of the community, political system, local government structure, political structure, dominant political affiliation, number of registered voters, power structure, formal and informal community leadership, formal community support systems, informal helping networks/mutual support and trusted community members, gatekeepers, opinion leaders, community historians, communication channels, inventories of citizen's associations and community organizations, inventory of capacities of individual community members, and groups of individuals.

SOCIODEMOGRAPHIC CHARACTERISTICS

Community Demographic Data

Population distribution by age, gender, race and ethnicity composition, social class, economic status, education levels, occupations, religions, marital status, gender ratios, socioeconomic data, employment status, neighborhood living conditions, value of housing, household living conditions, household crowding, indices of deprivation, levels of education, religion, nationality, and cultural characteristics, generational information, in-migration and out-migration, immigration status, trends of change in size and composition.

Social Demographic Data

Social attributes, social structure, community stability, social cohesiveness, civic engagement and pride, social networks, family and household characteristics, family values, family living patterns, community norms, customs and lifestyles, health-enhancing behaviors, values, attitudes, beliefs, opinions, social forces, cultural forces, religious beliefs, enrollment in government programs (including Temporary Assistance for Needy Families [TANF]), public assistance, food stamps, Supplemental Food Program for Women, Infants, and Children (WIC), Head Start, child care support, Medicaid, Children's Health Insurance Program (S-CHIP), vulnerable populations groups in community, quality of life, crime and security

Vital Events

Natality (births), fertility rates, life expectancy, mortality (deaths), marriages, divorces, population mobility.

APPENDIX D-2   EXAMPLES OF GOVERNMENT RESOURCES FOR HEALTH DATA

AGENCY FOR HEALTH CARE RESEARCH AND QUALITY (AHRQ), MEDICAL EXPENDITURE PANEL SURVEY (MEPS)

http://www.meps.ahrq.gov/

The MEPS collects data on the specific health services that Americans use, how frequently they use them, the cost of these services, and how they are paid for, as well as data on the cost, scope, and breadth of private health insurance held by and available to the U.S. population. MEPS is unparalleled for the degree of detail in its data as well as its ability to link data on health services spending and health insurance to the demographic, employment, economic, health status, and other characteristics of survey respondents. Moreover, MEPS is the only national survey that provides a foundation for estimating the impact of changes in sources of payment and insurance coverage on different economic groups or special populations of interest, such as the poor, elderly, families, veterans, the uninsured, and racial and ethnic minorities. The MEPS is resource designed to continually provide policy makers, health care administrators, businesses, and others with timely, comprehensive information about health care use and costs in the United States, and to improve the accuracy of their economic projections.

MEPS is the most recent in a series of medical expenditure surveys that began in 1977 as the National Medical Care Expenditure Survey and later became the National Medical Expenditure Survey (NMES). The last study in this series was conducted in 1987. This new survey provides critically needed updates to the 1987 data. The Agency for Healthcare Research and Quality (AHRQ), formerly called the Agency for Health Care Policy and Research, began fielding MEPS in March 1996. AHRQ conducts MEPS in conjunction with the National Center for Health Statistics (NCHS) and through contracts with Westat, a survey research firm headquartered in Washington, D.C., and the National Opinion Research Center, which is affiliated with the University of Chicago.

BUREAU OF THE CENSUS, DEPARTMENT OF COMMERCE

http://www.census.gov/index.html

U.S. Census 2000 http://www.census.gov/main/www/cen2000.html
Statistical Abstract of the United States http://www.census.gov/statab/www/

CDC, BEHAVIORAL RISK FACTOR SURVEILLANCE SURVEY (BRFSS)

http://www.cdc.gov.brfss/

The BRFSS is a state-based, ongoing data collection program designed to measure behavioral risk factors in the adult, noninstitutionalized population 18 years of age or older. Every month, states select a random sample of adults for a telephone interview. This selection process results in a representative sample for each state so that statistical inferences can be made from the information collected from the survey.

CDC, DATA2010

http://wonder.cdc.gov/data2010/

DATA2010 is an interactive database system developed by the Division of Health Promotion Statistics, National Center for Health Statistics, and contains the most recent monitoring data for tracking *Healthy People 2010*. *Healthy People 2010* contains 467 objectives that identify specific measures to monitor health in the first decade of the twenty-first century. Each objective includes a statement of intent, a baseline value for the measure to be tracked, and a target to be achieved by the year 2010. Objectives may include more than one measure. Each measure is shown separately in the database. Data for the population-based objectives may be presented separately for select populations, such as racial, gender, educational attainment, or income groups. The objectives are organized into 28 focus areas, each representing an important public health area.

Data are included for all the objectives and subgroups identified in *Healthy People 2010*. National data are available for all of the measurable objectives. State data are available for a subset of the measurable objectives. Sociodemographic data tabulated separately by race, Hispanic origin, gender, education or income, and selected other populations are available for all population-based objectives. All data in DATA2010 are the most recent available and may include revisions or corrections. Therefore some data may differ from data previously shown. DATA2010 is updated quarterly. Updates include new data years and possibly revisions to baseline data. Existing spreadsheets and technical information provide operational definitions for each *Healthy People 2010* measure. Users can obtain data for a single health objective, for all objectives within a focus area, for all objectives tracked by a particular data system, or for all objectives that target a specific population group (e.g., women, adolescents, or Hispanics). Users can also obtain data for the measures used to track the 10 *Healthy People 2010* Leading Health Indicators or the DHHS Steps to a Healthier U.S. measures.

CDC, NATIONAL NOTIFIABLE DISEASES SURVEILLANCE SYSTEM

http://www.cdc.gov/epo/dphsi/nndsshis.htm

In 1961, CDC assumed responsibility for the collection and publication of data concerning nationally notifiable diseases. The list of nationally notifiable diseases is revised periodically. For example, a disease may be added to the list as a new pathogen emerges, or a disease may be deleted as its incidence declines. Public health officials at state health departments and CDC continue to collaborate in determining which diseases should be nationally notifiable; The Council of State and Territorial Epidemiologists (CSTE), with input from CDC, makes recommendations annually for additions and deletions to the list of nationally notifiable diseases. However, reporting of nationally notifiable diseases to CDC by the states is voluntary. Reporting is currently mandated (i.e., by state legislation or regulation) only at the state level. The list of diseases that are considered notifiable, therefore, varies slightly by state. All states generally report the internationally quarantinable diseases (i.e., cholera, plague, and yellow fever) in compliance with the World Health Organization's International Health Regulations.

CDC, NATIONAL ORAL HEALTH SURVEILLANCE SYSTEM (NOHSS)

http://www.cdc.gov/nohss/

NOHSS is a collaborative effort between CDC, Division of Oral Health and the Association of State and Territorial Dental Directors (ASTDD) (http://www.astdd.org/), an affiliate organization of the Association of State and Territorial Health Officers. NOHSS is designed to help public health programs monitor the burden of oral disease, use of the oral health care delivery system, and the status of community water fluoridation on both a state and national level. NOHSS includes indicators of oral health, information on state dental programs, and links to other important sources of oral health information. NOHSS is designed to track eight basic oral health surveillance indicators as its main focus. This is a minimal set of indicators, to be expanded in the future, based on data sources and surveillance capacity available to most states. The Council of State and Territorial Epidemiologists (CSTE) and the Association of State and Territorial Chronic Disease Program Directors (ASTCDPD) were instrumental in developing the framework for chronic disease surveillance indicators, including these oral health indicators.

Data sources for NOHSS include national surveys (NHANES, NHIS, Fluoridation Census) and state-based surveys (BRFSS, YRBSS, PRAMS, ASTDD's Basic Screening Survey and annual State Synopses). Also, oral health maps are included in the NOHSS.

CDC, NOHSS, STATE ORAL HEALTH SURVEYS

http://www.cdc.gov/nohss/sealants/surveys.htm

Many states conduct periodic oral health surveys. Some states now use the BSS (Basic Screening Survey) protocol or similar protocols for their surveys. States can submit results from these surveys for inclusion in NOHSS. State data that meet criteria for inclusion in NOHSS are published on the NOHSS website.

The Basic Screening Survey (BSS) is a standardized set of surveys designed to collect information on the observed oral health of participants, self-report or observed information on age, gender, race and Hispanic ethnicity, and self-report information on access to care for preschool, school-age, and adult populations. The surveys are cross-sectional and descriptive. In the observed oral health survey, gross dental or oral lesions are recorded by dentists, dental hygienists, or other appropriate health care workers in accordance with state law. The examiner records presence of untreated cavities and urgency of need for treatment for all age groups. In addition, for preschool and school-age children, caries experience (treated and untreated decay) is also recorded. School-age children are also examined for presence of sealants on permanent molars. Edentulism (no natural teeth) is recorded for adults. States may use one or more of the surveys in the BSS to obtain oral health status and dental care access data for monitoring *Healthy People 2010* objectives. Training materials are provided with the surveys, and technical assistance from ASTDD on sampling and analysis is available to states undertaking these surveys using the standard protocol. BSS was developed by the Association of State and Territorial Dental Directors with technical assistance from CDC.

THE SYNOPSES OF STATE DENTAL PUBLIC HEALTH PROGRAMS

http://www2.cdc.gov/nccdphp/doh/synopses/index.asp

The Synopses of State Dental Public Health Programs collect oral health program information provided to the ASTDD annually by each state's dental director or oral health program manager. ASTDD, in conjunction with CDC, Division of Oral Health, presents that information with data from standard sources (U.S. Census, Department of Education, Bureau of Labor Statistics, etc.) on the State Synopses website. Each state has its own synopsis that contains state-specific information on demographics, oral health infrastructure, oral health program administration, and oral health program activities. An interactive national trend table aggregates that information to track changes over time. Maps display which states conduct each of 12 types of oral health activities and which states have full-time dental directors.

The State Synopses were developed and are maintained through a collaborative effort between the Division of Oral Health, CDC, and ASTDD.

CDC, NCHS, NATIONAL HEALTH AND NUTRITION EXAMINATION SURVEY (NHANES)

http://www.cdc.gov/nchs/nhanes.htm

Oral health data were collected in the NHANES (NHANES I, NHANES III, and NHANES 1999-2004).

NHANES I was conducted between 1971 and 1975. This survey was based on a national sample of about 28,000 persons between the ages of 1 and 74. Extensive data on health and nutrition were collected by interview, physical examination, and laboratory analyses. The sampling design of NHANES I did not include persons of Hispanic/Latin origin. NHANES III, conducted between 1988 and 1994, included about 40,000 people selected from households in 81 counties across the United States. To obtain reliable estimates, infants and young children (aged 1 to 5 years), older persons (aged 60 years and older), black Americans, and Mexican Americans were sampled at a higher rate. NHANES III also placed an additional emphasis on the effects of the environment upon health. Data were gathered to measure the levels of pesticide exposure, the presence of certain trace elements in the blood, and the amounts of carbon monoxide present in the blood. NHANES 1999-2004 began in April 1999 and is a continuous survey visiting 15 U.S. locations per year. Approximately 5000 people are surveyed annually. Oral health data from the current NHANES will be added to NOHSS when data from each phase of the survey become publicly available.

CDC, NATIONAL HEALTH INTERVIEW SURVEY (NHIS), NCHC, CDC

http://www.cdc.gov/nchs/nhis.htm

The NHIS is a cross-sectional household interview survey on the health of the civilian non-institutionalized population of the United States. The sampling plan follows a multistage area probability design that permits the representative sampling of households. NHIS data are collected annually from approximately 43,000 households including about 106,000 persons.

NATIONAL NURSING HOME SURVEY, NCHS, CDC

The National Nursing Home Survey (NNHS) is a continuing series of national sample surveys of nursing homes, their residents, and their staff. Nursing home surveys were conducted in 1973-74, 1977, 1985, 1995, 1997, and 1999. These surveys were preceded by a series of surveys from 1963 through 1969, called the "residence places" surveys. Although each of these surveys emphasized different topics, they all provided some common basic information about nursing homes, their residents, and their staff. All nursing homes included in this survey had at least three beds and were either certified (by Medicare or Medicaid) or had a state license to operate as a nursing home. The National Nursing Home Survey provides information on nursing homes from two perspectives—that of the provider of services and that of the recipient. Data about the facilities include characteristics such as size, ownership, Medicare/Medicaid certification, occupancy rate, number of days of care provided, and expenses. For recipients, data are obtained on demographic characteristics, health status, and services received. Data for the survey have been obtained through personal interviews with administrators and staff and occasionally with self-administered questionnaires in a sample of about 1500 facilities.

CDC, NATIONAL PROGRAM OF CANCER REGISTRIES—DATA COLLECTION AND SURVEILLANCE FOR CANCER CONTROL AND PREVENTION

http://www.cdc.gov/cancer/npcr/index.htm

State cancer registries are designed to (1) monitor cancer trends over time; (2) determine cancer patterns in various populations; (3) guide planning and evaluation of cancer control programs (e.g., determine whether prevention, screening, and treatment efforts are making a difference); (4) help set priorities for allocating health resources; (5) advance clinical, epidemiologic, and health services research; and (6) provide information for a national database of cancer incidence. Cancer registries collect information about the occurrence (incidence) of cancer, the types of cancers diagnosed and their locations within the body, the extent of cancer at the time of diagnosis (disease stage), and the kinds of treatment that patients receive. These data are reported to a central statewide registry from various medical facilities, including hospitals, physicians' offices, therapeutic radiation facilities, freestanding surgical centers, and pathology laboratories.

A few of these statewide registries also collect additional information on survival after the diagnosis and initial treatments. Data collected by state cancer registries enable public health professionals to better understand and address the cancer burden. Registry data are critical for targeting programs focused on risk-related behaviors (e.g., tobacco use and exposure to the sun) or on environmental risk factors (e.g., radiation and chemical exposures). Such information is also essential for identifying when and where cancer screening efforts should be enhanced and for monitoring the treatment provided to cancer patients. In addition, reliable registry data are fundamental to a variety of research efforts, including those aimed at evaluating the effectiveness of cancer prevention, control, or treatment programs.

CDC, NATIONAL VITAL STATISTICS SYSTEM (NVSS)

http://www.cdc.gov/nchs/nvss.htm

The National Vital Statistics System is the oldest and most successful example of intergovernmental data sharing in Public Health, and the shared relationships, standards, and procedures form the mechanism by which NCHS collects and disseminates the nation's official vital statistics. These data are provided through contracts between NCHS and vital registration systems operated in the various jurisdictions legally responsible for the registration of vital events—births, deaths, marriages, divorces, and fetal deaths. In the United States, legal authority for the registration of these events resides individually with the 50 states, two cities (Washington, D.C., and New York City), and five territories (Puerto Rico, the Virgin Islands, Guam, American Samoa, and the Commonwealth of the Northern Mariana Islands). These jurisdictions are responsible for maintaining registries of vital events and for issuing copies of certificates that record births (natality), marriages, divorces, and deaths (mortality).

CDC, PREGNANCY RISK ASSESSMENT MONITORING SYSTEM (PRAMS)

http://www.cdc.gov/reproductivehealth/srv_prams.htm

The PRAMS collects state-specific, population-based data on maternal attitudes and experiences prior to, during, and immediately following pregnancy. The PRAMS sample of women who have had a recent live birth is drawn from the state's birth certificate records. Each participating state samples between 1300 and 3400 women per year. Women from some groups are sampled at a higher rate to ensure adequate data are available in smaller but higher risk populations. Information is gathered by mail and telephone. Data collection procedures and instruments are standardized to allow comparisons among states. PRAMS allows CDC and state health officials to monitor changes in maternal and child health indicators (e.g., unintended pregnancy, prenatal care, breastfeeding, smoking, alcohol use, infant health).

CDC, SCHOOL HEALTH POLICIES AND PROGRAMS STUDY (SHPPS), CDC

http://www.cdc.gov/HealthyYouth/shpps/index.htm

The School Health Policies and Programs Study (SHPPS) is a national survey periodically conducted to assess school health policies and programs at the state, district, school, and classroom levels.

CDC, WATER FLUORIDATION REPORTING SYSTEM (WFRS)

WFRS is a water fluoridation monitoring tool for state and tribal water fluoridation program managers and oral health program directors or managers. This system requires special authorization for access. WFRS is the data source for the annual fluoridation information in the National Oral Health Surveillance System.

My Water's Fluoride

http://apps.nccd.cdc.gov/MWF/Index.asp
An internet site that provides information about the fluoridation status of local water system's fluoridation.

Oral Health Maps

http://apps.nccd.cdc.gov/gisdoh/
An internet site that provides water fluoridation status by state or county. Also, provides views of demographic characteristics of a selected state or county with more detailed water fluoridation information.
My Water's Fluoride, Oral Health Maps, and WFRS were developed and are maintained through a collaborative effort of the Division of Oral Health, CDC, and ASTDD.

CDC, YOUTH RISK BEHAVIOR SURVEY (YRBS)

http://www.cdc.gov/healthyyouth/yrbs/index.htm

The YRBSS is a CDC school-based survey conducted biennially to assess the prevalence of health risk behaviors among high school students. YRBSS includes national, state, territorial, and local school-based surveys of high school students. The school-based surveys use a cluster sample design to produce a representative sample of students in grades 9 through 12. Survey procedures are designed to protect the students' privacy by allowing for anonymous and voluntary participation.

CENTERS FOR MEDICARE AND MEDICAID SERVICES (CMS), MEDICAID STATISTICS AND DATA

http://www.cms.hhs.gov/medicaid/mcaidsad.asp

The primary data sources for Medicaid statistical data are the Medicaid Statistical Information System (MSIS) and the CMS-64 reports. The MSIS is the basic source of state-reported eligibility and claims data on the Medicaid population, their characteristics, use, and payments. The CMS-64 is a product of the financial budget and grant system. CMS resources include Medicaid Program Statistics (MSIS/2082 Report) and Medicaid/SCHIP Budget and Expenditure Information System (CMS 21, 37, 64 Reports—CMS 21, Detailed SCHIP Expenditure Information; CMS 37, Detailed Budget Information; and CMS 64, Detailed Expenditure Information).

HEALTH RESOURCES AND SERVICES ADMINISTRATION (HRSA), DATA AND STATISTICS

http://www.hrsa.gov/data.htm

Data and Statistics Resources include HRSA Geospatial Data Warehouse, Dental Health Professional Shortage Areas, Bureau of Primary Care Supported Health Centers, Uniform Data System, Child Health USA, Women's Health USA, MCHB Title V Information System, MCHB Projects Database, National Survey of Children with Special Health Care Needs, State Health Workforce Profiles, U.S. Health Workforce Personnel Factbook, Area Resource File (ARF) System

NATIONAL ASSOCIATION OF COUNTY AND CITY HEALTH OFFICIALS (NACCHO), NATIONAL PROFILE OF LOCAL HEALTH DEPARTMENTS (NPLHD)

http://www.naccho.org/project64.cfm

In its continuing effort to describe local public health activities, the National Association of County and City Health Officials (NACCHO) has conducted three nationwide studies of local public health agencies, the National Profiles of Local Health Departments Surveillance Series. These studies were funded through cooperative agreements between NACCHO and the CDC. As the national voice of local public health, NACCHO provides current, scientifically valid, informative, and useful data on the state of our nation's local public health infrastructure. A comprehensive, accurate description of the capacities and needs of local health agencies is critical to understanding the role they play in the nation's health system.

NATIONAL INSTITUTE OF DENTAL AND CRANIOFACIAL RESEARCH (NIDCR) AND THE DIVISION OF ORAL HEALTH, CENTERS FOR DISEASE CONTROL AND PREVENTION (CDC)—DENTAL, ORAL, AND CRANIOFACIAL DATA RESOURCE CENTER (DRC)

http://drc.nidcr.nih.gov/

The DRC serves as a resource on dental, oral, and craniofacial data for the oral health research community, clinical practitioners, public health planners, policy makers, advocates, and the general public. The DRC is co-sponsored by the National Institute of Dental and Craniofacial Research (NIDCR) and the Division of Oral Health, Centers for Disease Control and Prevention (CDC). The DRC includes:

(a) Catalog of Oral Health Surveys includes 300 surveys related to oral health and describes sample design, data collection methods, population studied or surveyed, geographic region, and references from the literature that contain statistics and summaries of the study or survey

(b) Archive of Procedures Related to Oral Health outlines 60 clinical indexes, questionnaires, and other methods of measuring oral health that have been used in oral health surveys. The Archives contains background information on the specific procedure or method, historic changes or well-established modified versions, references regarding the validity, reliability, and performance of the procedure, and listing of survey and studies using the procedure.

(c) Oral Health Questions in National Health Surveys is a searchable database of the text of oral health-related questions used in U.S. oral health surveys. Annual Report of Oral Health in U.S. is a compendium of oral health statistical data summarizing oral, dental, and craniofacial status, demographics, oral health services, health economics, and factors influencing oral health.

(d) NIDCR/CDC Dental, Oral, and Craniofacial Data Query System (DQS) is an on-line interactive data analysis tool that makes national oral health data readily available. The DSQ is a tool for viewing prepared tables or generating rapid statistical analyses of selected oral health data sets by queries to retrieve frequencies, percentages, and confidence intervals.

NATIONAL CANCER INSTITUTE (NCI), SURVEILLANCE, EPIDEMIOLOGY AND END RESULTS PROGRAM (SEER), NATIONAL CANCER INSTITUTE (NCI)

http://seer.cancer.gov/

The SEER Program of the NCI is an authoritative source of information on cancer incidence and survival in the United States. The SEER Program currently collects and publishes cancer incidence and survival data from 14 population-based cancer registries and three supplemental registries covering approximately 26% of the U.S. population. Information on more than 3 million in situ and invasive cancer cases is included in the SEER database, and approximately 170,000 new cases are added each year within the SEER coverage areas. The SEER Registries routinely collect data on patient demographics, primary tumor site, morphology, stage at diagnosis, first course of treatment, and follow-up for vital status. The SEER Program is the only comprehensive source of population-based information in the United States that includes stage of cancer at the time of diagnosis and survival rates within each stage. The mortality data reported by SEER are provided by the National Center for Health Statistics.

NCI staff work with the North American Association of Central Cancer Registries to guide all state registries to achieve data content and compatibility acceptable for pooling data and improving national estimates. The SEER Program is considered the standard for quality among cancer registries around the world. Quality control has been an integral part of SEER since its inception. Every year, studies are conducted in SEER areas to evaluate the quality and completeness of the data being reported.

The SEER team is developing computer applications to unify cancer registration systems and to analyze and disseminate population-based data. Use of surveillance data for research is being improved through web-based access to the data and analytic tools, and linking with other national data sources. For example, a new web-based tool for public health officials and policy makers, State Cancer Profiles, provides a user-friendly interface for finding cancer statistics for specific states and counties.

WHO GLOBAL ORAL HEALTH PROGRAMME

http://www.who.int/oral_health/en/

WHO ORAL HEALTH COUNTRY/AREA PROFILE PROGRAMME

http://www.whocollab.od.mah.se/

ORAL HEALTH PROFILES FOR COUNTRIES BY WHO REGION

http://www.whocollab.od.mah.se/expl/regions.html

Selected oral health indicators are tracked by the 39 nations in the Americas and include those reported by the United States. The Pan American Health Organization (PAHO) serves as the World Health Organization Regional Office for the Americas (AMRO) and leads this regional oral health surveillance effort on an international level. In addition, selected U.S. oral health indicators are incorporated into the World Health Organization (WHO) Country-Area Profile, and these contribute to the Global Oral Health Data Bank that tracks oral health on an international level through the WHO Global Oral Health Programme. The World Oral Health Report 2003: Continuous Improvement of Oral Health in the 21st Century—the Approach of the WHO Global Oral Health Programme is posted on the WHO website and reviews oral health from a global perspective.

APPENDIX D-3   SUMMARY OF DATA COLLECTION METHODS*

Method	Instrument	Cost and Time	Advantage
Document Study			
Review and evaluate existing documents or records describing past events or occurrences	Information abstracted from archival sources (raw data, datasets of summary data, printed reports); qualitative or quantitative data from public legislative bodies, governmental officials and agencies, private businesses, professional and community organizations, nonprofit foundations	$-$$ ⊕–⊕⊕	Data often readily available
Observational Field Study			
Assessment of actual events, objects, or people in "natural" setting	Assessors use checklist, evaluation forms, camera, tape recorder, rating scales, observation field notes. Qualitative approach with content or situational analysis	$$ ⊕⊕	Firsthand information
Windshield or Walking Tour			
Within community-designated boundaries, observers and recorders drive or walk in community areas at varying times of days and days of week to assess community activities, interactions, and events through observation, informal conversations, and interactions with community members	Observers and recorders document community characteristics and record information using observational guide, checklist, survey tools, notes, photos, audiotapes, videotapes; qualitative approach with content or situational analysis; results summarized and displayed through written narratives, tables, diagrams, slide and video shows, maps, collages	$-$$ ⊕–⊕⊕	Firsthand information
Mailed Survey			
Assessment conducted by mail; adaptations include questionnaire sent home with children from school, Fax survey, magazine or newsletter survey, or electronic survey (using networked computers or Internet)	Self-administered standardized, structured questionnaire with closed-ended and open-ended questions completed by respondent; quantitative approach with statistical analysis of responses	$$ ⊕⊕	Data can be collected from a large sample

*Consider assessment methods that can stimulate dialog, reflection, and action to improve community health.
$, Inexpensive; $$, moderate cost; $$$, expensive; ⊕, less time-consuming; ⊕⊕, moderately time-consuming; ⊕⊕⊕, very time-consuming.

Continued

APPENDIX D-3   SUMMARY OF DATA COLLECTION METHODS—cont'd

Method	Instrument	Cost and Time	Advantage
Telephone Interview			
Survey interview conducted by telephone	Interviewer reads structured interview schedule (standardized, questionnaire) with closed-ended and open-ended questions to respondent; quantitative approach with statistical analysis of responses	$$ ⏲⏲	Data can be collected from a large sample
Person-to-Person Interview			
Survey interview conducted face to face between a respondent and an interviewer	Structured interview schedule (standardized, questionnaire) with closed-ended and open-ended questions read to respondent by an interviewer; quantitative approach with statistical analysis of responses	$$-$$$ ⏲⏲– ⏲⏲⏲	Face-to-face communication allows for more in-depth information
In-depth Personal Interview			
Survey conducted face to face to learn about life history, events, and experiences	Interviewer uses open-ended, flexible, unstructured nondirective questions; transcriptions of tape recordings used for thematic analysis of content	$$-$$$ ⏲⏲– ⏲⏲⏲	Smaller sample with expanded perspectives
Screening Survey			
Rapid assessment using screening procedures	Standardized written criteria and measurements, measuring instruments, and protocols; cursory inspection provides crude estimates; quantitative approach with statistical analysis of results	$$ ⏲⏲	Practical and uniform information in a short time period
Epidemiologic Survey			
Extensive assessment using examination procedures, clinical samples, and clinical tests	Standardized written criteria and measurements, measuring instruments, and protocols; detailed planning of examination conditions, indexes, criteria, sampling approach, personnel training, data collection, data management, and analysis; quantitative approach with statistical analysis of results	$$-$$$ ⏲⏲– ⏲⏲⏲	More detailed information

APPENDIX D-3 SUMMARY OF DATA COLLECTION METHODS—cont'd

Method	Instrument	Cost and Time	Advantage
Asset Maps			
Geographic study and mapping that can identify patterns of community characteristics, physical assets, or settings of human activity and interactions	Input and display of data from existing sources or new data onto geographic map using simple materials (land use map and adhesives or pushpins) or detailed community planning and evaluation computer software (e.g., Geographic Information System [GIS] software) and other powerful tools for organizing location, distribution, and mapping of spatial data	$-$$$ ⏱–⏱⏱	Good overview and visualization of information
Inventories or Directories			
Documenting and cataloging of assets and capacities of individual community members or community resources, such as institutions, organizations, and associations	Identify, evaluate, and organize assets and capacities in a community and develop adequate mechanisms for linkages that can produce opportunities for action; such capacities may include assets owned or skills processed by individual community members; may also include sources of mutual aid, connections, and resources among institutions, organizations, and associations in a community	$-$$ ⏱–⏱⏱	Data often previously collected
Focus Group			
Guided group discussion provides information on a specific topic from a certain population group	Moderator leads guided group discussions among 5 to 12 individuals over 1/2 to 1 1/2 hours by using a series of open-ended questions on a pre-established discussion guide; transcriptions from tape recordings and written field notes of discussions used for thematic analysis of content	$$-$$$ ⏱⏱– ⏱⏱⏱	Varied and ample information

Continued

APPENDIX D-3   SUMMARY OF DATA COLLECTION METHODS—cont'd

Method	Instrument	Cost and Time	Advantage
Public Forum or Community Dialog Event			
Individuals or groups provide verbal input or feedback on specific issues	Moderator solicits, collects, and summarizes written comments or oral testimony; oral testimony recorded by tape recorder or court reporter to generate official record for analysis	$$ 🕐🕐	Firsthand and ample information
Community Visioning Process			
Groups of community stakeholders collectively develop shared vision of their community in the future	Through an interactive approach (retreat or workshop format), a skilled facilitator brings individuals together over one or more days and guides participants through vision process by posing questions and assisting participants to visualize the future community; small groups discuss visions and images; creation of document to reflect visions; follow-up meeting held to refine visions and to develop plan for incorporation of visions into community planning process	$$-$$$ 🕐🕐– 🕐🕐🕐	Broad with ample and varied input
Creative Assessment			
Community members document perceptions of community through creative means	Creative techniques and forums for expression (photography, film, theater, music, dance, murals, puppet shows, storytelling, drawings) used to convey wide range of perceptions of a community	$$-$$$ 🕐🕐– 🕐🕐🕐	Interesting and innovative

APPENDIX D-4   EXAMPLES OF INFORMATION FOR A COMMUNITY HEALTH ASSESSMENT

Community Health Measures	Examples
Health status (measurements of natality [births], morbidity [illness], and mortality [deaths])	**Birth statistics**: Age, parity of mother, duration of pregnancy, types of births (single, twin), complications of pregnancy, complications of birth, birth defects, birth weight (e.g., low), premature births, births to adolescent, older, or unmarried females
	Morbidity statistics: Incidence and prevalence of diseases, conditions, disabilities, or injuries (distribution, intensity, and duration), such as unintentional and intentional injuries, homicide, suicide, cancer, heart disease, diabetes, stroke, infectious diseases (communicable), HIV/AIDS, tuberculosis, STDs, mental illness, alcohol and drug abuse problems, occupational diseases, disability and decreased independence, developmental disabilities (e.g., cleft lip and/or palate, craniofacial anomalies), oral diseases or conditions (e.g., dental caries, periodontal diseases, oral injuries)
	Mortality statistics: Distribution of death rates by age, race/ ethnicity, sex, cause, geographic location, leading causes of deaths such as cancer (breast, colon, lung, oral), heart disease, stroke, homicide, motor vehicle injuries, suicide, unintentional injury, infant, neonatal, and postneonatal mortality
Health risks and protective factors (identification of patterns of behavioral and nonbehavioral factors)	**Self-rated (self-reported) general and oral health status**, recent poor health, days of work lost, days of school lost (e.g., because of dental problems or care), average number of unhealthy days in past month, satisfaction with quality of life and with public health, health care, and social service system
	Occupational risks and work disability
	Stress indicators and resources (drunk driving, robberies, assaults), access to drugs, recent drug use, alcoholic beverage outlets, gang problems, family violence (child abuse and neglect, spouse and elder abuse), major depression, self-esteem, alienation, discrimination, feelings of hope and despair, feelings of anger, social and family support, social and family resources (adaptation and cohesion), life events, stress (personal, family, job stress)

AIDS, Acquired immunodeficiency disease; HIV, human immunodeficiency virus; STD, sexually transmitted disease.

Continued

APPENDIX D-4   EXAMPLES OF INFORMATION FOR A COMMUNITY HEALTH ASSESSMENT—cont'd

Community Health Measures	Examples
Access to public health, health care and social service system (scope, adequacy, accessibility, and availability of services in a coordinated, integrated system)	**Levels of health knowledge, beliefs, attitudes, behaviors, practices, and skills** about self-care (toothbrushing with fluoride toothpaste and flossing) and health interventions, lifestyle diet (low in sugar), physical activity, health-related substance use (tobacco and alcohol), safety practices (seat belts, mouth guards), knowledge about location and availability as well as appropriate use of local health resources, services, programs, family health care expenditures
	Use of child and adult preventive health services: dental sealants, fluoride treatments, prenatal care in first trimester, immunizations for children and adults, Pap smear, mammogram, sigmoidoscopy for colon cancer screening
	Access to community preventive services (community water fluoridation) and public health services: Scope and adequacy of local health department covering essential public health services (including infrastructure and capacity measures, local voluntary health programs, operational health promotion and education programs in work sites, schools, and community) by health providers, numbers, types, locations, adequacy
	Access to facilities for personal health care: Assessment of numbers, types, location, adequacy of hospitals, emergency facilities, outpatient primary care, oral health, hearing, vision care, speech, physical, and occupational therapy, urgent care, mental health, alcohol and drug treatment programs, nursing homes, community health centers
	Access to health professionals: Adequacy and numbers of trained public health professionals and personal health service professionals with expertise and competence, levels of knowledge, attitudes, and behaviors, practices, and skills of public health professionals and personal health service professionals
	Access to health insurance and usual sources of health care: Comprehensive benefits with dental insurance and per capita spending (Medicare, Medicaid, State Children's Health Insurance Program [SCHIP], private insurance, Supplementary Security Income)
	Scope and adequacy of local social service programs in addressing basic human family and community needs

APPENDIX D-5   EXAMPLES OF PRIMARY DATA COLLECTION TASKS

PLANNING

- Determine scope and objectives
- Prepare protocols describing assessment plan
- Select data collection methods
- Establish criteria
- Determine sampling methods
- Obtain approval of authorities and processes
- Plan for personnel and physical arrangements
- Plan for data analysis phase (recording, managing, and analyzing data)
- Plan for data reporting phase
- Prepare budget
- Develop timetable of main activities and responsible staff
- Plan for referral process (for clinical findings detected in health survey)
- Plan and develop consent form
- Translate consent form
- Gain approval of consent form from Institutional Review Board
- Plan and develop data collection instruments
- Develop data collection protocols
- Plan data entry processes
- Plan quality assurance processes for data collection
- Plan and develop training materials for field team

- Plan and develop data collection and entry process (manual collection or direct data entry into personal computer)
- Translate data collection instruments
- Gain approval of data collection instruments from Institutional Review Board
- Pilot test consent form and data collection instruments
- Revise consent form and data collection instruments
- Obtain approval of revised consent form and data collection instruments from Institutional Review Board
- Draw sample
- Plan fieldwork and scheduling
- Purchase and organize supplies
- Initiate contact with data collection sites (work through established community networks or organizational structures)
- Organize logistics for data collection, including travel and site requirements
- Train field team
- Calibrate field team
- Implement pilot test of assessment

IMPLEMENTING

- Contact and recruit participants
- Gain consent of participants
- Record data
- Manage data

- Analyze data
- Maintain quality assurance processes
- Summarize findings
- Report findings

Selected Oral Conditions and Factors Influencing Oral Health That Can Be Assessed in Oral Health Surveys

SELECTED ORAL CONDITIONS OR FACTORS INFLUENCING ORAL HEALTH	EXAMPLES OF VARIABLES THAT CAN BE ASSESSED IN ORAL HEALTH SURVEYS
Clinical treatment needs	• Dental service needed by type of care (e.g., prevention, restorations, extractions, crowns, etc.) • Treatment urgency
Craniofacial anomalies, including developmental anomalies	• Cleft lip or cleft palate • Craniofacial anomalies • Oral malformations
Dental caries	• Coronal caries • Early childhood caries • dft, dfs, DMFT, DMFS • Gross loss of tooth structure • Pulpal involvement • Retained roots • Root caries • Untreated tooth (dental) decay • Restoration and Tooth Condition Assessment (RTCA)

- Significant Caries Index (SiC Index)—World Health Organization

Dental sealants

- Dental sealants on specific teeth (first molars, second molars, primary molars)

Dietary intake

- Healthy Eating Index
- Dietary recall and dietary intake questionnaire
- Food frequency questionnaire
- Food choices and dietary patterns
- Bottle feeding practices

Expense and payment source for oral health services

- Dental care expenses
- Dental insurance
- Medicaid

Fluoride

- Fluoride toothpaste use
- Community water fluoridation
- Fluoride supplements
- Fluoride treatments

Impact of oral health on daily living

- Acute pain
- Chronic pain
- Eating (e.g., trouble chewing or eating)
- Lost work, lost school days, activity change resulting from dental problems
- Masticatory function
- Mouth pain
- Orofacial Pain Assessment–orofacial pain questionnaire and orofacial pain examination
- Salivary function (e.g., dry mouth, Sjögren syndrome, xerostomia)
- Speech
- Swallowing
- Temporomandibular dysfunction (TMD)
- Temporomandibular Joint (TMJ) Assessment

Malocclusion

- Occlusion and occlusal traits
- Orthodontic treatment needs
- Dental Aesthetics Index (DAI)

Medications

- Medications prescribed for dental treatment

Oral and pharyngeal cancer

- Receipt of examination to detect oral cancer
- Oral cytology

Oral health knowledge, beliefs, opinions, attitudes, practices, behaviors, and skills	• Assessments of children, adolescents, and parents • Assessments of younger and older adults • Assessment of oral health care providers • Assessments of health care providers • Assessments of community stakeholders and policy makers
Oral health care providers	• Dental care provider information • Oral health care provider distribution • Oral health care provider training • Staffing of oral health care providers • Types of health care providers seen
Oral health care use	• Access to dental care (e.g., cost, travel, time, satisfaction) • Type of dental provider seen • Dental services by type (e.g., prevention, restorations, extractions, crowns) • Emergency dental care (e.g., traumatic injuries) • Dental care satisfaction • Frequency of dental visits • Last dental visit (indicating when) • Reason for dental visit • Reason for last dental visit • First dental visit • Frequency of dental visits • Number of dental visits • Usual source of dental care • Centers with oral health services • State and local dental programs
Orofacial injury	• Trauma • Accident • NIDR Trauma Index
Perceived oral health status and oral health–related quality of life	• Assessment of general oral health status • Global Oral Health Assessment Index (GOHAI) • Oral Health Impact Profile (OHIP) • Child Oral Health Quality of Life Questionnaire
Perceived treatment needs	• Self-perceived need for dental care
Periodontal diseases	• Alveolar bone loss • Community Periodontal Index (CPI) • Furcations

- Gingivitis
- Calculus (e.g., subgingival calculus or supragingival calculus)
- Gingival bleeding
- Gingival inflammation
- Loss of attachment
- Periodontal index
- Pocket depth
- Recession
- Tooth mobility

Preventive care

- Preventive care by clinician
- Preventive self-care (e.g., oral hygiene)

Primary/permanent dentition

- Cleaning
- Oral debris
- Oral Health Index

Soft-tissue lesions

- Mouth sores
- Oral herpes
- Oral lesions
- Oral ulcers
- Tongue lesions

Tobacco

- Cigarettes
- Smokeless tobacco
- Smoking cigars
- Smoking pipe
- Tobacco cessation counseling by dental professionals

Tooth loss/edentulism

- Tooth count
- Denture ownership and use
- Missing teeth
- Self-reported dentition status

BIBLIOGRAPHY

National Institute for Dental Research and Centers for Disease Control, Dental, Oral, and Craniofacial Data Resource Center (DRC): Catalog of Oral Health Surveys and Archive of Procedures Related to Oral Health. Rockville, Md, 2003.

National Institute for Dental Research and Centers for Disease Control, Dental, Oral, and Craniofacial Data Resource Center (DRC): Oral Health Survey Questions: A Compilation of Dental and Oral Health Questions Included on National Health Surveys. Rockville, Md, 2003.

Glossary

Abstract   A summary, confined to approximately 200 words, that concisely defines a study's purpose, methods, materials, and results; a brief description of the research, found at the beginning of a manuscript, designed to provide an overview of the study

Access   Assurance that conditions are in place for people to obtain the care they need and want

Administrator (Manager)   A supervisory role in which the dental hygienist directs and oversees oral health programs

Agent Factors   Biologic or mechanical means of causing disease, illness, injury, or disability, including microbial, parasitic, viral, and bacterial pathogens or vectors; physical or mechanical irritants; chemicals; drugs; trauma; automobiles; and radiation

Alternative Practice   A setting outside the private office in which the dental hygienist provides public health services

ANOVA (Analysis of Variance)   A commonly used test for parametrics; allows comparison among more than two means from different samples and compares interactions among the variability in multiple sample groups to the variability within groups

Assessment   A core public health function that includes the regular and systematic collection, assemblage, and analysis of data and communication regarding the oral health of the community

ASTDD (Association of State and Territorial Dental Directors) Basic Screening Survey   A survey used to assess need and referral for dental care; categories include (1) no dental care needed other than routine care, (2) early dental care recommended, and (3) urgent or emergency care recommended

Assurance   A core public health function in which agencies educate, support, and evaluate programs to ensure that the community's oral health needs are addressed

BRFSS (Behavioral Risk Factor Surveillance Survey)   A state-specific survey developed by the Centers for Disease Control and Prevention; structured questions are asked over the telephone to assess behaviors that influence health status; an oral health module assesses use of dental services

Calibration   Agreement of examiners who are involved in data collection with a set standard of performance

Change Agent/Consumer Advocate   A role in which the dental hygienist must have the knowledge and skills to work to promote change and advance people's health through legislation, public policy, research, and science

Chi-Square Test   The most commonly used nonparametric test; is used to analyze questionnaire data and to determine whether a relationship exists between two variables

Clinical Rotation   This curriculum-based activity is not necessarily associated with a service outcome and is designed primarily to benefit the student's learning. Students are assigned rotation through clinical experiences to enhance knowledge, skills, and expertise

Collaboration   The process of working together to accomplish a goal

Community   The public or group of people with common interests who live in a specific locality

Community Oral Health Assessment   A multifaceted process of identifying factors that affect the oral health of a selected population to determine resources and interventions for oral health improvement

Community Organization Theory   The idea of involving and activating members of a community or subgroup to identify a common problem or goal, to mobilize resources, to implement strategies, and to evaluate their efforts

Community Profile   A comprehensive description of the community, including items such as population size, geographic boundaries, community type, and physical conditions

Community Water Fluoridation   The addition of a controlled amount of fluoride to the public water supply with the intent of preventing dental caries in the population

Consultant/Resource Person   A role in which the dental hygienist acts as a liaison between the community and the dental profession to determine the appropriate programs and activities that will serve the needs of the community

Continuous Data   A type of collected information described as measurements made from a particular value, such as from temperature, scores on tests, or time; can be any value along a continuum

Control Group   The group of subjects in a study who do not receive the experimental treatment or intervention

Convenience Sample   A group of individuals who are most readily available to be subjects in a study

Correlation   A statistical method of determining whether a variation in one variable may be related to a variation in another variable

CPI (Community Periodontal Index)   An assessment of periodontal status of a population by grades of periodontal disease; measures gingival bleeding, calculus, and periodontal pockets

Cross-Cultural Encounter   Interaction with persons or communities of diverse populations

Cross-Cultural Communication   Effectively exchanging information with persons of diverse populations

Cultural Competence   Considerations that have an impact on the profession's responsibility to reduce the burden of disease for people of various cultures and backgrounds

Cultural Diversity   The degree to which a population consists of people from varied national, ethnic, racial, and religious backgrounds

Cultural Destructiveness   Attitudes, policies, and practices that are detrimental to culture, communities, and individuals

Current Status   State of affairs or position at the present time

Data   Pieces of information collected from measurements and counts obtained during the course of a research study

Data Collection   The process of gathering the information that can be used by the community to make decisions and set priorities

Demand   Health care services desired by the individual or community

Dental Public Health   The science and art of preventing and controlling dental disease and promoting dental health through organized community efforts

DHHS (Department of Health and Human Services)   A department of the federal government presiding over agencies that conduct oral health activities

Dental Health Professional Shortage Areas (Dental HPSA)   Geographic areas where the dentist/dental health professional to population ratio is low

Dependent Variable   The variable thought to depend on or to be caused by the independent variable; the outcome variable of interest

Descriptive Statistics   Used to describe and summarize data; determine information only about the sample being studied

Determinants of Health   Factors that interact to create circumstances and produce specific health conditions; can be classified as physical (environmental), biologic, behavioral, social, cultural, and spiritual

Diffusion of Innovations Theory   A concept that assesses how new ideas, products, or services spread within a society or to other groups or how innovations are adopted

Discrete Data   Collected information that is counted only in whole numbers

Disparities   Uneven distribution of the burden of disease (such as oral disease) throughout the population, especially in the poor, the elderly, and the disabled

DMFT, DMFS (Decayed, Missing, and Filled Teeth/Surfaces) Index   A survey used to count caries in the permanent dentition; dft and dfs are used to count caries in the primary dentition

Environmental Factors   Physical, sociocultural, sociopolitical, and economic components that interact with host and agent

Epidemiology   The study of the distribution and determinants of health-related states and events in specified populations and the application of this study to the control of health problems

Essential Public Health Services for Oral Health   Guidelines describing the roles of state oral health programs; used in the development and evaluation of public health activities at the state level

Ethics/Professional Ethics   The general science of right and wrong conduct; the code by which the profession regulates actions and sets standards for its members

Ethnocentrism   Judging others by one's own cultural standards

Evaluation   The method of measuring results of a program against objectives developed during the early planning stages

Experimental Group   The sample group of subjects in a study who receive the experimental treatment or intervention

Experiential Learning   An umbrella term that references various models of learning in which experience governs the learning process

Focus Group   Five to 10 members of the intended target audience who undergo group interviews lasting about 30 to 60 minutes; a moderator with structured questions guides the discussion

Follow-up/Referral   An essential component of assessment and screening; without further observation and referral for care, screening is ineffective

Framing Health Messages   A concept that relates to the cues (e.g., sounds, symbols, words, pictures) that signal how and what to think about an issue

General Supervision   Supervision of the dental hygienist in which the dentist does not have to be on the premises but the patient must be one of record or seen by the dentist previously

Goal   A broad-based statement of changes to take place from which specific objectives are developed

Health   Complete physical and social well-being, not merely the absence of disease

Health Belief Model   An assessment of perceptions of how susceptible one is to a health problem and whether one believes that recommended preventive behaviors will result in less susceptibility

Health Education   The process in which the client is encouraged to become responsible for personal oral health and is informed of scientifically based methods for preventing dental disease

Health Educator/Wellness Promoter   A role in which the dental hygienist works to prevent disease and to promote oral health through the presentation of scientific information

Health Promotion   A broad concept referring to the process of enabling people and communities to increase their control over the determinants of health and, therefore, to improve their own health

Health Security   The rights and conditions that enable individuals to attain and enjoy their full potential for a healthy life

Healthy People 2010   A document that contains national health objectives for prevention of disease and promotion of health

HIPAA (Health Insurance Portability and Accountability Act)   Regulations governing and protecting the rights and privacy of patients in health care.

Host Factors   Factors that affect a host's (a person's, an animal's, or a plant's) susceptibility and resistance to disease

Hypothesis   A statement that reflects the research question, stated in positive terms, and represents the researcher's prediction or opinion

Implementation   The process of putting a plan into action; monitoring a plan's activities, personnel, equipment, resources, and supplies

Independent Variable   The experimental treatment or intervention that is imposed on the experimental group

Index   A graduated numeric scale with upper and lower limits; scores correspond to a specific criterion for individuals or populations

Inferential Statistics   Used to draw a generalization between the sample studied and the actual population

Interrater Reliability Agreement of findings by two or more examiners

Interval Scale A scale of measurement that determines quantities; characterized by having order and equal distance between points on the scale

Intrarater Reliability Consistency of findings by one examiner with those previously recorded by the same examiner

Judgmental Sample A sample, provided through personal judgment, of subjects who are most representative of the population

Learning Styles The ways in which people collect and retain knowledge

Legislative/Policy Changes New or revised laws on health care that the dental hygienist as Consumer Advocate/Change Agent helps to create and implement

Mandala of Health Hancock's model of health of the human ecosystem

Mean Average of the group; a sum of all the values divided by the number of items

Median The exact middle score or value in a distribution of scores; when the total number of scores is even, the sum of the two middle scores, divided by 2, provides the median

MEPS (Medical Expenditure Panel Survey) Survey that reports on the number of annual dental visits for various population groups

Mode The score or value that occurs most frequently in a distribution of scores

Need Those services deemed by the health professional to be necessary after use of a variety of assessment and diagnostic tools and, perhaps, past experience

Network A system in which information about a common population is shared with other health professionals

NHANES (National Health and Nutrition Examination Survey) A national survey conducted in 1996 in which many aspects of oral health were measured

NHIS (National Health Interview Survey) A survey that asks questions about a person's health, including edentulous status

Nominal Scale A scale of measurement in which characteristics or numbers are assigned into categories by name only

Nonparametric Test A statistical test used when assumptions about a normal distribution in the population cannot be met or when the level of measurement is nominal or ordinal

Normal Distribution An assumption that approximately 68% of the population falls within 1 standard deviation (SD) of the mean, approximately 95% falls within 2 SDs of the mean, and 99% lies within 3 SDs of the mean

Null Hypothesis An assumption that there is no statistically significant difference between the groups being studied

Objective The desired end result of program activities, described in a measurable way; more specific than a goal

Oral Health Coalition A cooperative effort on the part of many individuals and organizations to build systems and to develop programs that improve community oral health

Oral Health Education A learning experience directed at assisting people in preventing oral disease

Oral Paper   A method of presentation of a topic

Ordinal Scale   A scale of measurement that orders data into categories in rank order; the space between these categories is undefined

Organizational Change: Stage Theory   A statement of how organizations pass through a series of stages as they initiate change; organizational structures and processes influence workers' behavior and motivation for change

Parameter   A term relating to numeric characteristics of the population

Parametrics   A technique used when data include interval or ratio scales of measurement; best used when the sample is large and randomized and the population from which the sample is taken is normally distributed

Pilot Study (Trial Run)   A preliminary study performed in preparation for a major study

Planning   An organized response to reduce or eliminate one or more problems

Planning Cycle   A model commonly used in public health practice that provides a basic flowchart of steps in process to assess, plan, implement, and evaluate

Pluralistic Systems   Numerous, distinct health care delivery systems that coexist simultaneously

Policy Development   A core public health function in which laws are planned and developed to support community oral health issues

Population   The entire group, or whole unit of individuals, having similar characteristics to which the results of an investigation can be generalized

Poster   A method of presentation of a topic

Power Analysis   A determination of how many subjects are needed to provide significance; calculated using a specific statistical formula based on what an examiner hopes to observe in a specific number of subjects

Practicum/Internship   This activity is typically longer than a clinical rotation and is designed to benefit the student. The student may be assigned to work in a particular specialty area for an entire academic quarter or semester.

Primary Prevention   Services that are used to prevent a disease before it occurs; this level includes health education, avoidance of disease, and health protection

Professional Ethics   The code by which the profession regulates actions and sets standards for its members

Public Health   The science and art of preventing disease, prolonging life, and promoting physical health and efficiency through organized community effort

P Value   A declaration of how likely it is that a study could have come to a false conclusion; the probability that the obtained results are due to chance alone

Qualitative Data   Information that reflects the quality or nature of things that cannot be numerically measured or analyzed

Qualitative Evaluation   A determination of why and how (e.g., why did people participate in the activity, and how do they intend to change their parenting behaviors?)

Quality of Life   Characteristics of living that are affected by a person's health status; oral disease restricts activities at school, work, and home and often diminishes one's quality of life

Quantitative Data   Information that is objective and measurable; can be expressed in a quantity or amount (such as the number of children with dental sealants or the rate of dental caries in young children)

Quantitative Evaluation   A determination of how many (e.g., how many people increased their knowledge of the causes of early childhood caries?)

Random Sample   A sample in which each member of a population has an equal chance of being included, thus preventing the possibility of selection bias by the researcher

Range   A measurement of the difference between the highest and lowest values in a distribution of scores

Ratio Scale   A scale of measurement that not only has all the qualities of nominal, ordinal, and interval but also has an absolute zero, such as age, height, and weight

Refereed Journal   A journal in which articles have been reviewed by an editorial board of peers

Reflection   Critical thinking and critical expressions about the Service-Learning experience and the specific encounters. The aim of reflection is to draw meaning from the experience.

Reliability   Consistency and stability of the data collected in a study

Researcher   A role in which the dental hygienist uses scientific methods to acquire knowledge on topics relevant to

serving the needs of the public's oral health

Risk Management   A phase that suggests that risks can be managed with organizational influence. An affiliation agreement between the service providers and the organization being serviced would be an example.

Round Table Discussion   Method of presentation of a topic in which the participants sit in a circular pattern and discuss issues relevant to the topic

Sample   A portion or subset of the entire population

Sealant   A plastic resin material applied to the occlusal surfaces of molars and premolars; an effective primary preventive strategy

Service-Learning   Service-Learning (SL) is an example of an experiential learning method. SL is a jointly structured learning experience in which the course learning objectives (LO) and the community partner's service objectives (SO) are deliberately combined for mutual benefit.

Service Provider/Clinician   A role in which the dental hygienist assesses oral health needs and provides treatment

Shortage Areas   Localities where the dentist-to-population ratio shows an unmet need for oral health

Social Learning Theory   The idea that people learn through their own experiences by observing the actions of others and the results of those actions

Social Marketing   Use of effective advertising tools from commercial marketing to influence a valued health behavioral change

Social Responsibility A broad term encompassing professionalism, personal and professional ethics, and the role of a profession in the context of the greater society

Stages of Change Theory The idea that change is a process or cycle that occurs over time rather than as a single event

Standard Deviation The positive square root of the variance

Statistics Numeric characteristics of samples

Status State or condition

Stratified Sample Random selection of subjects from two or more subdivisions of the population

Systematic Approach to Health Improvement Framework describing the interrelated determinants of health, including the goals and objectives necessary to improve health

Systematic Sample Selection of subjects by including every nth person in a list

Table Clinic Method of presentation of a topic

Tailoring Messages A concept in which specific cues are used to make messages meaningful for a specific individual

Target Population The people from whom information is being collected and to whom the researcher would like to generalize the findings of a study

Technical Assistance The use of the professional skills and knowledge base to provide guidance to nondental community members interested in developing preventive programs

Theory A set of interrelated concepts, definitions, and propositions that present a systematic view of events or situations by specifying relations among variables to explain and predict the events or situations

Trend Inclination or direction on a particular course over a period of time

t-Test A test used to analyze the difference between two means

Type I (Alpha) Error Based on statistical results, the researcher rejects the null hypothesis when it is true

Type II (Beta) Error Based on statistical results, the researcher accepts the null hypothesis when it is actually false

Validity The degree to which an instrument measures what it is intended to measure

Variable A characteristic or concept that varies, or differs, within the population under study

Variance A method of measuring the way in which individual variables are located around the mean; a common technique of measuring interval and ratio variables

Volunteerism Activity where students provide a service to the community and the major benefit is for the community. This activity is not necessarily associated with an academic course.

Index

Page numbers followed by f indicate figures; t, tables, and b, boxes.